THIS DYNAMIC BOOK

... is aimed straight at the heart of every citizen of the United States, the country where coronary disease is the master killer of our adult population.

In clear and straightforward terms, the author describes what a heart attack is, who is likely to have one, and why. He explains that the Prudent Diet, an important weapon against the blood excesses our over-abundant, over-rich diet brings on.

Every serious reader of this book—and that should be every American—will come away with a clear understanding of the major factors in heart attacks—*and what can be done to prevent them!*

HEART ATTACK:

ARE YOU A CANDIDATE?

ARTHUR BLUMENFELD

▲ PYRAMID BOOKS   NEW YORK

HEART ATTACK: ARE YOU A CANDIDATE?

A PYRAMID BOOK
Published by arrangement with Paul S. Eriksson, Inc.

Pyramid edition published March, 1971

Library of Congress Catalog Card Number: 64-17749

Printed in the United States of America.

PYRAMID BOOKS are published by Pyramid Publications
A Division of the Walter Reade Organization, Inc.
444 Madison Avenue, New York, New York 10022. U.S.A.

This book is dedicated to the
medical scientists of the
AMERICAN SOCIETY FOR THE STUDY
OF ARTERIOSCLEROSIS,
and to all the scientists throughout the world,
whose medical researches have done so much
in the battle to curb the coronary epidemic.

Contents

Introduction

This book is a welcome contribution to the general effort now under way to alert the public to the dangers it faces in the widespread occurrence of pre-senile coronary atherosclerosis.

There are differences of medical opinion as to the relative importance of the various causative factors presented herein. There is no doubt, however, that the author's insistence on the possibility and necessity of prevention of coronary disease receives my wholehearted support. I agree with the important point made in the book that it is almost never too late to mend one's ways, even to stop smoking.

By bringing to the public's attention the great contributions being made today by medical scientists throughout the world, this volume gives new hope that the American people can improve their chances for good health and a longer life through exercise, a more frugal diet, and a more positive outlook for the future.

Among the features of the book which are especially noteworthy is the documentation of facts well known to those of us who are constantly seeing patients from all over the world. We are cognizant of the fact that wherever people live prosperously they tend in some way to abuse their prosperity and to develop serious atherosclerosis earlier in life. Enough medical research is presented in the book to make it evident and increasingly clear that over-nutrition today is the most serious type of malnutrition. The harm being done to us by physical indolence is shown in many ways. Truly we have become slaves to our machines instead of being their masters.

Finally, let me call attention to the section in which it is noted that when we delay or prevent coronary atherosclerosis we also delay or prevent atherosclerosis elsewhere, which includes the circulation to the brain wherein are

located both our mental activities and our very soul or
personality.

If this book succeeds in calling the public's attention to
these problems, it will have served a worthy cause. It is
up to physicians everywhere now to help blaze the path
to the maintenance of health as well as to the diagnosis
and treatment of disease.

PAUL DUDLEY WHITE, M.D.

Boston, Massachusetts

Preface

If the United States Department of Agriculture were to announce tomorrow that the nation's supply of beef cattle is threatened by a disease which could kill half of them, the people, the press and Congress would immediately clamor for action against so dire a threat.

And if the United States Department of Health were to warn the nation than an epidemic was imminent, and of such serious magnitude that it threatened to kill a large percentage of the adult population, almost all medical research would undoubtedly be drafted into an unprecedented drive to find a remedy.

The irony of our age is that although advances in science and technology have eliminated the possibility of such announcements, these same advances have resulted in changes in our environment which could be the cause of a new epidemic which now menaces, in their prime years, a large percentage of our adult males.

The name of the disease is neither strange nor new. It is *heart attack*.

There is no hue and cry about it—no panic or hysteria—because most laymen as well as many doctors have convinced themselves that heart disease in our day and age is inevitable. The public especially has the defeatist attitude that prevention is unattainable or impractical and that all anyone can do is to hope for a cure when heart attack does strike.

The purpose of this book is to show that, *although there is real reason for concern, prevention of the disease is now possible.*

The plan of the book is simple. It tells what heart attack is, what causes it, and what you *yourself* can do to prevent it.

No miracles are reported in this book. No drugs are pre-

11

scribed, no special cure or magical formula. It simply brings together well-documented evidence from which inevitable conclusions can be drawn.

A question has frequently been put to me: "Is your interest in this subject due to your having had a heart attack?" The answer is "no."

I am an inventor and an electronics engineer, but I have always been interested in matters of health as well. As a scientist, I have spent all of my adult life examining information in order to arrive at reasonable and accurate conclusions.

Some ten years ago, evidence began to pile up that heart attack might be preventable. During this past decade, the public has been virtually bombarded with information on atherosclerosis, cholesterol, fats, and various kinds of frightening statistics. At least once a week newspapers could be counted on to report the pros and cons of various scientific discoveries and theories about heart attack. The result has been confusion and indecision.

Many books and hundreds of articles have been written on the subject. The material prepared by doctors has necessarily been written from particular and specialized points of view. The material written by professional writers and reporters has been overpopularized and does not examine the rapidly accumulating evidence objectively.

During the ten years that I have been preparing this book, I have examined medical books, hospital records, encyclopedias and medical journals without number. I have corresponded with research scientists throughout the world, and visited many of them. I have attended conferences and medical conventions devoted to heart attack and its prevention. I have read virtually every report of medical importance in the field.

Research is still going on all over the world but I feel that the time has come to bring the available verified knowledge to public attention in this form . . . without exaggeration and without sensationalism.

How did I come to undertake such a task? About thirty years ago I invented the Reflex Loudspeaker—the kind you see on top of all sound trucks, in airports, stadiums, etc.

In 1937 a small factory named University Loudspeakers was set up to manufacture and sell this particular speaker as well as others which I developed. In time, the company expanded until it employed several hundred people in our factories both here and in India. In the early years, as a result of my interest in health, we set up a medical clinic where examinations for employees were conducted once a week by Dr. Anton Gorelic who was interested in preventive medicine and heart-attack etiology. We also distributed free vitamins, books and pamphlets on health.

In the early Fifties, as the rate of heart attack continued to climb, I began to feel the urgency of bringing to as many people as possible the facts of heart-attack prevention. A series of lectures for friends and business associates was arranged. The data used in these lectures were part of the material I had planned to use in an illustrated booklet on the subject. The talks were well received but did not fully accomplish their purpose. From the reactions of the audiences, it was apparent that it was not going to be easy to convince the public to make changes in its way of life and diet, despite known scientific evidence of harmful effects on the arteries and the heart. Before any changes were made, proof of necessity would have to be overwhelmingly convincing and irrefutable. The small booklet I had planned now seemed inadequate and was put aside.

I concentrated, instead, on the current medical journals which covered my desk each morning, as well as on many of the earlier medical researches. A highly organized business and efficient group of executives and associates enabled me to devote a good part of the day to this work.

By 1958, I had reached the decision to write a book. . . .

The need for concentration on prevention has been emphasized by the world-renowned heart specialist, Dr. Paul Dudley White, who says: ". . . I am sure that the most important development in the next decade will not be in the diagnosis or treatment of heart disease, but in its *prevention* . . . This is the aim—or should be. If we are content simply to improve our diagnostic acumen and our therapeutic triumphs, we will get nowhere in the long run."

Dr. White and his colleagues throughout the world have already supplied the basic research data necessary to provide the foundation for an adequate prevention program. This program has been generally accepted by the majority of heart researchers and cardiologists.

But prevention will not be possible until we all become aware of the importance of the tremendous amount of research already done. I am now convinced that the American public, because of the legitimate skepticism of some, and the obstinate self-indulgence of others, will not accept and adhere to the urgently needed heart-attack-prevention program unless they individually have a full understanding of all the facts compelling its adoption.

A year ago, in order to test the acceptability of a thoroughly detailed and documented story, a wide survey was made of reader reaction to an early version of this book.

The results of the survey showed that readers welcomed all the factual material, and I was encouraged to add still more evidence to the final version which required another year for completion.

In its present version, then, the book brings the reader right up to the very frontiers of current scientific knowledge.

It is my earnest hope that it will achieve its purpose: the prevention of heart attack.

ARTHUR BLUMENFELD

May, 1964.

CHAPTER ONE

Why Adult Male Americans Are Prime Candidates For Heart Attack

Face these shocking facts:

The chances are better than two-to-one that, directly or indirectly, the adult male American will die of heart disease.

What's more, the odds against him have been increasing year by year. And still more alarming is the fact that the rate of increase in these unfavorable odds is greater among younger men.

Fortunately, recent research on the problem of heart disease from all over the world offers reassurance that there are ways for the individual to reverse these appalling odds.

But first consider the facts.

In the great cities and outposts of modern civilization, heart disease has been rising ominously. In recent years, the rate of heart attack has tripled in England and Norway, quadrupled in Scotland. But nowhere in the world has it risen to the astronomical heights found today in the United States.

"A pressing concern of our time is the frightening increase in the incidence of clinical coronary artery disease," states Dr. Richard Gorlin of the Harvard Medical School.

"Westernized communities," declare two eminent professors of medicine, Dr. H. Gordon and Dr. J. F. Brock, of the University of Capetown, "are experiencing an epidemic of . . . heart disease.

England's leading epidemiologist, Dr. J. N. Morris, adds somberly: "Coronary thrombosis is the scourge of Western civilization."

What is "coronary thrombosis"?

The serious obstruction of the small blood vessels called

coronaries, which feed directly to the muscular part of the heart, is called "coronary disease." When the flow of blood through any of these coronary arteries is blocked by "deposits" that substantially narrow the channel, the heart can no longer function normally. When the blockage reduces the blood supply critically, a heart attack may occur, with the result that small parts of the heart may actually "die," thus permanently ceasing to function. The most serious type of heart attack, "coronary thrombosis," occurs when a blood clot forms in one of the partially blocked coronary arteries.

This, then, is coronary thrombosis, the modern epidemic that Dr. Morris calls "the scourge of Western civilization."

Nowhere throughout the Western world is the effect of this epidemic more severe than in the United States.

In 1960, the National Office of Vital Statistics reported that "these [heart and artery] diseases resulted in over 900,000 deaths—more than 55% of all deaths [including accidents, suicides, and 'childbirth-related' deaths] occurring in the United States."

Eliminate the deaths caused by accidents and suicide (about 7%) and those related to childbirth (about 11%) and the adult heart-disease fatality rate assumes its true proportion to other *adult diseases*, about 70%.

This book deals only with the atherosclerotic diseases, which—according to Dr. R. Puffer in the *Bulletin of the World Health Organization*—account for three out of four heart disease deaths. Therefore the final toll of heart attack and related disease amounts to about half of all the adult deaths.

But fatalities are only one part of the havoc wrought by heart attack. For every person who dies of a heart attack, there is one, or more, who has survived, but is still under the constant menace of a fatal attack. Currently, there are many millions of such victims, and the number is growing.

Consider the testimony of one of our foremost clinical cardiologists. In November 1962 Dr. A. M. Master estimated in his report, in *Diseases of the Chest*, that from 5,000 to 10,000 coronary occlusions (heart attacks) are occurring daily in this country.

When did this "epidemic" first strike?

In 1870, New York City's most prominent physician, Dr. Austin Flint, wrote that he had rarely seen angina pectoris (pains caused by coronary artery disease) in his practice, and that as many as five years had passed without his having seen such a patient. Heart attack was then a "medical curiosity."

In fact, it was not until 1912, after Dr. James Herrick of Chicago had diagnosed his first six cases, that he was able to give to American doctors the first comprehensive report dealing with all the events of a heart attack. For ten years this report was practically ignored, but by the late 1920's the medical world was beginning to take notice of this new problem.

Since then the constantly increasing rate of heart attack has become the subject of grave concern in the editorials of medical journals. Many of our most prominent medical authorities have commented on the year-by-year increase observed in their own individual practices. These authorities include Sir Maurice Cassidy in England and Dr. Paul Dudley White, Dean of American cardiologists, who says, "The strict truth is that cardiovascular disease has increased to astronomical heights."

But there is still a group of scientists—cardiologists, clinicians and others—who remain skeptical. These scientists question the validity of the statistics which show increases in the death rate from coronary disease. They "explain away" the increase by our longer life span and the improved diagnostic skills of physicians.

The surest way to decide this question is to reexamine autopsy reports covering a long period that deal with the dissection and inspection of coronary arteries.

Fortunately, Dr. Henry M. Parish, seeking a project for additional postgraduate medical research, decided to conduct just such an examination. He finished the project in 1959 and in September, 1961, his report appeared in the *Journal of Chronic Diseases.*

To eliminate possible errors of medical diagnosis, Dr. Parish searched the actual autopsy data at the hospital connected with the Pathology Department of Yale University, which described the coronary blockage in 2,731 men. "The autopsy descriptions," said Dr. Parish, "were just as complete for 1935-1944 as they were for 1945-1955. The methods of examining the coronary arteries and recording the results remain consistent."

If the coronary dissection data in the autopsy records indicated that coronary blockage has increased in recent years, this would show that the increase in coronary artery disease was *real* and not to be attributed to greater diagnostic skill.

What did Dr. Parish find? Comparing closely matched age groups of accident victims in 1940 and 1950, he discovered that there was an *increase* in artery blockage. About 60% more cases in the later period had severe blockage in their coronary arteries.

WHY CORONARY THROMBOSIS IS INCREASING MOST RAPIDLY IN YOUNGER MEN

These startling statistics tell only part of the story. Heart attack is affecting more younger men in each succeeding generation.

Dr. David Spain, head of the Department of Pathology of New York's Beth-El Hospital, made autopsy comparisons of age-matched men who had died during a period of twenty years. In December, 1960, the disturbing facts were printed in the *American Journal of the Medical Sciences*.

Dr. Spain's work, an accurate comparison of the exact condition of coronary arteries, covered a longer period than that of Dr. Parish's. It proved that similar age groups in the more recent period were much worse off than their predecessors. Specifically, Dr. Spain's data showed that present-day forty-year-olds have more artery blockage than the fifty-year-old group of the previous generation.

And the rise was not limited to this age group. In *every age group* the coronary arteries showed *worse blockage* compared to a ten-year-older group of the previous generation.

The graph of coronary incidence continues to climb, and youth no longer affords the protection it once did. *The Lancet,* the "official" British medical publication (November 26, 1955), flatly states: "Young people . . . below the age of 40 . . . are affected much more than formerly."

A research team headed by Dr. Henry Shanoff found data of a similar nature in families with a history of heart disease. In these families attacks occurred at progressively earlier ages in succeeding generations. The pattern was that the heart attack in the offspring struck *two decades earlier* than in the parent.

Dr. Shanoff was not the only one to find evidence of the earlier incidence of heart attack in succeeding generations. Dr. S. A. Levine in the July 1963 issue of the *American Heart Journal* tells about a group of fathers whose heart attacks occurred at an average age of 61 years. Their sons were stricken with heart attack at an average age of 48. Other surveys have shown the same tendency of heart attack to occur in younger men.

The Cardiovascular Clinic at the University of Texas has one special advantage for the study of this rapidly changing picture. The clinic is unique in that it has had the same personnel for the past twenty-five years; therefore its standards of diagnosis, as was stated in their report, had remained constant. And what did this unusual research team discover?

They found that twenty-five years previously coronary heart disease had been comparatively rare, that the rate of incidence has been steadily increasing, and that, during this same twenty-five years prior to their report in 1953, the rate had skyrocketed from 2% to 16%.

The most alarming news for today's younger men comes from the world-famous Mayo Clinic, located in the town of Rochester, Minnesota, where two-thirds of all deaths in that small city are subject to autopsy by Mayo pathologists. From a five-year survey of almost every death of medical interest, a research team headed by Dr. Ralph E. Spiekermann, in January 1962, revealed that in a community without equal in the nation for the quality of its medical service, the percentage of deaths from coronary was greater among the younger men (age group, 30-64) than among older men (age group 64-100).

Dr. R. M. Drake of the California Department of Health had clinically examined thousands of men for coronary disease and found that in the under sixty-five age group the number of coronary cases was 50% higher than in the over-sixty-five age group (*American Journal of Public Health*, April, 1957).

What precisely are *your* chances of a heart attack?

Does the fact that you seem to be in good health, based on a full cardiac examination, exempt you from the dangers shown in the statistics?

"We still have the serious problem," warns Dr. Howard Burchell of the Mayo Clinic, "of an individual assured by

a competent cardiologist that he had a normal heart . . .
and yet died that day of acute myocardial infarction [heart
attack]. We must suspect coronary disease in many of our
adult population even when they do not give a history . . .
or a clue . . . to its presence."

The causes of heart attack may be building up, without
the patient or the physician being aware of it. The eminent
heart authority Irving S. Wright stated in 1960 that, "Anyone seeing enough autopsies cannot avoid being impressed
by the numerous scars in the heart muscle produced by
former infarctions [attacks] that were so mild they were
never recognized clinically."

Heart attack is not a sudden visitation from out of the
blue. It only seems so. Coronary disease is a *hidden* disease,
increasing the blockage year by year, *secretly*. Until the
blockage reaches the danger point, there are no telltale
signs and you are in apparent good health.

What most people think is *the* cause of a heart attack is
only the last straw that breaks the back of an overburdened
cardiovascular system.

Drs. James M. Jett and S. M. Grundy of Baylor University have recently made a statistical study of all the
heart attacks, the "silent" unfelt damages as well as the
known, in a large group of autopsies. Their statistics show
that by age sixty-five almost three out of every four of all
known myocardial infarctions (heart attacks) have already
occurred.

But this ratio, of three-out-of-four heart attacks before
sixty-five, is not an inevitable fate. This ratio *can* be lowered. Medical science has found ways by which heart
attack can be set back for years, and in many cases actually prevented.

THE HEART ATTACK—BLOW-BY-BLOW
DESCRIPTION OF A MENACE
THAT STRIKES WITHOUT WARNING

The basis for the heart attack is coronary artery blockage. Although the heart is a complicated organ, it is only
necessary to become acquainted with its external arteries
to learn about heart attack. The simplified picture below
shows these arteries and the arrows illustrate how the blood

flows from inside the heart pump (dotted arrow) to the aorta and the two main coronary arteries.

The great aorta artery arching out of the top of the heart carries the blood to all parts of the body. Imagine the body as a machine. In it the aorta functions as an enormous pipe, carrying the fuel without which the body could not function.

"But," it might be asked, "the heart muscle is part of the machine, too. How does *it* get *its* fuel?"

The heart muscle is not fueled directly by the blood in its chambers. But observe the two main coronary arteries branching off from the base of the aorta. They are the side pipelines that carry the blood, by means of the still smaller branch lines shown in the diagram, directly to all the muscles of the heart.

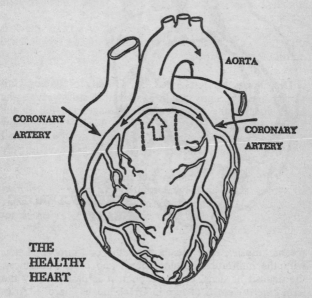

AORTA

CORONARY ARTERY

CORONARY ARTERY

THE HEALTHY HEART

What you are looking at is a picture of a healthy heart with clear coronary arteries. The blood can flow smoothly through them and can keep the heart muscles pumping steadily and efficiently.

But what if these side pipelines became clogged and blocked? Blockage in the coronaries means that the amount of blood reaching the heart muscles is reduced. When the blood supply is reduced below a certain point, the affected parts of the heart muscle can no longer function. When a section of heart muscle stops functioning, a heart attack and even death may result.

Medical science has several names for the combination of substances which block the arteries. *Atheroma* is the term for the soft fibrous and fatty deposit which clogs the arteries during the early stage of blockage. *Athero* in Greek

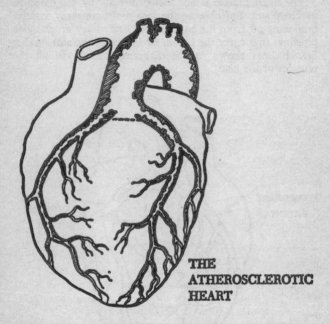

THE
ATHEROSCLEROTIC
HEART

means "mush"; *oma* means "growth" or "tumor." Later, with the infiltration of more fibrin and other substances, the deposit hardens, at which point it is described by the term *atherosclerosis* (*sclero* in Greek means "hard"). Arteriosclerosis, an older and more general name for *all* types of arterial illness, is now considered too general a term and so is gradually falling into disuse.

In the healthy artery, as shown in the illustration, the amount of blockage is negligible. But as can be seen in the illustration of the atherosclerotic artery, the deposits have narrowed the channel through which the blood flows. It is the degree of blockage that determines whether or not the heart muscles will receive enough blood to continue to function.

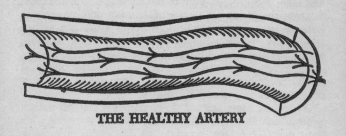

THE HEALTHY ARTERY

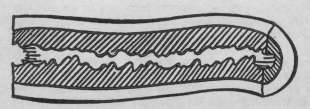

THE ATHEROSCLEROTIC ARTERY

The coronary arteries are small, the largest no wider than a thin soda straw. For a menacing condition to arise, only a small quantity of atheroma need be present.

The blockage grows silently, insidiously. There is no way of knowing how much atheroma is accumulating inside the arteries until it is too late.

People often ask: "Is there no warning before the blood supply to the heart begins to get dangerously low?"

In some parts of the body, such as the legs, a reduced blood supply to the muscles can cause *localized* pain sensations. But in the heart there are no nerves which can specifically localize the pain.

However, pain *can* result from insufficient blood to one of the muscles in the heart, only this pain is not felt directly *in* the heart, but is "referred"—perhaps by some little known mechanism via nerves in the spinal cord—to muscles in the chest, neck and arms. This pain is known as *angina pectoris. Angina* means "pain," *pectoris* means "chest muscles."

Does this mean that all chest pains are due to artery blockage? Far from it. Pain in the chest is one of the most frequent complaints the doctor hears. Many chest pains, for instance, are due to calcifications between the ribs and to other types of non-coronary disorders. However, because of the advanced extent of coronary artery blockage present in the average middle-aged man, every suspicious pain should be reported to the physician for analysis as a possible symptom of coronary disease.

One of the complaints of the physician is that the patient is often unable to be sufficiently helpful in describing his chest pains. The more accurate the description, the easier it is for the doctor to be certain whether or not the pain is of coronary origin.

In the early stages, and quite frequently in the very late stages of coronary disease, it is the patient's ability to help the doctor by means of a clear description of his sensations which is of most value. Laboratory or electrical instrument tests are too often of no use in the diagnosis of this hidden ailment. Physicians have commented that the patient's ability to give a good and complete history of all his pain sensations—and the situations that caused them—is more valuable than all the other tests and physical examinations combined.

One important feature characterizing the pain of angina is that it often moves or "radiates" from the chest to the left arm, and at times to the right arm, the neck and many other parts of the body.

A second feature is that the pain is rarely indicated by pointing to a specific region. Most frequently if a gesture is used, it is made with the flat palm of the hand or even both palms on the chest. Sometimes the sensation is so general that no gesture can be used to indicate the pain.

A third feature is that of time. The pain of angina rarely lasts less than thirty seconds or longer than thirty minutes.

A fourth very important feature is the *type* of pain. The pain of angina is frequently described as a deep sense of pressure, a vise-like squeezing or constriction in the chest region. There may be a feeling of choking, of anxiety, of anguish. As a matter of fact, the Greek word *anchein,* from which angina is derived, contains all these meanings.

With these distinctive sensations may come dizziness, weakness in the arms, and even perspiration. Men will frequently ignore and even conceal these symptoms, in the wishful hope that their cause is insignificant. When the pain comes, the individual may attempt to deal with it by himself. If it came on walking, he stands still. If it came while lying down, he may stand up. But since statistics show that coronary blockage is almost universally present in the middle-aged American male, a "head-in-the-sand" behavior is dangerous.

Any type of pain which may cause suspicion of angina, no matter how slight, definitely should not be ignored, and the sensations should be described to the physician immediately.

The purpose of this suggestion is not to make hypochondriacs of American middle-aged men, but to focus attention on a very critical condition in this country.

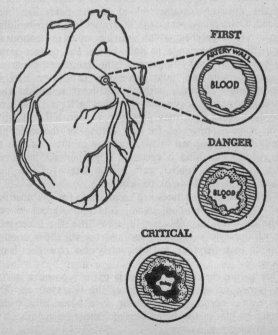

THREE STAGES OF ARTERY BLOCKAGE

Dr. Oglesby Paul and his group of cardiologists who made a five year study of coronary disease at the Hawthorne Works of the Western Electric Company have concluded that "of particular importance is the link between a history of any type of chest discomfort and the later recognition of coronary disease. This finding confirms what many clinicians have observed."

However, a diagnosis of angina by the doctor should not result in fatalistic pessimism. There is medical evidence that some of the damage causing the angina is reversible. Some of the atheroma in the artery can be slowly cleared away. And most important, the formation of additional deposits of atheroma can be prevented.

Although the angina symptoms, if heeded, can save a man's life, the heart-attack victim doesn't always receive that warning. Angina does not occur in a large percentage of the cases of coronary heart disease.

The accompanying diagram shows in a simplified form, how the flow of coronary blood to the heart has been reduced. Over many years, the atheroma has been building up in layers or patches, which indicate separate "episodes." Frequently the blockage is built up to the danger point with the victim totally unaware of the dangerous situation. Actually a man can have coronaries with over half of their capacity blocked, without the least sensation that anything is wrong. Even his physician, after all the most up-to-date heart tests, may give him a clean bill of health.

The stage is now set for the climax of the coronary tragedy. It may happen in the next few minutes, or it may take years. One thing it certain: If proper action is not taken, the time is sooner, rather than later, for the final disaster of the heart attack to occur.

What specific substances are responsible for the obstruction? Their names: cholesterol, fats and fibrous tissue. As the obstruction builds up, little by little, the inner passage of the artery becomes too narrow to allow enough blood to get through to adequately nourish the heart muscle.

This severe narrowing, which is called *coronary occlusion,* is one of the basic causes of the heart attack. The other cause, *coronary thrombosis,* is a blood clot which completely blocks the inner passage, most frequently at a point of severe narrowing.

Heart attack may vary in intensity from the mildest,

which is often mistaken for another illness, to the most serious, which results in instantaneous death. Statistics vary but at least three out of five cases of heart attack do not result in death. Frequently two or three attacks occur before the final one. The sensations felt during the attack are similar to those of angina, but usually they are far more painful and prolonged. After an attack, victims have often remarked that they had the sensation that "death was near."

Although the pain of the heart attack is felt instantly, the permanent damage does not appear until some hours later. Here's what happens: the occlusion (or thrombosis) in a coronary branch shuts off the blood supply to one area of the heart, whose muscles are affected very much like a city upon which an atom bomb has been dropped. As the illustration shows, in the immediate area of the blockage everything has been wiped out, and at some distance, there is partial damage.

The central area around the blocked artery actually dies. The scientific name for the disaster just described is *myocardial infarction.*

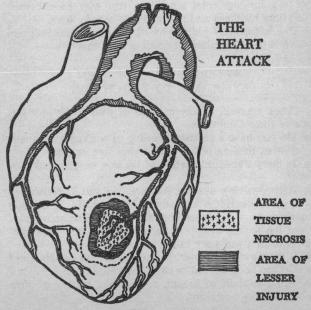

THE HEART ATTACK

AREA OF TISSUE NECROSIS

AREA OF LESSER INJURY

After the attack, a natural "repair mechanism" goes to work, eventually turning the dead tissue into a fibrous scar which binds together the rest of the functioning muscle. The stricken heart is now "repaired"—although less efficient.

Sometimes this myocardial infarction, this tissue death, will occur silently, without a heart attack, without any pain—no sensation at all. This is the "silent" heart attack.

A "silent" heart attack usually means that a very small branch of the "coronary artery" has been shut down and that the area of tissue death has been very small. But the combined effect of several of these unfelt heart damages will finally call attention to the now apparent tragedy. These silent attacks are the most important cause of another common heart ailment, *heart failure*.

After the heart attack and the formation of scar tissue, there are two possible courses. The first is to permit the existence of the same environmental conditions that originally caused the artery blockage. This attitude will almost inevitably lead to further artery blockage.

The second course, which is the prudent one, is to seek out the environmental conditions that may have caused the artery blockage and to attempt to change them.

This is the basic philosophy of the Prevention Program which is to be explained in detail in later chapters.

ARTERY BLOCKAGE—TEN SYMPTOMS TO WATCH FOR

Check yourself, or any member of your family, for just one of these symptoms:

● Do you have a persistent feeling of weakness, coldness, numbness, tingling or burning in your toes or feet?

● Is there a small ulceration of the skin on your ankle or foot?

● After walking a short distance, do you experience a feeling of heaviness or fatigue in the calf? When you continue to walk, does the discomfort turn into pain? Does the feeling disappear soon after you stop walking?

● Is there a white arc in the iris of your eye?

● Is there a clouding over the lens of your eye (a cataract)?

● Do you have blurred or darkened vision?

● Are you short of breath, so that you must stop often when walking hurriedly?

● Do you have head noises? Dizziness? Light headedness? Sudden spells of partial deafness? Ringing in the ears? Vertigo?

● Have you experienced a brief fainting spell or blackout?

● Do you seem to be losing your mental grip? Are there increasing periods of confusion, loss of memory? Are you beginning to lose the ability to distinguish between the significant and the insignificant?

A "yes" answer to any one of these questions may be a symptom of atherosclerosis in one of its many forms. For atherosclerosis is not only a disease of the *coronary* arteries. It can affect *any* artery in the body, and wherever it strikes, a localized form of the disease occurs. A blackage in the ear artery can cause deafness. Atheroma in an eye artery can lead to blindness. And when these deposits clog the arteries of the brain, the result may be senility and stroke. What in the past was considered a separate disease is now known to be a local effect of the general atherosclerotic condition. Dr. Irving S. Wright, the eminent cardiologist, sums up the contemporary medical view:

"One of the most important changes that has taken place in medicine is the concept that we shall no longer look upon disease of the coronary arteries as a manifestation of heart disease, or strokes as a manifestation of brain disease, or senile diabetes as a manifestation of pancreatic disease, or intermittent claudication [leg pain] as Buerger's Disease . . . but that we should look upon these disorders as chance manifestations of a generalized process of atherosclerosis or clogging up of our arteries."

Let's take a closer look at some of these specific local forms of atherosclerosis, beginning with the ear.

Have you ever had a "ringing" in your ear when no bell was actually ringing? In past years this seemed to occur only among the aged, but today this symptom occurs with increasing frequency in younger people. According to Dr. Ferenc Torok of Rumania, it's the first symptom of atherosclerosis of the arteries of the inner ear.

Deafness and vertigo, as well as "ringing," is attributed by Dr. Noah D. Fabricant to atherosclerosis of the arteries of the labyrinth, that part of the ear that governs our sense of balance.

According to Dr. H. Droller's report in the *Journal of Laryngology and Otology,* of nearly five hundred elderly persons studied, in those cases where vertigo was present the major cause was found to be artery blockage.

Sudden deafness as a symptom of this same type of artery blockage was described by Dr. O. Erik Hallberg of the Mayo Clinic in his report "Sudden Deafness and Its Relation to Atherosclerosis."

It is possible that artery blockage is responsible for a large part of the affluence of the American hearing-aid industry.

However, the ear is not the part of the body most affected by atheroma. To the legs goes this dubious honor. The arteries of the legs bear the added pressure of all the body fluids above them. The blood pressure is therefore higher in the lower limbs than in the rest of the body, and this causes increased deposits of artery blockage in the legs.

When severe blockage occurs in the legs, it is recognized by a specific symptom, "intermittent claudication," sometimes referred to as "angina pectoris of the legs." The word claudication comes from the Latin verb, *claudicare*, to limp. After the victim walks a short distance, a feeling of heaviness or fatigue develops in the leg. Pain comes with continued walking. Standing still for a few minutes relieves the pain, which returns after walking is resumed. Atherosclerotic deposits in the arteries of the leg, thigh, or lower abdomen have prevented supplies of blood sufficient to fuel the extra work of walking from reaching the leg muscles. From the lack of blood comes the heaviness, fatigue and a "vise-like" pain.

When diminished blood circulation occurs in the vessels feeding the legs, another distressful condition may occur: an ulcer near the ankle.

Of very special concern to the physician treating diabetics is the diminished arterial circulation due to atherosclerosis, especially in the feet and toes. This condition may necessitate the amputation of toes, or even of a leg, should the lowered blood supply cause gangrene.

Atherosclerosis affects not only the ears and the toes. Between these extremes of the body's geograply lie all our vital organs, any one of which can suffer a disaster when enough atheroma blockage forms in the arteries that feed them. But, most often, atheroma strikes the more vulnerable coronary arteries first, and because of an eventual fatal heart attack, a man will never learn of the dangerous deposits accumulating in the arterial life-lines of his stomach, pancreas, kidneys, or liver.

Artery blockage in the digestive system results in "angina of the stomach," which is recognized by pains following even an ordinary meal. Artery blockage to the pancreas is a frequent cause of "senile" diabetes. An increasing and all too frequent result of artery blockage to the kidneys is high blood pressure, which completes a vicious cycle by causing further artery blockage.

Blood vessel blockage in the lungs is of a different type, and is usually a result of blood clot (thrombosis) in the large veins of the legs which breaks loose and lodges in the small veins of the lungs.

A large percentage of all blindness is due to diabetic artery blockage in the tiny vessels in the eyes. Dr. C. H. Pope, who studied the chemical composition of this blood vessel blockage, found it to be mainly of fat-like deposits.

Heart failure, although frequently a result of artery blockage, should not be confused with heart attack. Heart failure is the result of an imbalance in the pumping action between the left- and right-side pumps of the heart. This imbalance may be due to various disorders, but its major cause is a series of small and frequently "silent" or unnoticed heart attacks due to coronary artery blockage, which weaken the muscles of one side of the heart, causing the imbalance.

While the heart attack is not accompanied by any social stigma, the clogging of the arteries in the brain is quite a different story. A man's brain is the seat of his personality, of his essential self. With the destruction of one small part of his brain, his whole behavior pattern may change, and he will no longer be the same person.

Few of us would admit that something, no matter how slight, has interfered with the normal functioning of our mental processes. Yet atherosclerosis of the brain arteries occurs frequently, and can lead to mental deterioration, emotional derangement, senility and stroke.

The most dramatic of these atherosclerotic symptoms is the stroke. It causes sudden paralysis of some part of the body: In an instant the features are distorted, the leg muscles no longer respond, the eyes go blind, the hearing vanishes, or the tongue is stricken mute. But despite its lightning-like occurrence the stroke is actually slow in coming. It's the crippling climax of a long atherosclerotic development.

A stroke occurs when the blood supply to some part of the brain is cut off or reduced to an insufficient trickle. When a part of the brain is put out of action, the muscles, nerves and organs it controls are paralyzed. It's as if a switch were suddenly turned off.

Fortunately, nature has anticipated the clogging of brain arteries and evolved an intricate system of protection. No part of the brain is supplied by a single direct arterial lifeline. There is, instead, an intricate network of alternate routes of crisscrossing pathways. A true stroke can only occur when *all* the lifelines to a brain area are blocked, and this takes a long time. What may occur is the clogging of one route, then another, then another—until the blood supply fails and a stroke occurs.

Is there any way of knowing whether this is happening? Yes, there are many warning signs.

Some of these signs are *physical*. Long before a stroke there may be a feeling of dizziness and light-headedness. There may be numbness, tingling and weakness in the extremities. The vision may blur or darken. Head noises and a general sense of confusion are other possible warning signs.

Not only does the United States rank first in heart attacks, but now it is also becoming famous for a new symptom referred to by Dr. P. Wertheimer of France as the transient "little stroke" of the Americans.

Dr. W. C. Alvarez and Dr. H. A. Schroeder in their reports have frequently referred to these symptoms as "strokelets."

This problem is now so prevalent, that the United States Public Health Service found it necessary to issue a free pamphlet titled "Little Strokes." The most significant section is subtitled, "Younger Persons May Have Little Strokes." As can be seen from the following quotation, the pamphlet emphasizes the difficulty of correct diagnosis. "A little stroke might show itself only by a few minutes of confusion, a passing dizziness, a thickness of speech for a few hours . . ."

But blockage of arteries in the brain does not always bring on these noticeable symptoms.

Atheroma blockage in the brain arteries may instead be the cause of progressive mental deterioration. There may be a lessened ability to face a challenge or to handle new situations. At first the events of yesterday are forgotten, then the events of years ago. The mental and emotional horizons may contract little by little, until eventually the world is filled only with one's own ego. This is the sad picture of atherosclerotic senility.

Senility, we now know, is not a normal condition of old age. It's a disease—a local manifestation of atherosclerosis. Many aged men have not only escaped senility, but have been active to the point of genius even in their nineties. Goethe finished the second part of his *Faust* after seventy. Bernard Shaw was still writing in his nineties. On the other hand, when atherosclerosis of the brain is severe, even a middle-aged man can experience the symptoms of the senile.

In *The American Journal of Psychiatry*, Dr. D. Rothschild points out that among the young, when atherosclerosis of the arteries of the brain occurs in a poorly balanced personality, mental disease is likely to result. Many chronic psychoses, Dr. Rothschild concludes, are atherosclerotic in origin.

The Russian medical scientist, Dr. A. L. Myasnikov, in his book, *Atherosclerosis*, points out that when the arteries feeding the cortex of the brain are blocked, our mental inhibitions become weakened. The result is that personality trends formerly kept under unconscious control may now go unchecked. A man who was thrifty now becomes miserly. If he was strict, he becomes rigid and cruel. Good-natured before, he becomes overcomplacent. Senile behavior, the sudden excessive fault-finding, the torrid temper, the chronic irritability, are now easier to understand.

Based on the recent findings that "strokelets" occur in younger men, there is increasing possibility of premature senility in the coming years.

This serious situation calls for intensified research. "In all the recent excitement about coronary heart disease," writes Dr. Walter Alvarez of the Mayo Clinic, in *Geriatrics*, "there has been great need for a study designed to show how often atherosclerosis of the vessels in the brain parallels that of the vessels in the heart . . . Every big department of pathology ought to have someone working on this problem."

Fortunately, the same prevention program found by

medical research to prevent heart attack will also prevent artery blockage in every part of the body, including the brain. The following chapter will introduce one of the main phases of the whole prevention program—a change in diet.

CHAPTER TWO

The World's Most Important Public Health Document

THE AMERICAN HEART ASSOCIATION REPORT ON HEART-ATTACK PREVENTION

There now exists clear evidence that the unhappy situation presented in the foregoing chapter can be remedied. During recent years scientists from all over the world have made important discoveries concerning the causes and prevention of the coronary epidemic.

In 1959 the outstanding heart-research specialists connected with the American Heart Association recognized the urgent need of an *official* medical digest and analysis of the vast accumulation of data on coronary prevention. The AHA appointed a committee of six eminent heart specialists to make such a study and to report their findings.

The committee immediately went to work, and all the existing published data on the subject was studied, scrutinized, and weighed by them. As a result of this study a report was published which ranks among the world's most important public-health documents. The title of the report was: "Dietary Fat and Its Relation to Heart Attacks and Strokes."

This report may well mark a turning point in medical history. It was considered of such significance that it was published simultaneously in two of the country's foremost medical journals, the *Journal of the American Medical Association* and *Circulation*, which is the official medical journal of the American Heart Association.

The essence of the report is that, ". . . *the reduction of fat consumption with reasonable substitution of polyun-*

saturated fat for saturated fats, is recommended as a possible means of preventing atherosclerosis and decreasing the risks of heart attacks and strokes."

This recommendation is, in effect, an authoritative medical recognition of the need to change our eating habits.

But can we rely on this report alone to motivate the necessary changes in the eating habits of present-day America? The answer, unfortunately, is—*no*. The diet of the average American is intricately bound up with his family background, cultural customs, and acquired tastes and habits. To expect these ingrained traits to be modified by any one document, however authoritative, would be naive.

Ideally, the man to initiate dietary change is the family doctor. He is most qualified to adjust the anti-coronary diet to the particular physical and psychological needs of each patient. And he also possesses the authority to give full information on how to prevent coronary disease.

Yes, *prevent*—for every medical authority agrees that the best way to combat coronary heart disease is through prevention. But prevention, according to the AHA report, entails a change in diet, a voluntary abandonment of old eating habits and an assumption of new ones. Therefore it will not be accomplished unless one *wants* to accomplish it, and a person may not relish the thought of such a change until forced by necessity or convinced by a full understanding of the prevention program.

Ultimately, it will be the doctor who is going to recommend the change to a low-fat diet on an individual basis. But the task of educating the public at large to the threat of coronary disease and directing people to coronary health is complex and arduous; it demands patience and constant repetition. It calls for the ability to translate medical terminology into easy-to-follow explanations and instructions.

All this takes additional time. And as we well know, with our population continually growing, time is one commodity the general practitioner is unable to spare.

Consequently, the American doctor is not able to do all of the educational and motivational work involved in the coronary-prevention program. Frequently, he can do no more than give a pointed warning.

Most patients contribute to the difficulty of the problem by coming to the physician confused, badly informed and unmotivated. Their dietary patterns are already fixed, and they resist changing them. Medical literature contains many complaints by general practitioners deploring the situation. Patients are so firmly attached to the old rich diet that the harassed doctor, with an overcrowded waiting room of patients clamoring for attention, cannot cope with the time-consuming task of motivation.

By the time the patient reaches the consultation room he should already be convinced of the necessity of dietary reform and inclined to follow the doctor's latest scientific dietary advice.

It is for this reason that the American Heart Association has made its report available for public distribution by the physician in booklet form.

Only a few paragraphs of the AHA's report—*"Dietary Fat and its Relation to Heart Attacks and Strokes"*—are reprinted here. Other parts and many of the references are dealt with in other chapters of this book. In reading the paragraphs presented here, it should be remembered that the report is the work of six leading heart authorities, and as a whole has the endorsement of the American Heart Association.

The six authorities are:

IRVINE H. PAGE, M.D., *Chairman, Director,* Research Division, Cleveland Clinic Foundation.

EDGAR V. ALLEN, M.D., *Senior Consultant* in Medicine, Mayo Clinic.

FRANCIS L. CHAMBERLAIN, M.D., *Clinical Professor of Medicine,* University of California School of Medicine.

ANCEL KEYS, Ph.D., *Director,* Laboratory of Physiological Hygiene, University of Minnesota.

JEREMIAH STAMLER, M.D., *Director,* Heart Disease Control Program, Chicago Board of Health.

FREDERICK J. STARE, M.D., *Professor of Nutrition* and *Chairman* Department of Nutrition, Harvard Medical School.

The following excerpts are the paragraphs which contain the highlights of the report:

"What Types of Research Relate Diet to Atherosclerosis?"

"Many years ago a scientist fed cholesterol and other types of fat to rabbits. The blood cholesterol content increased and the rabbits developed atherosclerosis; that is, cholesterol and other fatty substances were deposited in the walls of the arteries. Many other animal species have been found to behave similarly. These animal experiments indicate that diet may be an important cause of atherosclerosis.

"Global studies have shown that dietary habits of human populations differ. Evidence gathered from many countries suggests a relationship between the amount and type of fat consumed, the amount of cholesterol in the blood and the reported incidence of coronary artery disease."

*   *   *   *   *

"Study of diets in the United States indicates that they usually contain large amounts of fat which account for approximately 40-45% of the calories. In contrast, many populations in other parts of the world—for example, large groups in Asia, Africa and Latin America—eat food containing barely a third as much fat. The concentrations of cholesterol in the blood of such groups are much less than in those consuming the excess calorie and high-fat diets, and some reports indicate that heart attacks are correspondingly fewer."

*   *   *   *   *

"Third, the blood cholesterol concentration may also be reduced by controlling the amount and type of fat in the diet without altering caloric intake. Not all fats in the diet have the same effect on the amount of cholesterol in the blood. In the usual diet eaten in the United States, a large part of the fat is of the saturated type. Too much of this type of fat tends to increase the cholesterol in the blood. Considerable amounts of saturated fat are present in whole milk, cream, butter, cheese and meat. Coconut oil and the fat in chocolate also have a high content of fats of the saturated type. Most shortenings and margarines have less than half as much saturated fat, and the common vegetable oils have still less. When the intake of saturated fats is reduced, blood cholesterol levels usually decrease."

"In contrast to the above food fats, many natural vegetable oils, such as corn, cotton and soya, as well as the fat of fish, are relatively low in saturated fats and high in fats of the polyunsaturated type. When these fats are substituted for a substantial part of the saturated fats without increasing calories, blood cholesterol decreases."

The essence of the above paragraphs is this: *the relation of saturated and unsaturated fats and their effect on the amount of blood cholesterol is the key to the prevention of heart disease.*

The American Heart Association's historic document was published in 1961. But animal fat as a possible cause of coronary heart attack had been suspected decades ago. Why, then, did official medical science wait so long before placing its seal of approval on a discovery involving the health and life of every person in the Western world?

Before scientists release any conclusive data directly to the public, they check and recheck repeatedly. It is easy to understand why scientists, particularly the medical scientists, take these extraordinary precautions.

In essence, the dietary recommendations of the American Heart Association's report are similar in many respects to the Prudent Diet, which was designed by Dr. N. Jolliffe for his New York City Anti-Coronary Club. The Prudent Diet will be explained in greater detail in later chapters.

In the pages that follow, we will highlight the research data used by the American Heart Association Committee in its 1961 report and also the medical research which has been made public since the report.

Although there have been voluminous reports of important research on the causes of artery blockage in animals, this book is mostly concerned with studies conducted on human beings. Paradoxically, the events which provided the early data on which a life-saving prevention program could be based, occurred during the darkest days of World War II. This is the subject of the following chapter.

CHAPTER THREE

Hidden Dangers in Our Diet

AN UNEXPECTED LIFE SAVING DISCOVERY BY MEDICAL SCIENTISTS

Where do the substances that form the atheroma—the cholesterol, the fats, the fibrous tissue—come from? How are they deposited on and in the artery walls?

The American Heart Association report makes it clear that saturated fats in our diet may constitute one of the important causes of artery blockage. Some of the background material for the report was furnished by one of the most dramatic and unusual nutritional experiments ever made. It was an experiment on a colossal scale observed by scientists all over the Western world. The laboratory was Europe during and after World War II.

Our story, however, really begins in 1932 with the publication of a medical report that also was to make history. Its author, Dr. Wilhelm Raab, Emeritus Professor of Medicine at the University of Vermont, was at the time a heart specialist in Vienna. The title of his paper was: *"Dietary Factors in the Origin of Arteriosclerosis and Hypertension."*

Dietary factors? Why were *dietary factors* suspected? Dr. Raab knew that during World War I the incidence of atherosclerosis and heart disease had dropped. And during the same period, the consumption of eggs, milk, butter and meat had also dropped. Was there a connection?

A large body of medical evidence linking fats to atherosclerosis, studied not only through animal experiments, but also through experiments on human subjects, had been reviewed in Dr. Raab's report. The positive evidence seemed very impressive. But Dr. Raab still called for additional research.

"It is the main purpose of this treatise," he wrote, "to stimulate an internationally organized statistical study of the problems of arteriosclerosis . . . with particular consideration . . . to the . . . named . . . dietary factors."

Dr. Raab's call for the great nutritional experiment went

unheeded. But in less than ten years the situation changed. Suddenly the great nutritional study was in full swing. However, it was not arranged by scientists but by the accident of war.

From the day the Panzers knifed their way through Poland, the food supply of every man, woman and child in Europe was affected. The ration card permitted only a bare supply of "luxury" foods. At that time doctors noticed the statistical relationship between the decreased incidence of heart disease and the war-imposed low-egg, low-milk, low-butter and low-meat diet. In every country in war-torn Europe, doctors observed that the percentage of deaths from coronary heart attacks was falling.

For example, in the municipal hospitals of Rotterdam, during the depth of the wartime deprivation diet, only six coronary deaths were recorded for the year 1945. The prewar annual average had been thirty-five. This made Dr. H. E. Schornagel conclude that, "The decrease in coronary is closely related to the nutritional intake . . . particularly to a diet which had been rich in fat."

Drs. Sivertssen, Stuart and Godal compared the percentage of heart-disease patients entering St. Joseph's Hospital in Porsgrunn, Norway, during the prewar and war years. The prewar coronary percentage, during the period of a high-fat diet, was 3% of the total hospital admissions. During the war years, when the fat intake was low, the coronary percentage was reduced to half. Dr. I. Vartianen of Finland, comparing the number of coronary attacks in his country from 1936 through the war years, concluded that the *minimum rate of coronary attacks occurred in 1944, the year when fat restriction had its maximum effect.*

And from Russia came further evidence. "During the blockade of Leningrad in 1941-42," wrote Dr. K. G. Volkova in Moscow's *Clinical Medicine,* "a marked reduction was found in the incidence of angina pectoris and coronary occlusion."

The lean diet the Russians fed their German prisoners produced the same effect. Dr. G. Schettler, a world-renowned German cardiologist, worked as a prison doctor in a Russian POW camp, where he was permitted to perform autopsies. He was amazed, he told a symposium at the New York Academy of Science in October, 1961, to discover that, "On hundreds of autopsies, there was very little evidence of any atherosclerosis." He attributed this to "the effects of the low-fat diet given the German prisoners of war by the Russians." Dr. Schettler added that, "In Germany in the final years of World War II, I was told by my colleagues, it was difficult to obtain examples of individuals with atherosclerosis for demonstration to the medical students."

The effects of the restrictions of the war years were also felt in Japan, despite the already low Japanese coronary rate, and Dr. Shunio Okinaka of the Tokyo University Medical School has reported that at the height of the fat deprivation, there was a drop to half the already low prewar rate.

The beneficial effects of the ration cards were felt even in the United States. The rising death rate from diabetes showed a definite drop during all of World War II. Diabetes, as will be shown later, is an important cause of coronary disease.

To many scientists these findings gathered from all over the world offered conclusive proof that the original high-calorie, high-fat diet was a major cause of atherosclerosis. But others wanted to see whether the change back to the prewar diet would raise the coronary-heart-disease rate to prewar levels.

With the war over, recovery, prosperity and the old rich diet supplied the data. Phase II of the great nutritional experiment was under way. Consider, for example, those prisoners of war under Dr. Schettler's care in Russia. What happened to them once they were back home and again on a high fat diet? "In these same soldiers from the POW camps—dozens of cases of coronary developed," Dr. Schettler told the author. "I diagnosed them myself."

This is dramatic evidence, and it is supported by long columns of statistics. Professor Fritz A. Pezold, for example, reviewed the data from over 6,000 Berlin autopsies, and found that directly after the war, when the proportion of fat calories in the average German diet was a low 8%, evidence of severe coronary blockage was found in five out of ten autopsies. But later when they had partially returned to the fat of the land and the average consumption of fat was up to 30% of the calories, severe coronary blockage was evident in eight out of ten.

More proof came from Dr. Schornagel who continued his investigation in Rotterdam beyond the war years. With the return to the "normal" high-fat diet, coronaries zoomed.

By 1950, the rate was as high as it had been in 1940—
over five times higher than at the low point of the wartime
low-fat diet!

Dr. Hugh M. Sinclair, world-famed British nutritionist,
addressing the Newspaper Food Editors Conference in
New York City, supplied an independent corroboration:
"Let me illustrate the importance of dietary fats . . . .
When we introduced wartime rationing in 1940, the rise
in heart disease was temporarily halted. But then it started
up again in 1943—[not long] after the introduction of
American lend-lease."

As eggs, butter, milk and meat found their way again to
the tables of Europe, death rates from coronary rose to
prewar levels and eventually exceeded them. At St. Joseph's
Hospital in Porsgrunn, Norway, where the percentage of
coronary patients to total admissions had dipped during the
war years from a prewar 3% down to 1½%, in 1948 it
was up to 2½%, in 1951 to 5%, and in 1954 to 7%.

Had the great nutritional experiment corroborated Dr.
Raab's prediction of 1932? There was no question about
it in the minds of any of the medical scientists reporting on
the relationship between fat intake and coronary. *Increase*
your fat intake, the statistics indicated, and you increase
your chances of atherosclerosis. *Decrease* your fat intake
and the possibility of a heart attack declines.

One source of fat was to receive special notice from
some of the doctors. The incriminating statistics seemed
to point particularly to eggs. Dr. E. Malmros of Sweden
investigated this theory with a complete statistical analysis.
The decline in coronary in Sweden during the war years
was attributed by him especially to a drop in egg consumption. Besides fat, another substance—cholesterol—is known
to contribute to atheroma. Eggs are the richest food source
of this substance. Dr. Malmros was convinced that a reduction of cholesterol-rich foods in the diet is directly associated with a decline in deaths from coronary.

Drs. Axel Strom and R. Adelsten Jensen of the University of Oslo in Norway were in agreement with Dr. Malmros. From their country's Ministry of Supply they
obtained data on the estimated annual consumption,
between 1938 and 1948, of the main sources of cholesterol:
milk, cream, butter, cheese and, of course, eggs. They
correlated this information with the drop in coronary, and

found that the decline in death rate due to coronary paralleled the decline in consumption of cholesterol-rich foods. Was this proof that diet cholesterol was a major cause of coronary heart disease? "Not certain proof," commented Strom and Jensen, but they added "we have . . . been unable to find an alternative explanation of this remarkable decline."

Fats, cholesterol . . . was the cast of the coronary tragedy complete? Or would the wartime nutritional experiment unmask still another villain? Remember that there are two converging roads leading to a heart attack: first, the piling up of atheroma in the walls of the coronaries, diminishing the blood supply below the minimum level necessary for the heart muscles to survive, and second, thrombosis, complete blockage caused by the blood clot.

What did the wartime nutritional experiment indicate about rich foods and the clotting of blood in veins and arteries? The answer lies in the records of the surgeons, who are most vitally concerned with the prevention of internal blood clots. In the critical period following an operation a blood clot may form, seriously threatening the patient's recovery.

From the report of Germany's Dr. A. Werthemann: "Decrease in incidence of blood clots in veins during World War II . . . was possibly due to the deficiency of the blood-clotting elements in a fat-poor diet."

From Norway's Dr. Jens Dedichen: "The mortality from circulatory diseases in Norway showed a marked decrease during the last World War." And his data show an equally marked *increase*—of 300%—in venous blood clots at the Riks Hospital in Oslo after the war.

From Switzerland's Dr. Eisenreich: "The relationship between fat consumption and venous thrombosis formation [blood clots in the veins] has been noted."

From Austria's Drs. Zeithofer and Reiffenstuhl: "From clinical studies, it is known that the frequency of thrombo-embolic disease [clots in the veins] decreases during periods of poor nutrition. . ."

From Holland's Drs. Van Unnik and Straub: "During World War II the frequency of thrombosis and embolism greatly decreased in the Netherlands."

The evidence was unanimous. Foods *can* affect the clotting of the blood. The foods suspected by the wartime medical experts were the same foods found to cause atherosclerosis—excessive amounts of eggs, milk, butter and other animal fats.

The great nutritional experiment was over, and it pointed to a possible method of conquering the coronary-heart-disease epidemic. War had deprived the Europeans of excess calories, excess saturated fats and excess cholesterol. Why not voluntarily eliminate these excesses from our present diet? Or would our general health suffer if we did so?

This question has been answered by many medical authorities. Says Dr. Folke Henschen of Sweden: "On the other hand supply of vitamins was adequate. People grew thin and complained bitterly about this, but it was no doubt beneficial for their health, at least in Sweden; as a matter of fact, the Swedes have never in their history been so healthy as during the years of food restrictions."

In this chapter there have been listed many reports citing the benefits of a sparse low-fat diet in reducing coronary disease, heart attack, and thrombotic blood clots. In addition to these reports, many more have appeared supporting the evidence presented here.

Is this then the complete story of the effects of all the wartime deprivations? Nothing has been said about the wartime lack of sugar, refined foods or cigarettes. There is no doubt that these restrictions also had beneficial effects, as will be seen later in our discussion of the complete prevention program.

From the research of the European medical men, as well as the American medical scientists who have studied this field, come their two guiding principles:

● Whenever a group of people are placed on a diet low in fats, calories and cholesterol, we may expect a decrease in coronary artery blockage and heart attack.
● Whenever a group of people are placed on a diet much higher in fats, calories and cholesterol, we may expect a much higher incidence of coronary disease and heart attack.

VITAL DIET FACTORS
REVEALED IN ASIA AND AFRICA

One method of obtaining data for the study of coronary heart disease is to note its relative incidence in different countries and to observe how it affects groups of people living under different environmental conditions. The ideal countries for this type of study are those in which there is a great disparity in the incidence of heart attack. Since the United States has the highest rate of the entire world, the countries in which heart attack occurs least frequently are the best places for comparative study.

A veritable "scientific mine" of this type of data is located far from our medical laboratories. It is found in the economically less-developed areas of the world, among the peoples of Africa, Asia, and Central and South America.

It has long surprised medical scientists that although the coronary epidemic was increasing in the Western countries, the so-called "backward peoples" seemed to be virtually immune to heart attack. The significant difference in their way of life that seems to account for this "immunity" lies in their diet, frugal where ours is lavish. But diet is not the only item to be considered. Differences in cultural patterns including stress, exercise and even heredity must also be taken into account.

The earliest reports come from China. In 1925, Dr. F. Oppenheim of Shanghai had investigated coronary disease among the Chinese. At the hospital to which he was attached, Dr. Oppenheim analyzed 100 autopsies. Among these he found only four cases of atheroma, and of these three were moderate and only one was "pronounced." Two years later, Dr. J. H. Foster made a study of angina pectoris among 4,000 Chinese patients in Changsha. After four years of study, he did not encounter a single case.

As the coronary epidemic increased in the West, the difference between the rates of heart attack among Western and non-Western people became more evident. For example, in 1958, Dr. C. L. Tung of the Shanghai Sixth People's Hospital reported that out of 200 heart cases of all types—mostly rheumatic heart disease and high blood pressure—only four had coronary disease. Dr. Tung attributed the superior coronary health of the Chinese to ". . . the low cholesterol of normal Chinese. Fats constitute less than 15% of our diet . . ."

In 1957, Dr. T. H. Wang had reported in the *National Medical Journal of China* that the Chinese did become afflicted with coronary atherosclerosis, *but it occurred twenty years later in life than in Western men.*

In 1946, Dr. P. E. Steiner of the U. S. Army, conducting autopsies on 150 Japanese civilians in Okinawa, found only seven cases of atherosclerosis, none of them severe. His summary stated that the Okinawans were ". . . amazingly free of degenerative diseases of the cardiovascular system." He also noted that the everyday diet of the Okinawans consisted generally of sweet potatoes, rice, vegetables, soybeans and very little meat—an extremely low-fat diet. On this diet Dr. Steiner found the Okinawans well nourished and physically well developed.

In his *Chinese Lessons to Western Medicine* which had appeared in 1941, Dr. I. Snapper, now Director of Medical Education at the New York Beth-El Hospital, wrote: "The rarity of coronary thrombosis in North China is the more striking because the increase . . . in America is appalling . . . The rarity of arteriosclerosis is proved by scores of middle-aged patients—showing hardly any atherosclerosis at autopsy."

After several years of research at a large Chinese hospital, Dr. Snapper, searching for symptoms of coronary heart disease, found but one victim. He attributed the freedom from coronary in China to the low-calorie, low-fat diet.

But it was by the recognition of a new factor that Dr. Snapper firmly established his name in medical history. He was the first to put the spotlight on the *kind of fat* used in the Chinese diet. According to Dr. Snapper's reports, it was the *unsaturated* vegetable fats that were a major factor in their low rate of heart attack.

As far back as 1938, Dr. Snapper had realized that in coronary disease, the *type* of fat is just as important as the amount of fat. In a recent book, *Bedside Medicine*, Dr. Snapper reasserts his early conclusions that the virtual nonexistence of coronary disease in China is attributable to the Chinese diet. He further states that this diet helps to neutralize certain of the thrombotic or clotting factors in the blood. What other discoveries Dr. Snapper would have made in China will never be known, for, at the height of his research, the Japanese invasion forced him to return to the United States.

In the meantime, other medical investigators familiar with the problem of atherosclerosis were making similar studies among the African peoples. The Bantu of Uganda, for example, have lived for untold generations on a sparse

but wholesome low-fat diet. Would they reveal a low rate
of heart attack? From 1930 to 1956, Dr. H. C. Trowel of
Uganda performed 6,500 autopsies on Bantu men and
women without uncovering a single instance. "In the African population of Uganda," reports Drs. Shaper and Jones
in *The Lancet*, (October 10, 1959), "coronary heart disease is almost non-existent."

So far all the studies cited have in a sense been one-
sided, that is they have dealt only with *single groups* of
subjects. Actually there's only one way to arrive at valid
conclusions, and that is to study a number of Americans
and Bantus, corresponding in age, sex and general health,
and then to examine the conditions of their coronary
arteries. Scientists call this process, *matched controls,* and
it is the most accurate method of medical investigation.

True, it is impossible to match up *all* factors. Stress is
undoubtedly different and greater in the Americans, less in
the Bantu. The effects of the stress factor will be analyzed
later in this and other chapters.

A matched control method was used in 1961 by Dr. R.
F. Scott of the United States and Dr. R. N. P. Davies of
Uganda. In 200 autopsies of matched Africans and Americans, they looked for the comparative amount of blockage
in the coronary arteries. Their findings indicated that in
half of the Americans, a number of the vital blood channels ot the heart muscle had become blocked, causing myocardial infarction. In almost all of the 100 Bantus, the
coronary arteries were extraordinarily "clean." Where
deposits existed, they were present mainly in the arteries of
70-year-olds.

Dr. J. B. Hannah, physician for a Northern Rhodesian
mining company, made an autopsy study of the intima,
the inner lining of the coronary arteries, of similar-aged
adult Europeans and Africans. One sentence from his
report should serve to convey his impressions: "It was
interesting to compare the stretchable smooth grey intima
of these African vessels with the unyielding ochrous
intima of specimens from like-aged Europeans."

Two South African doctors, J. Higginson and W. J.
Peppler, employed the same method of matched controls
in the early 1950's, in an effort to determine the comparative percentage of severe coronary-obstructing growths
among Americans and Africans. In the over-60 age group,

this figure was four times greater for Americans, and in the 40-59 age group it was *eight times greater*.

Examining matched-age groups for coronary obstructions, Dr. J. Wainwright reported in *The Lancet* (February 18, 1961) that in all three age groups under investigation (40-50, 50-60, 60-70), the Bantu showed only a minor amount of obstruction. But in the "matched" Europeans, Wainwright found considerable amounts of atherosclerosis accompanied by complications and by ulcerations covering large areas of the coronary arteries.

From his own autopsy data, Dr. M. I Sachs, a South African pathologist, demonstrated that one out of two Bantu in the 40-to-60 group possesses absolutely "clean" arteries; but among matched-age group Europeans, the ratio is only one out of fifteen.

In 15,000 consecutive admissions to a Bantu Hospital in Southern Rhodesia, as reported in the *West African Medical Journal* in 1952, not a single case of coronary heart disease was encountered. Similarly, in 1954 a low incidence of the disease among the natives of the West Coast of Africa was reported in *Transactions of the Royal Society of Tropical Medicine and Hygiene*.

So exceptional is the occurrence of coronary disease among Africans that the *East African Medical Journal* (Oct., 1956) devoted a special paper to the first case diagnosed: *A Case History of Heart Disease in an African* by H. C. Trowell and S. A. Singh.

The following important question was asked of Dr. Bronte-Stewart, Professor of Medicine at the University of Cape Town: "Is it not possible that the lean diet of the Bantu is responsible for malnourishment and ill health?" "Quite the contrary," he replied. "They are a strong people. Some of their best war dancers are men in their sixties and seventies, and war dances are strenuous performances."

Dr. A. R. P. Walker of South Africa who has conducted many nutritional experiments among the native Bantu and European inmates of the Johannesburg prison has observed that "On these black and white prisoner groups, certain motor fitness tests have been carried out; the Bantu seem virtually inexhaustible . . . in comparison to the white prisoners."

Although the Bantu people consume less protein and calcium (their diet contains no milk) than Westerners think is needed for vigorous health, Dr. Walker says that in all probability this proves that *our* "minimum" requirements for these essentials are *excessive*. Lack of protein is a problem in the Bantu diet, but *Nutrition Reviews* (September, 1958), has the following to say: "Chemical analysis shows 30% more protein in the milk of the Bantu mother than in American mothers on a higher protein diet. Also the [Bantu] milk failures are much lower than here . . ."

What are the effects of the calcium "deficiency" among the Bantu? *Nutrition Reviews* reports rickets to be uncommon, teeth perfect, and bones more than the "normal" Western strength.

Whatever the difference of opinion about the adequacy of their diet, some of the Bantu people are certainly subject to malnutrition in early childhood, resulting in the well-known illness, "kwashiorkor," a protein-deficiency condition which results in liver disease.

The existence of this illness in some of the Bantu has raised the suspicion that their freedom from heart attack was related to the liver disorder. Dr. Walker has examined the problem and states that, "The relative freedom of the Bantu from coronary occlusion [heart attack] is due primarily to their diet and not to liver disease and abnormality, although the latter may confer additional protection to a small proportion of the adult population."

At this point it is important to refer to a survey on artery blockage in a group of Africans found to be totally free of kwashiorkor conducted by an investigating group which included Dr. Paul Dudley White.

The examinations were made using the Albert Schweitzer Hospital in Central Africa as the study center. The conclusion made by Dr. White was that "coronary disease as far as we could determine was nonexistent."

Additional interesting observations were that, "As compared to the classically emotionally tense, physically soft, overfed, hyperlipemic white American male candidate for coronary thrombosis, these Africans are different in every respect. Most of them are remarkably easy-going, they tend to be hard and thin, and their diet is sparse and lean."

"Calories derived from fat comprise only 18 per cent . . . the daily per capita intake of animal fat is well under [one third of an ounce]."

India and Japan have also been under scrutiny. In 1961, Dr. K. S. Mathur, of the Sarojini Naidu Medical College of India, compared these two underdeveloped countries and their low-calorie, low-fat diets with the United States, employing data utilizing age-matched groups. His charts showed the low incidence of arterial atherosclerosis in India and Japan. A pattern of extremely slow growth of coronary blockage, similar to that in the Chinese, was apparent. His charts are corroborated by the conclusion of a group of Japanese and American pathologists led by Dr. Ira Gore of the Massachusetts Hospital: "The onset of [coronary] intimal disease occurs approximately two decades later in Japan and progresses thereafter at a much slower rate."

To sum up so far, the main areas comprising the natural laboratories of Asia and Africa have been studied. Every age-matched autopsy analysis which compared these people with their Western counterparts has shown a vastly greater incidence of arterial blockage among the Western peoples. And the paramount cause of this high incidence was considered to be the Western luxury diet.

In the Americas there are also natural laboratories among the underprivileged economic groups. The low rates of coronary disease in Indians subsisting on frugal, low-fat diets in Mexico and Guatemala is a matter of medical record. Dr. Marcos Roitman of the Dos de Mayo Hospital in Lima, Peru, in a study of over 10,000 clinical cases, states that "the complete absence of myocardial infarction in the Indian race was striking."

This mention of race brings up the questions referred to earlier—heredity, stress and exercise factors in these peoples.

In Central America important research regarding the possible connection of heredity to atherosclerosis was carried out by Dr. Jack P. Strong of the Louisiana State University of Medicine in collaboration with Dr. Carlos Tejada of Costa Rica. In age-matched groups from the United States and Costa Rica, the two researchers studied the atherosclerotic index, employing a complex scientific method of evaluating the extent of coronary blockage. Americans reached the danger point in their atherosclerotic index by age fifty and consistently fell within the extremely dangerous, high-index range during their sixties.

The Costa Ricans, on the other hand, never crossed

the danger-zone index, even at age sixty-five. The pattern of the fifteen-year coronary precocity of Americans had again emerged, this time in comparison with the Costa Rican group.

What is the significance of these findings? Dr. Strong and Dr. Tejada answer: "Since Costa Ricans and New Orleans whites are both principally of European extraction, racial factors are unlikely to be . . . responsible." In other words, heredity was ruled out.

What then *did* cause the difference? "Of possible . . . factors, diet appears at present to be one of the most important." The diet of the average New Orleaner contained 40% fats, while the low-income Costa Rican diet contained only 12% fats.

There is one country which provides an almost ideal laboratory for the study of atherosclerosis. This country is Israel, which has a twofold advantage for this study: first, the highest per-capita ratio of doctors to patients; and second, a continuous influx of Jewish groups "immune" to heart attacks, arriving from backward areas of the Near East.

Two such groups have been under continuous study, the Yemenite Jews of Arabia and the Atlas Mountain Jews of North Africa. These Jews, prior to their arrival in Israel, had been living for two thousand years on the same frugal, low-calorie, low-animal-fat diet. Both groups, when they arrived in Israel, showed the same low rate of coronary disease exhibited by the other non-coronary peoples of Africa and Asia.

These previously isolated and almost ethnically pure groups have since partially adopted the Israeli diet, which is much higher in calories and animal fats. If the low coronary rate were truly a hereditary trait, these two groups should have been protected against coronary attacks even after a change in diet. But medical evidence shows no such protective effect. Within twenty years on the Israeli diet, the coronary rate of the Yemenite Jews was almost equal to the prevailing Israeli rate.

Medical scientists have not yet gathered enough evidence on the absence of "civilized" stress as a factor among the coronary-free peoples of the world. But certain studies—made for other reasons—can throw light on this problem.

Let us set up the conditions of an ideal test: First, find

a group of people free from stress but living on a high animal-fat diet. Other conditions should be the same as among non-Western, non-industrialized people: outdoor life, exercise, etc. If stress were the primary factor, then we should find comparatively little coronary disease, even on a high saturated-fat diet.

A "natural" setup closely simulating such ideal experimental conditions existed in the stress-free Melanesian islands of the South Pacific, studied by American doctors during World War II. On these islands the coconut is sometimes the food staple. The coconut is rich in a fat which, strangely enough, is of an exceptional kind. Its chemical composition is equivalent to that of animal fat. On the islands where the coconut is abundant and where it is used as a major source of food, the Melanesians are actually living on a diet almost as harmful as that of the West.

The actual basis for the investigation of this special area had as its origin a logistic problem during World War II, when the American Army in the South Pacific needed native labor to maintain its bases. Health inspection was important, and the most serious of the disabilities found, strangely enough, included atherosclerosis of the legs and heart failure, as well as coronary disease.

Yet even though "civilized stress" is almost non-existent among the Melanesians, Dr. A. S. Hyman in the *Annals of Internal Medicine* for May, 1945, reports that "Arteriosclerosis was prevalent . . . coronary disease common . . . cardiovascular disease almost as frequent as among Americans and Europeans."

The absence of stress did not protect the Melanesians, although it did help slightly to reduce the severity of the disease. While chronic coronary heart disease was common, it occurred without the pain of angina. Dr. Hyman reported that myocardial infarctions (heart attacks), when they came, were "silent." The Islanders died as the result of an accumulation of many small "silent" attacks, which eventually caused heart failure, rather than of the more dramatic heart attack.

Dr. Hyman's report, "Heart Disease in the Jungles of the South Pacific," impressively presents the substantiating data from this unusual natural laboratory. Additional evidence of the effect of coconut fat as a major dietary cause of coronary among a comparatively stress-free population comes from the cardiologists of India, where, for economic reasons, many of the people have been using the inexpensive coconut oil as a staple.

States Dr. Padmavati of India in *Japanese Circulation Journal* (May 1961): "We find the incidence of coronary artery disease in all parts of India is low compared to the U.S.A., England or Sweden. We have found that the incidence is highest in those parts of India *which consume coconut oil.*"

Two years ago, returning from a medical convention, I was lucky enough to be able to spend a week in the most ideal of all the stress-free islands, Tahiti. During my stay, I made a few medical inquiries at the lovely municipal Hôpital de Papeete concerning cholesterol levels and coronary disease among the Tahitians.

The data on cholesterol was obtained from Dr. Chastel who was in charge of this work. On a proportional basis, he said, there were many Tahitians with a high cholesterol level. And heart attack? Of the five cases in the past year, four were Tahitians, one an American.

What was the cause of the heart attacks? Dr. Chastel's opinion was that some of the Tahitians were extremely fond of the pigs which were fed on the high-saturated-fat coconut scraps. This diet, for those of the Tahitians who could afford to indulge in it, was almost as bad as our Western diet.

Dr. A. R. P. Walker was the medical witness at an unusual diet experiment in South Africa which seems to sum up the story of the world's coronary-free people. Oddly enough, in this apartheid country, long-term white prisoners in a Johannesburg jail were integrated with the Bantu prisoners and fed the Bantu diet. Because of previous research, Dr. Walker was not surprised to find that all clinical evidence of coronary disease symptoms in the white prisoners gradually disappeared.

In Dr. Walker's opinion, "The only certain known way . . . to ward off death from coronary occlusion . . . is by adoption of the pattern of diet . . . consumed by the Bantu and similar populations . . ."

Dr. K. T. Lee of Albany Medical College found heart attack among the very low-fat-diet Koreans, "sufficiently rare . . . that they are reported at medical meetings . . . infarcts have been seen in upper class individuals . . . the amount of fat they ingest [over 17%] is near or slightly beyond the amount tolerated by man . . ."

The lessons learned from the World War II data, as well as the corroborating evidence from Africa, Asia, Central and South America, is very ably summed up by Dr. Paul Dudley White in his Convocation Address at the 1963 Annual Meeting of the American College of Cardiology:

"Wherever in the world people eat richly of calories and animal fat as nearly all of us do in the U.S.A., there we find much atherosclerosis; wherever in the world people are optimally nourished or undernourished, there is much less atherosclerosis."

The next section will discuss two other "experiments" that are currently in progress in the United States, involving men living on a diet extraordinarily high in calories, fats and cholesterol. The implications of these "experiments" are now becoming clear and steps are being taken to remedy the situation which is shown to lead to increased artery blockage in the young men and to coronary thrombosis in the older men.

INSIDIOUS FIFTH COLUMN
IN THE MESS HALL

Wanted
Volunteers to test a special diet suspected of being the primary cause of heart disease in the adult American male. Young men only.

This "ad" never appeared. No true laboratory experiment of this sort was ever carried out on human beings. And yet, because our Federal government has a dual problem on its hands, the basic conditions for this experiment are actually in operation in the U.S. Army today.

Our government must build and maintain the high morale of millions of young volunteers, draftees, career enlisted men and officers. Serving "good" food helps build morale.

The government must also dispose of the surplus butter, eggs, and other products stored by its farm program. Thus, two problems are being solved by reducing the surplus food to "enrich" the army diet.

Public Law 690 was enacted by the 83rd Congress to provide an increased allowance of dairy products for the Armed Forces. In compliance with this law it has been the policy of the Quartermaster General to allow up to 22 ounces of milk per ration *in addition* to the milk included in the Master Menu, *already extremely high* in calories and animal fats.

What is the effect of this high-calorie, high-saturated-fat diet on artery blockage? Ordinarily, after two years of this diet, the G.I. is released. And without autopsies, the results remain hidden.

But autopsies were performed on 300 American casualties during the Korean War. Three Army medical officers, Drs. W. F. Enos, R. H. Holmes, and J. C. Beyer, were assigned the task of post-mortem determination of the extent of coronary blockage in the casualties, men averaging twenty-two years of age, who, to all outward appearances, had been in good health.

Here is their report from the *Journal of the American Medical Association*: One out of every ten of these "healthy" young men had a section of his coronary artery blocked by more than 50%, and one in four had a 20% blockage.

The condition had gone unnoticed. It had caused no trouble. But it was there, working secretly, silently, toward a possible future heart attack.

What had caused this condition? " . . . Basic factors, such as diet must be present," concludes the Army medical team in their report "Coronary Disease Among United States Soldiers Killed in Action in Korea."

The reactions were not long in coming. After the announcement, headlines appeared:

"HEART DISEASE" DISCOVERED IN G.I.'S KILLED IN ACTION"

"YOUNG MEN HAVE HEART ILLNESS"

"3 OUT OF 4 YOUNG SOLDIERS SHOW CORONARY LESIONS"

For a day . . . public shock and scientific amazement. And then . . . silence and public apathy. The G.I. menus remained as before. But along with the Enos group a few other responsible U.S. medical military officials were very much concerned about this new insidious "fifth-column" that had been discovered in the Army.

From a military point of view, even if only one soldier out of a hundred were vulnerable to a heart attack, he would constitute a potential military threat. Suppose this one coronary-prone man were at the controls of a strategic aircraft? It was a grave risk the Air Force could not afford to ignore.

With the Korean War over, the possibility of mass autopsy analysis no longer existed. Where could two interested military doctors, Drs. W. M. Glantz and V. A. Stembridge of the Armed Forces Institute of Pathology, begin their researches? Since they were particularly concerned with heart attacks among pilots, they decided to examine the coronary arteries of pilots who had died in actual crack-ups.

Among the pilots involved in the crack-ups for which no definite mechanical cause could be assigned, 6% exhibited severe coronary blockage. And in 2% of the cases, the pilot had suffered a proven heart attack. In more than 200 cases of military aircraft fatalities—average age, 28—the autopsies revealed almost the same degree of coronary blockage as was present among the Korean casualties.

The same problem also exists in the British Air Force. This was revealed by an excessive number of cases of "white arc" in the iris of the eyes of their pilots. "White arc"—a cholesterol deposit—is an indication of atherosclerosis. Among *aged* Canadian Indians, subsisting on a low-fat diet, Dr. H. M. Sinclair of Oxford found *no* white deposits. But, among *young* British and New Zealand pilots, fed the regulation British Air Force, high-fat diet, the tell-tale "white arc" showed up clearly in one out of ten cases.

In the United States this condition, medically known as "Arcus Senilis," is no longer a disease of the senile. According to Dr. J. S. Andrews of the Harvard University Medical School, "Arcus is present in all persons past middle age." There is even serious discussion at the present time of a separate category to be labeled "Arcus Juvenilis."

So important had heart attack become to U.S. Air Force medical experts that they arranged a symposium on it in 1954. At this symposium the diet question was emphasized by Harvard's world-famous authority, Dr. Frederick J. Stare, whose opinion was: "If the Air Force wishes to keep its pilots from developing atherosclerosis, it should not furnish the usual 3,500 to 4,000 calories in its mess." And in regard to animal fats Dr. Stare stated that, "since most American males consume over a hundred grams of fat (3½ oz.) daily, a restriction to 70 grams (2¼ oz.) a day will be effective . . . and after a period of adjustment tolerably palatable."

The problem of coronary artery blockage in our young fliers was also investigated by Dr. Ashton Grabiel of the U.S. Naval School of Aviation Medicine. He ruled out stress as a causative factor, saying that "We have no evidence that flying stress leads to early appearance of heart disease." Dr. Grabiel then recommended "service-wide revision of the present high animal-fat diet, eliminate hard [animal] fats from the diet . . . and, to a judicious degree, substitute oils."

Authoritative medical investigators such as Enos, Glantz and Stembridge, Stare and Grabiel, as well as many others, had been warning the U.S. Army and Air Force to revise their menus. But to date their warnings seem to have been ignored. The result is that we are still continuing "the traditional air force high-fat, high-calorie diet designed to develop large body build and aggressive energy . . . *troops that are tigers.*" With this one sentence Colonel William Preston of the U. S. Air Force *Military Medicine* (March, 1962) injects a note of irony into the grim situation.

And in the same publication, Colonel W. J. Walker, chief cardiologist of Walter Reed Hospital, who is a strong advocate of a new streamlined low-fat menu, states: "Atherosclerosis is the leading cause of death from disease in active-duty personnel in the U.S. Army." And the average age of death from this cause, according to his statistics, is only forty-three years.

The problem today, of course, exists not only in the Army but is nation-wide. Drs. Enos, Holmes and Beyers, the pathologists who discovered the artery blockage in our young soldiers, have since then been investigating young men for excessive amounts of blood fats, which they regarded as a major cause of atherosclerosis. In March, 1962 this team of pathologists published a statement which should alert the entire nation to this problem.

"The fact that atherosclerotic lesions . . . in the coronary arteries cause significant luminal narrowing [artery blockage] in a majority of young white adult American male subjects . . . [is] . . . one of the most serious cardio-vascular problems in the United States today."

There are, however, some straws in the wind which indicate a possible change in attitude of those responsible for feeding the Army. One indication is the fact that a "Supervisors Course for Army Hospital Dietitians," which was held in June 1963 at the Walter Reed Army Institute of Research, included a lecture by Dr. W. J. Walker on "Dietary Factors in Atherosclerosis." Another indication is that the temporary 1962 revision in meat grading standards has already been made permanent for the U.S. Army. It gives the "Grade A" rating to the leanest beef and the lowest rating to the fattest beef.

THE MILK ULCER DIET
PRESCRIPTION FOR A CORONARY?

Most animals on a high-fat diet develop atherosclerosis. In 1908, Dr. Ignatovski of the Russian Imperial Military Academy fed milk and egg yolks to rabbits and observed the severe atherosclerosis that resulted. Medical research data on tens of thousands of fat-and cholesterol-fed laboratory animals have since supplied striking proof linking diet to atherosclerosis. No lack of proof—concerning *animals*. But is there experimental evidence of harmful effects of such a diet on *humans?*

The story of the U.S. Army and Air Force diet is the story of an "experiment" on a mass scale, but on young men. And during this short period the young men showed the same evidence of artery blockage as that detected in the fat-fed laboratory animal for an equivalent period.

The Army's "experiment" stops when the average youthful G.I. is returned to the civilian population. To find out if people get the same severe artery blockage as laboratory animals, it is necessary to study an older group as well.

Such a group does exist among peptic-ulcer patients who have been fed the Sippy ulcer diet. To understand this diet we must go back to the early days of the medical treatment of peptic ulcer.

In 1912, four years after Ignatovski's pioneering experiments on rabbits, Dr. Bertram W. Sippy first made public his method of treating peptic ulcer, which consisted mainly of hourly feedings of milk and cream. Now, fifty years later, Dr. David J. Sandweiss of Detroit's Mt. Sinai Hospital asks. "Having employed the modified Sippy ulcer diets for 50 years, with their high saturated fats and low polyunsaturated fat content, have we exposed our ulcer patients to arteriosclerotic heart disease while treating their ulcers?"

The answer to Dr. Sandweiss' provocative question can be found in the research of Dr. M. Plotz, which he reported in the March 1949 issue of the *Journal of the American Medical Association*. This was a detailed analysis of ten coronary patients who were also afflicted with a peptic ulcer. All ten, after seven months on the Sippy ulcer diet, died of heart attack.

Dr. Plotz was one of many investigators who had gone back to the data on the Sippy cases after the connection between high-fat diet and coronary disease had become more than a suspicion. The significance of the data on these ten cases remained unnoticed in the autopsy files until Dr. Plotz analyzed them. In the years between 1949 and 1960 a number of studies were made of ulcer patients living on the Sippy Diet. The most thorough study of these Sippy cases was made by Dr. R. D. Briggs of Washington University Medical School. He and his associates enlisted the aid of fifteen hospitals in this country and in England, who supplied data on coronary disease in patients with ulcers *on* the Sippy Diet, and also in patients with ulcers of similar severity, but *not* on the Sippy Diet.

The first objective of Dr. Briggs was to find if the ulcer or the condition inducing the ulcer was a possible cause of the coronary. He found the answer by comparing the incidence of heart attacks in the ulcer group with that of a *non*-ulcer "control" group. The figures for patients with ulcers, but *not* on the Sippy Diet, matched those for patients without ulcers—the incidence of heart attack was the same. *The ulcer itself had no influence* on the rate of heart attack.

But did the Sippy Diet contribute to a rise in heart attacks? Dr. Briggs next matched the incidence of heart attacks in the non-Sippy-Diet ulcer group and the Sippy-Diet ulcer group. Here are the results from the ten American hospitals: for patients with ulcers *not* on the Sippy Diet, the incidence of heart attack was 15%; but for patients with ulcers *on* the Sippy Diet, the incidence of heart attack was 36%! In England almost the same high ratio of coronary disease in ulcer patients on the Sippy

Diet, compared to non-Sippy-Diet ulcer patients, was observed.

The results of Dr. Briggs' analysis make it clear that heart attacks were induced through the use of the Sippy Diet.

There is, according to Dr. Winston R. Miller, a type of atherosclerosis called *iatrogenic* (*iatro* means "doctor," *genic* means "induced"). Dr. Miller explains in *Minnesota Medicine* (May, 1957): "We Americans eat more fat than any other people, and we American physicians are prescribing . . . ulcer . . . diabetic . . . and even some reducing diets which contain more fat than the average population consumes. Diabetic and ulcer patients as a group have an incidence of atherosclerosis roughly twice that of the general population . . . It is not likely that we have contributed to this astounding mortality rate by our diet prescriptions?"

Let Dr. Sandweiss sum up the evidence: "Milk had been advocated from the earliest times and used throughout the centuries in the treatment of the peptic ulcer. The milk-cream-egg diet was . . . popularized by Sippy in 1915. Ever since, many physicians, we included, have used these diets in the treatment of ulcer patients. Even the convalescent ulcer diets have a high fat . . . content. In fact, interval feedings of milk, of milk and cream, of eggs, and of custards and puddings are frequently prescribed . . . with the hope of preventing ulcer recurrences . . . But . . . a high intake of fat may cause . . . coronary atherosclerosis . . . The question occurred whether . . . it is proper to continue this high-fat dietary regimen for ulcer patients . . ."

Among the animals, the rat is probably the most resistant to diet-induced "heart attack." Dr. W. Stanley Hartroft and his group have published many reports on this problem. Finally they did discover a special diet very high in saturated fat and cholesterol which gave "heart attack" even to the rat. To the charge that this diet was "unnatural" Dr. Hartcroft replied in *Archives of Surgery:* "The therapeutic dietary regimen Sippy used in some cases for the treatment of peptic ulcers is probably the diet consumed by man which most closely resembles the experimental infarct ["rat heart attack"] producing diet."

Dr. David J. Sandweiss has published data which shows that the Sippy ulcer diet brings on heart atack at a much earlier age than in the general population.

What is the way out? Continue the high-fat diet to try

to cure the ulcer, with the high risk of a heart attack, or eliminate the Sippy Diet and permit the patient to suffer from the peptic ulcer? Could the dilemma be resolved?

Dr. Sandweiss delved deeper: "Recent studies incriminate the saturated . . . [animal] fat content of the diet . . . point an accusing finger at high *saturated* fat diets and the . . . high incidence of coronary atherosclerosis in ulcer patients . . . An analysis of the fat contents of our own hospital's ulcer diets emphasizes the sizable amounts of *saturated* fats to which the ulcer patient has been subjected for years . . ."

The dilemma *could* be resolved. The solution became clear: "For those ulcer patients who have a . . . history of coronary heart disease," Dr. Sandweiss concluded, "we have reduced saturated fat . . . increased unsaturated [vegetable] . . . fat . . ."

Let us again review the two guiding principles established previously: (1) Whenever a group of people are placed on a *diet low in fats, calories and cholesterol,* we may expect *low incidence* of coronary atherosclerosis and heart attack; (2) Whenever a group of people are placed on a *diet high in fats, calories and cholesterol,* we may expect a much *higher incidence* of coronary atherosclerosis and heart attack.

The validity of the first principle was clearly shown during World War II. The validity of the second principle was demonstrated by the Korean War autopsies, the United States Air Force studies, and the high-fat, stomach-soothing, artery-blocking ulcer diet.

The dietary factor in heart disease has been established not only by these studies but by many other recent researches to be described later in this book. But first let us take a look at some of the other factors which contribute to the annual toll of heart attack.

The four *non-diet* factors most frequently mentioned are:

- The *stress* of modern society
- The *lack of exercise* due to mechanization
- The effects of *heredity*
- The protection of women due to their *sex.*

In the next chapter all four will be considered. It will be found that they all affect the arteries through the same "key" factor, and this in turn will simplify formulation of a Prevention Program.

CHAPTER FOUR

Stress . . . Exercise . . . Heredity . . . Sex

WHAT IS YOUR "STRESS-CORONARY PROFILE?"

I have an intense, sustained drive to get ahead.	YES...	NO...
I'm anxious to reach my goals, but I'm uncertain what those goals are.	YES...	NO...
I feel a need to compete and win.	YES...	NO...
I have a persistent desire for recognition.	YES...	NO...
I always seem to be involved in too many things at once.	YES...	NO...
I'm always racing the clock, constantly on edge about meeting deadlines.	YES...	NO...
I have an inner drive to speed things up, get things done faster.	YES...	NO...
I'm extraordinarily alert mentally and physically.	YES...	NO...

How many times did you answer "Yes" to the questions above? Each "Yes" helps complete a special picture of the coronary type. Scientists call this kind of a picture a "profile." The more "Yes" checks, the more *positive* your coronary profile. If you answered "Yes" to all eight questions, you have a 100% positive coronary-profile.

Dr. Meyer Friedman, Director of the Harold Brunn Institute in San Francisco, reported in association with Dr. H. Rosenman, in the *Journal of the American Medical Association,* (March 21, 1959), "Intensely ambitious men who drive themselves in work or play and race to meet deadlines are particularly susceptible to angina pectoris and coronary occlusion."

Dr. Friedman, who is recognized as the leading medical authority on stress and heart attack in this country, arrived at his conclusion after studying two selected groups of subjects with opposite emotional attitudes. *Group A* was made up of men who answered "Yes" to all the stress attitude questions—men with 100% *positive* coronary profiles. *Group B* was made up of men who answered "No" to those questions—men with 100% *negative* coronary profiles.

And what were the findings: Coronary heart disease occurred much more frequently in Group A than in Group B.

Even before the Friedman-Rosenman findings were published, the connection between stress and coronary had been accepted as a fact both by the medical profession and the public. The phrase, "take it easy, you'll get a heart attack," had become a familiar expression. There was little doubt in anybody's mind that stress and heart attack went hand in hand.

At this point two questions need to be answered. First, where in our society do we find Dr. Friedman's highly stressed Class A individuals, and second, what are the specific physical effects of this high stress on the blood.

SURPRISING REVELATIONS
ABOUT PEOPLE UNDER STRESS

If we take the entire country as our "laboratory," we shall find that Class A stress individuals will not always be found where most people expect them to be. They are not always in the top executive group, the presidents and the managers. The Class A stress individuals are also frequently found in the lower ranks.

A team of scientists headed by Drs. J. M. Mortensen and T. T. Stevenson, reported in *Archives of Industrial Health,* that among insurance and telephone employees, the *highest* rate of coronary incidence was among the clerical force and the *lowest* rate occurred in the top executive personnel.

In one large company, Drs. R. E. Lee and R. F. Schneider examined the rate of heart attack in men in the executive group and also the rate in the non-executive group; they found ". . . no increase in incidence of . . . atherosclerotic disease in the executive class."

These unexpected results were supported by the findings of Drs. C. A. D'Alonzo and Sidney Pell, who conducted "a . . . study of acute myocardial infarction among employees of the DuPont Company." (*The Journal of the*

American Medical Association, February 11, 1961.) Among salaried employees, they reported, the higher the levels of responsibility, the lower the incidence of coronary disease.

And what about data based on income? Dr. D. M. Berkson and his associates of the Department of Medicine at Northwestern University classified all deaths due to atherosclerosis in Chicago according to the victim's earnings. They discovered that, as earnings rose from lowest to highest, deaths from atherosclerosis went down 10%!

What then, is the truth about the so-called stressful occupations and coronary heart disease? On the one hand, there's the universal belief, backed by the scientific work of Friedman and Rosenman, that in individuals subject to high stress there's a relatively high incidence of coronary. On the other hand, there are the findings of Mortensen, Schneider and others that among the high-echelon groups, whom we assume to be under great stress, there is no relative increase of coronary.

Which report is right? The answer is—both.

What the Mortensen-Schneider type investigators *did* discover was a stress-afflicted group where few suspected it existed, in the lower echelons of our industrial society, among clerks, laborers, craftsmen, technicians and minor white-collar workers. Perhaps it's due to the American way of life, which sets up high goals for many at all levels, but only allows a few of the most ambitious and able individuals to reach them. Among the lower-income groups, there are many who have adopted aggressive patterns (discovered by Dr. Friedman in his Class A stress group) in their great drive to strike it rich.

Among all high stress individuals there can be found a type of behavior which seems best suited to meet the financial and other goals they set for themselves. Dr. Friedman says that it is almost impossible to induce a change in the internal stress patterns of the most highly stressed Class A individuals; the actual or expected "success" rewards are too great.

Evidence that too many of us are under too much stress comes from a surprising souce, a dental specialist. This is what Dr. Ralph H. Boos told the Southern California State Dental Association: "Americans are gnashing their teeth away. It's a modern phenomenon, this teeth grinding, due to the great increase in worries and tensions being experienced by modern man."

And how many Americans are doing it? "Nine out of ten," said Dr. Boos. Then he added that our national teeth-grinding habit is so severe, it's cutting the life of our teeth by 50%.

In addition, the grinding and clenching, which often goes on in sleep as well, wears out the jaw-hinge and results in the "I-can't-bite-an-apple" jaw-muscle injury, curable only by removal of stress. It is significant that Dr. Friedman and Rosenman had noted in their positive-stress-profile personalities such physical habits as hand and jaw clenching and teeth grinding.

As a matter fact, Dr. Friedman finds it possible to recognize the class A type stress personality on the sole basis of a short interview. Since many individuals will not answer the "stress questionnaire" objectively, it was necessary to rely on observations of (1) restlessness (2) a sense of time urgency and (3) certain types of "motor traits," or what the stress research workers call "motorization of hostilities," in order to properly evaluate the stress classification of the individual.

Since "Class A" stress is a contributory factor in heart attack, it should be eliminated. But how can we eliminate a condition which for many Americans has become as much a part of life as the air they breathe? Are most of us, then, doomed to the stress-triggered high rate of heart disease?

No. Because there *is* a way of nullifying the effects of stress.

At this point it is necessary to answer the question posed earlier in the chapter. How does stress exert its effects in coronary artery blockage?

Let us look for the answer in the puzzling behavior of the blood cholesterol levels. Doctors had come to look upon blood-cholesterol data as one of the indicators of coronary health. In some patients, however, cholesterol values varied greatly. What was behind the strangely shifting cholesterol values?

In the laboratories of the College of Medical Evangelists in Claremont, California, a research team headed by Dr. John E. Peterson, found the answer. He discovered excessive cholesterol variations in some students under observation. When these students were taking their examinations, Peterson reported, in the August, 1960, issue of *Circulation,* their *average* blood cholesterol went up 16% over base values!

Blood cholesterol rose during examination periods, which are periods of *stress*. Now the relation of stress to coronary disease through the increase in blood cholesterol became clearer.

Peterson's findings are supported by other investigators who have linked the upsurge of blood cholesterol with the incidence of stress. For example, around income-tax time, it has been noted by numerous medical-research groups, that cholesterol levels of accountants are temporarily higher.

Since cholesterol, as will be shown later, is carried in the blood stream only inside microscopic fatty-globules, could one logically assume that, under stress, the number of these globules increases? Dr. Vincent P. Carroll and his associates set out to find the answer. Their findings were that "Elevations in . . . cholesterol associated with periods of stress were confined largely to the beta [fatty globules] . . ." (*Circulation,* October, 1961).

There is another fatty globule in the blood which is known as the chylomicron. In 1960, Dr. G. H. Becker of the Michael Reese Hospital added to the picture of the effects of stress on the fatty blood globules. His investigation showed that the stress of fear doubled the amount of chylomicrons in the blood after a fatty meal and kept them in the blood twice as long as under normal conditions.

The conclusion is inescapable: stress does cause damage in the blood by increasing the amounts of (1) Cholesterol (2) Beta fatty globules and (3) Chylomicron fatty globules.

It has been known since Dr. Canon's pioneering experiments that stress causes blood to have a greater tendency to clot. Since then dozens of researches have confirmed this fact. But it is only in recent years that experiments showed this clotting tendency to be related to the stress-induced release of fatty globules into the blood.

However, will stress bring about atherosclerosis *when men are on a rational Prudent Diet, such as modern medical science proposes?*

Laboratory experiments have not yet been conducted

along these lines on human beings. But there have been some excellent experiments performed on animals, which point to the possible answer.

In 1959, Dr. Herman N. Uhley together with Dr. M. Friedman, who was introduced earlier, reported the results of their work on rats exposed to stress. One group of rats was fed an atherosclerosis-producing high-saturated-fat diet; another group was fed the same diet but was subjected to stress by repeated electrical shocks. In ten months, both groups showed raised levels of blood cholesterols and blood lipids (fatty globules), but the amount in the high-stress group was double that of the non-stress group. However, the important evidence is that *on a non-atherosclerotic diet,* stress did *not* cause a rise in either cholesterol or in other blood lipids. Similar experiments with rabbits showed identical results. In animals at least, diet proved to be a protection against the harmful effects of stress.

The work of Dr. M. E. Grover, originally conducted for the U. S. Air Force, also gives some excellent data on the relation between stress, cholesterol and heart attack. He kept accurate individual records of the blood cholesterol levels and stress conditions of the Air Force personnel in his care, over an extended period of time.

Other investigators have already linked high blood cholesterol to atherosclerosis, but Dr. Grover's research showed that fluctuations in the cholesterol levels also characterized the most coronary-prone airman.

What caused the wide variation in cholesterol levels? Stress!

Dr. Grover found that when one of his men, already afflicted by high cholesterol, carried out orders of a hostile commanding officer, his cholesterol level increased; and that when another airman was engaged in tense political activities, his high blood cholesterol mounted even higher. And that when one of his USAF patients had problems with his incompatible wife, the soaring blood cholesterol registered the stress he experienced.

Dr. Grover's research showed that individuals with high blood cholesterol, who are also subjected to the severe cholesterol-level fluctuations caused by intolerable stress, were the first ones in the group to be affected by coronary heart disease.

The eminent heart specialist, Dr. Henry I. Russek,

cardiovascular consultant to the United States Public Health Service Hospital at Staten Island, New York, has also studied the relation of stress to heart attack. Dr. Russek's conclusion is that, "While there is abundant evidence that a high-fat diet predisposes population groups to coronary artery disease, it appears equally clear that in persons so disposed, emotional stress, more than any other factor, compounds this susceptibility . . . A high-fat diet and a stressful mode of life must be deemed a highly lethal combination."

In addition, according to Dr. Grover, one of the ways that stress exerts its harmful effects is through compulsive eating. Many other medical authorities are of the same opinion. For instance, Dr. Sprague in 1958 has stated that, "It seems likely that emotional tension results in eating, drinking and smoking in many individuals as compensation for anxiety, and I believe it is through this indirect mechanism that stress has its influence on coronary disease."

Dr. Russek, in addition to other research in this field made a comparative survey of the diet habits of ten young victims of coronary attacks, who had been under prolonged emotional stress before their attack. In comparing their diets with that of a control group, more than twice as many of the young heart victims had used an "unusually rich" diet, compared to those in the control group.

Medical opinions are divided as to how much of the present day coronary damage is caused by stress compared to that caused by inactivity combined with a rich fatty diet. It is possible for instance, that a high rate of coronary will occur in a country low in stress and high in physical activity, yet living on a rich fatty diet?

Proof that this indeed is a fact can only come from a modern country with a minimum of Western stress, but still living on a rich Western diet. One European country which meets this specification is Finland. This mainly agricultural nation has drawn comment from many medical scientists for its relative absence of modern socio-economic stress. But its high-calorie, high-saturated-fat diet is accompanied by a blood cholesterol level which is as high as that in the United States.

Dr. M. J. Karvonen of the University of Helsinki, at a symposium on atherosclerosis in London in 1962, remarked that Finland seems to have almost as great a rate of coronary deaths as the United States. The absence of stress is not a protective factor among people like those in Finland living on a high dairy-fat diet.

Now consider the reverse situation: What will happen if the high-fat diet is removed while the high stress remains? In the opinion of Dr. Russek, with the fat base removed, high stress will not have the foundation needed to influence atherosclerosis. Dr. Russek's conclusions are: "In the United States where prodigious amounts of fat are ingested, emotional factors appear to be far more significant in coronary heart disease than the actual excess of dietary fat itself."

"Nevertheless, since no acceleration of atherogenesis [growth of artery blockage] has been observed in 'stressed' populations subsisting on a low-fat diet, it must be recognized that 'stress' can exert its devastating effects only when superimposed on excess [fat] molecules in the circulating [blood]."

One additional note is needed to complete the stress story. The American Heart Association invited Dr. Friedman to report his latest research on stress and heart attack to the 1963 Minneapolis Symposium on Coronary Disease. His data showed that in the most stress-affected 10% of the population, those who are in the class A stress category, the blood cholesterol and all the fatty globules were definitely elevated. There was no doubt that their high rate of heart attack was due to the effects of stress on their blood lipids.

After his report, the question was put to Dr. Friedman, "What do you do in your clinic with these unfortunate class A stress individuals?"

His answer was, "It is almost impossible to get them to change their stress pattern, so it is necessary to place them on a low-saturated-fat diet."

HOW EFFECTIVE IS EXERCISE?

According to a recent news interview, Dr. Paul Dudley White said that "the chief danger of automobiles isn't from accidents, but from the fact that they take people off their feet." Dr. White relates this to coronary disease by adding that, "The sedentary life and the wrong diet are the two most important causes for this kind of heart trouble."

The former president of the American Heart Association, Dr. Howard B. Sprague, comments: "Prosperity is causing too many Americans to become spectators, making them lazy and allowing them to get fat. Hardly anybody works any more as we used to think of work. Hardly anybody plays any more either. We watch TV or ride in cars, or go to the movies. We just aren't burning up our fat."

The result is that each year, if the average American weighed himself, the scale would show an increase of two to three pounds. Now, at forty-five, he is fifty pounds heavier than at twenty-five. With each pound of added weight, brought on by gradually decreasing physical activity combined with an unchanged high-fat, high-calorie diet, the blood cholesterol rises year by year.

That exercise does cancel the harmful effects of a rich diet can be seen from the reports of Harvard's Dr. G. V. Mann. His experiments in 1955 proved that even doubling the daily food intake caused no increase in the blood cholesterol when *enough energy was expended in muscular activity*.

This fact did not come as a surprise. Back in 1921, Dr. Rakestraw, writing in the *Journal of Biological Chemistry*, reported a decrease in blood cholesterol after physical exertion. But in 1921, the role of blood cholesterol in atherosclerosis was not well known, and Dr. Rakestraw's discovery was ignored.

Thirty-five years later, Dr. Ancel Keys and his associates at the well known Physiological Laboratory in Minneapolis extended Rakestraw's work with an interesting experiment. They measured the blood cholesterol increase after breakfast in sedentary men and in men who took some exercise. The blood cholesterol rise among the sedentary group was significantly higher. By 1956, the coronary danger of excess blood cholesterol had already been established, and Dr. Keys could conclude: ". . . these results suggest a reason for part of the difference in susceptibility to coronary heart disease between active and inactive men."

With this in mind, Dr. Lawrence A. Golding, director of the Exercise Physiology Laboratory at Ohio State University, set about discovering to what extent blood cholesterol could be reduced by exercise. In April, 1962, he announced that daily exercise could reduce blood cholesterol by as much as 25% in one year. But since the diet was not restricted, the exercise required was very strenuous: a mile and a half run, 30 laps in the swimming pool, 35 pushups and 55 situps.

It is not necessary to exercise this vigorously as part of the prevention program. A moderate amount of exercise will be found sufficient to normalize blood cholesterol provided calories are watched and the diet fats are properly selected and consumed in moderation.

The importance of exercise in controlling blood cholesterol has been proven by many studies of groups who do not have the "benefits" of our mechanized civilization, among whom a high-calorie, high-fat diet was counterbalanced by the heavy work required in their difficult daily existence.

One example is the Finnish lumberjack, who eats three times as much of the same high fat diet as his city counterpart, yet still has the same blood cholesterol level. In this case his work energy output is as enormous as his appetite.

It is now clear that a high-calorie, high-saturated-fat diet is not the only factor responsible for high blood cholesterol. Exercise is of great importance. It is only in the highly mechanized and physically inactive Western countries that the worst effects of a rich diet are felt.

Exercise may be a potent factor in the prevention of heart attack as evidence from many parts of the world shows.

From England Dr. Morris Crawford reports in the *British Medical Journal* that heavy exercise was found to be very effective in cutting down the toll of coronary heart disease.

In Israel, on the collective agricultural settlements (kibbutzim), there is a single communal dining room for all, regardless of occupation. Dr. Daniel Brunner of Tel Aviv reported to an American Heart Association Convention that the rate of coronary disease among sedentary workers in these settlements was three times as high as among hard working laborers. "Therefore, it was possible," he said "to single out physical activity due to daily work as a factor in the prevalence of coronary heart disease."

Dr. J. N. Morris sums up the situation in the *British Medical Journal*. Based on 3,800 autopsies, his conclusion is that ". . . men in physically active jobs have less coronary heart disease during middle age, what disease they have is less severe, and they develop it later than men in physically inactive jobs. Physical activity of work is a protection against coronary heart disease."

In the United States the results are not as clear-cut. Dr.

H. L. Taylor working at Dr. Ancel Keys Physiological Laboratory made an extensive survey of railroad workers. He found that the sedentary workers had almost double the amount of heart attacks in comparison with the most active outdoor workers of the same age. But this difference does not seem to exist in most of the other studies of active and sedentary groups in this country.

Indeed, Dr. J. M. Chapman of Los Angeles has uncovered statistical evidence that the most active workers in the civil services in California had the same amount of coronary disease as those doing medium or light work.

Similarly, Dr. D. Spain's autopsy studies of 1960 had shown that in every age group active and sedentary workers had the same amount of atherosclerosis.

Why did these three American reports differ so widely from those coming from other areas?

One answer is that in our increasingly automated economy, the difference in energy output between an "active" and a sedentary worker is markedly less than between corresponding groups in Europe. In other words, the "active worker" in the United States is no longer very active. Hence the statistics reveal negligible differences in both blood cholesterol and coronary disease between active and inactive workers.

Another reason for the seemingly low protective effect of exercise in this country is our excessively rich diet. In the opinion of Dr. A. M. Adelstein of the University of Manchester, "In communities where incidence of atherosclerotic heart disease is high, the casual [diet] factor tends to swamp any protective influence that may be exerted by exercise . . ."

Even though at present the benefits of exercise may be obscured by our harmful diet, a defeatist attitude would be extremely unwise. The solution on a national and individual basis is both to increase our physical activities and correct our diet simultaneously.

Another protection which exercise affords against heart attack is through the stimulation of the collateral circulation. When there is danger of coronary blockage, exercise can widen the narrow bypaths, the back-road coronary blood vessels in the affected section of the heart, so that the blood can bypass the obstruction. Dr. R. W. Eckstein said at the Convention of the American Heart Association, in 1956 that, "Exercise does far more for the stimulation of the collateral circulation than anything medicine or surgery can offer."

"LOAFER'S HEART"

Dr. Wilhelm Raab of the University of Vermont College of Medicine, who served as the American member of an international team of scientists formed to study this problem, has accumulated evidence pointing to the lack of physical exercise as a contributory cause of atherosclerosis. For our non-exercising, motorized population, he has coined the phrase, *loafer's heart*. "Lack of exercise is a threat to Western civilization," was his conclusion when he addressed the meeting of the American College of Physicians in Chicago in 1959. "It is not the so-called 'athlete's heart' which should be considered abnormal, but rather the degenerating, inadequate *loafer's heart*."

One of the major concepts which Dr. Raab now emphasizes is that there are two main factors which determine the onset of a heart attack. One is the extent to which artery blockage has reduced the flow of blood to the heart muscle. And the second is the state of efficiency or the oxygen requirement of the heart muscle. The usual heart attack is a combination of a diminished blood supply due to a blocked artery and an inefficient heart muscle that requires even more than a normal blood flow for its minimum oxygen supply.

The problem of general health and its effect on heart muscle efficiency is still another related factor. In the prevention program all three factors must be improved.

Dr. Raab has visited every country in Europe to study the physical exercise methods used to combat the problems raised by the "diseases of civilization and prosperity." He concludes: "The superindustrialized, physically immobilized American people are more in need of such public health-protection policies than any other people, and the financial resources of the United States far surpass those available in the countries abroad which have been pioneering in this field for years."

In his book *Organized Prevention of Degenerative Heart Disease* he shows that although there are 2,928 preventive reconditioning centers in Europe, there is not even one in the United States.

In 1932, Dr. Raab had called for the great nutritional experiment. Now, thirty years after having correctly anticipated the diet solution to the basic cause of coronary disease, he is calling for a new mass trial, this time of exercise for the "loafer's heart."

CAN HEART ATTACK BE INHERITED?

With more than half of our adult male population suffering from atherosclerosis, the chances are that some one in your family—a father, brother, uncle or cousin—has had a heart attack. If this has happened, the thought must have occurred: *does it run in the family?*

The answer is—yes. But it is not quite that simple. Although heart attack does run in some families, is it a disease passed down from one generation to another in the genes? Or is there some other factor that accounts for the high incidence of heart attacks in coronary-prone families?

Many studies have been made of coronary-prone families. But they have been statistical studies, concerned only with tracing the incidence of heart attack from generation to generation.

An exception is the study conducted by a group of researchers from the University of Modena, in central Italy, who were looking for the reasons behind the statistics. The head of the project, Dr. G. P. Vecchi, wasn't satisfied merely to decribe *what* had happened. He wanted to find out *why* it happened.

The subjects of Dr. Vecchi's experiment were twenty-seven families with "a positive heredity and family history of coronary atherosclerosis." For comparison Vecchi selected both a local group of "normal" families, and in addition a second normal control group from the town of Rofrano located in southern Italy where the diet is frugal by comparison with that in central Italy.

Dr. Vecchi found that among the "hereditary" families the coronary incidence was *high*. In the so-called "normal" group it was *medium*. In the southern frugal-diet normal group it was *low*.

Then Dr. Vecchi correlated these findings with the amount of fat in the diet:

In the "hereditary" coronary group, the proportion of dietary fat was 55%.

In the "local normal" control group, dietary fat reached as high as 32%.

But the frugal-diet normal control group, was *low* both in coronary disease and dietary fat which was only 22%.

What's more, where atherosclerosis was highest, saturated-fat intake was highest. Where atherosclerosis was lowest, saturated-fat intake was lowest.

From this study came Dr. Vecchi's conclusion: It was not heredity in the Modena families that made them atherosclerotic. What was passed on from generation to generation was the high-saturated-fat diet.

Corroborating evidence comes from Canada's Dr. J. F. Mustard. This internationally renowned expert on blood-clotting research examined the thrombotic effects of a high-fat meal upon three groups of human subjects: those already afflicted with atherosclerosis; those not yet afflilicted but coming from "hereditary atherosclerotic" families; and a normal control group.

One phase of Dr. Mustard's research is of special interest for our study. Dr. Mustard was able to determine the amounts of saturated fat in the diet of each group by recording the number of times such fat was eaten each week. The chart based on his findings showed that the total number of saturated-fat units for the atherosclerotics was 144. The "normals" from the families with "hereditary" atherosclerosis consumed 134 units, nearly as much. But the saturated-fat intake of the normals was markedly lower, being only 114 units.

It is now clear that the "normals" whose families were already afflicted with "hereditary" atherosclerosis consumed almost as fatty a diet as the actual victims of atherosclerosis. Once again the dreaded family "hereditary" trait had been shown to be merely the persisted-in family dietary habit of overeating saturated fats.

Unfortunately, the researches of Drs. Vecchi and Mustard are the only "hereditary" studies correlated with diet research recorded in medical literature. Can we, then, rule out heredity as the prime cause of atherosclerosis on the evidence of just two experiments? But we need not make such a choice. There is further relevant evidence that can be used to fill the gaps in our knowledge.

There have been surveys relating a "positive family history" for coronary disease to the amounts of cholesterol and fatty globules in the blood. Dr. M. J. Albrink reported in 1962 that the men she studied, whose families had a higher than "normal" coronary history, also had higher blood cholesterol and higher blood fats than controls from normal families.

But are these differences in blood lipids "inherited" from their "coronary-prone" ancestors?

Dr. D. R. Bassett of the National Heart Institute, made a survey on this subject in 1962. He found that the cholesterol and blood fats and the *relative weight* were all high in young males from atherosclerotic families.

His conclusion was that "this may represent a behavior pattern acquired from the parent and may account for the higher [blood] lipid values and the greater relative weight."

In his recent book *Atherosclerosis* Dr. Campbell Moses states that, "almost all the data on familial factors [concerning coronary disease] relate to the occurrence of diabetes, hyperlipemia, hypercholesteremia, obesity and hypertension." It will be shown later that *all* these diseases can be influenced by the Prudent Diet.

This material sums up all the published medical data on "family hereditary tendencies" that pertain to the prevention of atherosclerosis. Since this data implicates diet and blood lipids as important factors in "hereditary tendencies," the whole problem may be clarified if we study the effects of changes in diet in large groups with a uniform hereditary background. Dr. J. N. Morris, the eminent British epidemiologist, calls such studies "hereditary in environment."

An excellent "laboratory" for this study is Israel, where three groups with distinct dietary habits can be studied. These groups are: (1) Yemenite Jews recently arrived from Arabia; (2) Yemenite Jews who have lived in Israel 20 years, and (3) European-born Israelis.

The Yemenite Jews, having dwelt apart in central Arabia for about 2,000 years have, in effect, become one large "family" and can be considered to possess a uniform heredity. Their diet was a frugal one, low in calories and total fats and containing almost no dairy or animal fat.

The blood-cholesterol values of the Yemenite Jews on their arrival in Israel were in the low range of 140-155. But after they had lived in Israel for 20 years and partially adopted the Israeli diet, their cholesterol level rose to 155-200.

These figures are taken from a study conducted by Dr.

M. Toor and his group (*Lancet,* June 1, 1957). The same study further shows that European Jews in Israel, accustomed to a Western-type diet, have Western averages of blood cholesterol readings.

To sum up so far, Dr. Toor has studied three groups and has shown a step-by-step increase of saturated fats in the diet paralleled by an increase in blood cholesterol. His final conclusion is based on the mortality rates from atherosclerosis in each group at age 65:

Newly arrived Yemenite Jews _____ 6%
Twenty-year settled Yemenite Jews _____ 24%
European-born Israelis _____ 36%

Again, coronary disease was shown to be closely related to diet and blood cholesterol and not to heredity.

Dr. Toor made another comparative study of 75-year-old men, European Israelis vs. Yemenite Israelis who still clung to their old frugal diet. The study showed a blood cholesterol index of 176 for the Yemenites and 211 for the Europeans. Also, there were three times as many atherosclerotic Europeans as there were atherosclerotic Yemenites. "Diet," concluded Dr. Toor, "is positively related to the incidence of atherosclerosis."

Other "heredity in environment" surveys have been made on ethnic non-coronary groups who have moved away from their homeland. All have shown that the migrating group tends to develop the coronary tendency of the host nation and that the change in the atherosclerotic pattern is always preceded by a change in diet.

The Japanese, for example, have an exceptionally low rate of coronary heart attack, due to their low-saturated-fat diet. But as they migrate across the Pacifiic, their coronary rate rises. It is higher in Hawaii than in Japan, and much higher in the States than in Hawaii. In Hawaii the Japanese have adopted a partially Westernized diet; on the mainland they live on a full Western diet.

Another important "heredity in environment" story is told by Dr. Paul Dudley White in *Annals of Internal Medicine* (November, 1958). Dr. White's work began in the Naples region of southern Italy. There, with a low-calorie diet containing only 20% fat, mostly unsaturated, the coronary rate was found to be extremely low—3%. But Dr. White's study of age-matched men who had moved from

Naples to Boston, and who had subsisted for years on a "normal" United States high-saturated-fat diet, showed a shocking transformation. As the fat in their diet had risen from 20% to 40%, the incidence of heart attack had jumped from 3% to 18%.

One particular characteristic makes Italy well-suited for the study of "heredity in environment." Its long narrow shape divides the country into many areas, each of which boasts a traditionally different diet.

Starting with a frugal low-saturated-fat diet at the "heel" of the Italian "boot," there are regions of increasingly rich diets, including one which is particularly rich in saturated fats in the Bologna region, which is the "hog belt" of Italy.

Among the medical specialists who have been studying the heart attack problem in Italy for many years is Dr. Vittorio Puddu of Rome's Ospedali Riuniti. After many years of research concerning the wide variations in heart-attack rate in different areas of Italy, he published his findings in the *American Journal of Cardiology* in September 1962.

Dr. Puddu's final conclusion was that there is a close relationship between diet fat and heart attack and, further-more, that, "The average level of blood cholesterol and the frequency of coronary heart disease vary in a parallel fashion in the various geographic regions and are higher in persons having a high consumption of fats."

There have been many other reports of non-coronary groups considered by some scientists to have a "hereditary protective factor," who on migrating to affluent areas where a high-fat diet was customary, would invariably lose their "hereditary protection."

One such case was noted by Dr. C. D. Langen in his "Clinical Textbook of Tropical Medicine." According to his personal clinical observations, the coronary-free Chinese who emigrated to the Dutch East Indies, and there adopted the high fat diet of the European colonists, now became much more frequent victims of coronary disease.

Migration Studies charting the changes in day-to-day food patterns are not the only means of demonstrating the role played by diet in coronary rates of people with similar hereditary background. Drs. Keen and Rose of St. Mary's Hospital in London obtained data on a group of twenty-eight atherosclerotic patients and then compared their diet with that of a group of matched controls. The diet of the controls was found to contain fewer calories and less saturated fat.

While the results of Keen's and Rose's work were interesting, it was their method of study that had important implications. It led to a new concept: Any two groups can be studied, no matter what their social, cultural or economic background, provided proper controls are used.

In this respect England, with the far-reaching effects of its once rigid socio-economic caste system, provides a good "laboratory." At the bottom of the status ladder is the unskilled and the semi-skilled worker; at the top, the managerial, professional and leisured groups; in-between, the skilled worker and the white-collar worker.

Data on British men between twenty and sixty-four, gleaned from Dr. Bronte-Stewart's report in the April, 1959 *Post-Graduate Medical Journal*, shows these relative rates of coronary heart disease, which are based on the average for the group as a whole.

Professionals	50% above average
White Collar Workers	10% above average
Skilled Workers	4% above average
Unskilled Workers	15% below average

As clear-cut as the economic and social class distinction in England was the food-consumption pattern of each class. The lower classes who couldn't afford to buy rich foods or to over-eat, got along on a minimum amount of eggs and dairy products. On the upper rungs of the status ladder, there is a greater income and with it, more consumption of richer foods.

Here is D. H. W. Fullerton's statistical analysis in the *Proceedings of the Royal Society of Medicine* of the tie-in between earnings, fats and calories:

	GRAMS FATS	DAILY CALORIES	PERCENT FAT
Highest Incomes *(Professionals)*	136	3240	38%
Intermediate Incomes *(White Collar)*	121	3120	35%
Lower Incomes *(Skilled Workers)*	99	2800	28%
Lowest Incomes *(Partly Skilled Workers)*	72	2320	27%

The statistical link between coronary rates and food habits was so obvious that Dr. Fullerton could only conclude that ". . . the figures so far show a striking parallelism between dietary fat and [the] higher incidence [of coronary heart disease] in the professional classes."

Adds Dr. Bronte-Stewart: "In Britain the occupational mortality statistics could be related to the fact that the amount of dairy fats and other animal fats constitutes one of the most important social class differences in the dietary habits of man."

Obviously, within one people of the same general racial background, the high-calorie, high-saturated-fat diet was the determining factor in the incidence of atherosclerosis.

Certainly, Drs. Fullerton and Bronte-Stewart were well aware that the beneficial effects of exercise on some of the lower-income workers contributed to their low coronary rate. They also knew that stress may have played a part. But they insisted on the dietary factor as the dominant cause of the clear-cut, class-by-class progression toward an increased coronary rate.

This research was based on nutritional surveys made about fifteen years ago. Since that time there have been many social and economic changes in England, and at present a new nutritional "experiment" is now in the making. Dr. J. N. Morris gave a hint of this latest development at a Royal Society of Medicine lecture; ". . . the poorer third or half of the nation has probably been eating much more fat in recent years; and this may be associated with the increase of [coronary] heart disease among them."

Unlike England, the United States possesses an over-abundance of food, so much so, in fact, that the government must buy surplus butter and eggs. Even the lower economic classes in the United States can afford to indulge in a high-fat diet.

Can we then expect to find much difference in the rate of coronary heart disease among economic classes based on variations in diet? The statistics answer "no." In the United States every economic group, from lowest to highest, is afflicted by the same high rate of coronary disease and heart attack.

Although coronary heart disease is not a true chromosome-linked hereditary disease like hemophilia, each of us *may* be born with some predispositions toward or protections against atherosclerosis Some scientists believe that

men with certain types of physical make-up are less liable
to the disease than others. Statistically it is known that the
big-boned, heavy-set man is more likely to become a heart-
attack victim than the thin man of slight stature.

With almost 50% of adult male fatal illness caused
directly or indirectly by coronary disease, there are certain
to be many families who have more than a "normal" share
of heart attack. This now leads to the concept of a "hereditary tendency."

However, in 1923 when Dr. J. T. Wearn studied the
situation, the data led to a different conclusion. After
studying a group of nineteen cases of heart attack at the
Peter Brent Brigham Hospital in Boston, Dr. Wearn remarked in the *American Journal of Medical Science* that
"Coronary thrombosis with infarction of the heart as a
clinical entity is a condition which is generally classed
among the rarities of medicine."

What was the cause? Dr. Wearn did not know, but he
went on to say: "Heredity was dismissed at once, for there
was only one instance of sudden death in a previous
generation."

But today it is easier for doctors to err concerning the
role of heredity in atherosclerosis This was shown by the
recent reanalysis of a supposed hereditary-coronary experiment. In 1957, Dr. Ernest P. Boas and Dr. Frederick H.
Epstein of the Sidney Hillman Health Center in New York
investigated the prevalence of coronary heart disease among
Italian and Jewish workers chosen at random. Motivating
the research was the once prevalent notion that Jews, by
heredity, are more prone to heart attack than Italians. The
findings seemed to substantiate this view, for the corresponding coronary rates were 6½% for the Italians and
15% for the Jews.

Boas and Epstein felt they could attribute the higher
rate of heart disease among the Jewish workers in part to
diet and in part to heredity. But they weren't sure. There
was another factor, they thought, the mythical "third
factor" that cropped up so often in the medical literature
of that period, an "unknown, yet-to-be-discovered" primary
cause that if once found, would serve to disprove the
dietary explanation.

What was that unknown factor? The answer actually lay
concealed in the published Boas-Epstein data. After publication, other scientists studied the facts as reported by this

research and solved the riddle of the "third factor." The fat in the Jewish diet was mostly saturated, the fat in the Italian diet was mostly unsaturated.

In 1959 the conclusion reached by the scientists reviewing the Boas-Epstein data was this: the "third factor" was the saturated-unsaturated fat *ratios*. The higher rate of heart attack among the Jewish workers was *not* caused by heredity, but by diet.

In many discussions of the origin of coronary disease, heredity is still mentioned as a possible primary cause, but no valid data has yet been presented to substantiate this claim. The opinion of Dr. Edmond A. Murphy of the Johns Hopkins School of Medicine is that, "this field is at present in a confused state." And he goes on to conclude his report on hereditary factors in heart attack with the following eloquent summation:

"There is a tendency to fatalism where genetics is concerned. If we are convinced that this disorder originates in our genes where *we cannot get at them* we may abandon attempts to prevent atherosclerosis, eating our eggs for breakfast, drinking our fifth of Bourbon after dinner, and allowing our muscles to waste from sloth. If we take the stand that we are masters of our fate, perhaps we can achieve some success in combating this worst of all curses from Pandora's Box."

Actually, there is one "hereditary" situation which is definitely related to artery blockage and heart attack. It is well known that *women* are protected from coronary disease.

The next section will explain why this is so and how the knowledge of this fact helps the whole prevention program.

HEART ATTACK PROTECTION IN WOMEN

Up to now we have concentrated on the problem of coronary disease in men. In Western countries the incidence of heart disease is much greater among men than women. Therefore most of the medical experiments in this field, including autopsy as well as clinical and other tests, were conducted on men.

An examination of the data on women, however, is of great importance. It may, in fact, yield clues to new ways of preventing coronary disease in both men and women. For if, on the whole, there is less atherosclerosis among women of Western nations than among Western men, there must be *something* that protects the women.

Just how do the sexes differ in regard to their relative rates of coronary heart attack?

The first difference is that in Western countries, between the ages of forty and seventy, the incidence of coronary heart attack among women is a third of that among men.

The second difference is that in Western countries, the ratio of male to female coronary heart attacks is not consistent but varies with age.

After a study of 1,000 autopsies performed at the Edinburgh Royal Infirmary in 1955, Drs. M. P. Oliver and G. S. Boyd compiled these statistics:

- In the age group 40 to 50, the coronary heart attack ratio was *7 men to 1 woman.*
- In the age group 50 to 60: *5 men to 1 woman.*
- In the age group 60 to 70: *2 men to 1 woman.*
- And in the age group 70 and over: *1 man to 1 woman.*

Dr. Campbell Moses in his book *Atherosclerosis* describes his study of artery blockage in men and women who died of causes *other* than *coronary disease.* During the 30-40 age range the coronary arteries of men are very much more "blocked" than those of women of similar age. In the 40-50 group the difference is less. During the 50-60 and 60-70 decades, the amount of blockage slowly becomes equal; and when they are over 70, many women have arteries which are even slightly more blocked than those in the men.

Apparently, whatever protection women possess seems to decrease with age until, late in life, the disparity in the incidence of coronary heart attack between the sexes disappears.

Here, then, are the two major differences. What are the reasons for them?

Medical research has shown that a high rate of coronary disease is related to high blood-cholesterol levels. If this finding is true in general, we should discover that the cholesterol levels of women are *lower* than those of men. And this is exactly what we do find. In Western countries the blood-cholesterol levels of women are definitely lower than those of men. This explains the first difference, the fact that between the ages of forty and seventy, the incidence of coronary heart attack among women is a third of that among men.

Now for the second difference. We should expect that, as the incidence of coronary in women increases, their blood cholesterol will also rise. This also is exactly what the experimental evidence demonstrates.

In women blood cholesterol usually remains low until they reach thirty-five. Only then does it begin to climb. Their blood cholesterol equals the male level at the age of forty-five and soon rises above it. At the age of sixty, women actually have *higher* cholesterol levels than men, and they maintain these higher levels for the rest of their lives.

"But," you now might ask, "if, after age forty-five the woman's blood-cholesterol level surpasses the man's, why isn't the incidence of coronary heart attack among women, at that time, higher than in men?"

Look at it this way. Compare life to a boxing match. In the man, the body blows dealt by high cholesterol come early in the fight, softening him up for the eventual coronary knockout. The man of Western civilization has been receiving body blows from excess blood cholesterol for fifteen to twenty years longer than the woman. By the time the woman's blood-cholesterol begins to hit the danger zone, the man is already "exhausted" and ready for the knock-out blow. But since the woman is just beginning to receive these softening-up punches, she can last longer.

We now can go on to consider just what protects women from the swift rise in blood cholesterol that afflicts Western men. The clue lies in the age range at which the women's blood-cholesterol level rises so suddenly. The rise occurs between the ages of thirty-five and fifty, the time of the menopause, when secretion of the female hormone lessens.

Is the loss of the female sex hormone responsible for the rise in high blood cholesterol? The answer is: *yes.*

One of the means used by scientists to study the effect of sex-hormone deprivation in women is to observe what occurs in women whose ovaries were removed by surgery. In previous years this operation was performed far too frequently. Now, due to the recent findings concerning sex hormone and coronary heart attack, doctors realize that a total hysterectomy can result in the serious "side effect" of depriving the patient of her hormone protection against coronary heart disease.

Here are the facts as reported in 1959 by Drs. Oliver and Boyd in *The Lancet*. Nine times as many women suffered heart attacks after both ovaries were removed as those who had only one ovary removed. With one ovary remaining, at least *half* the natural hormone protection was left.

From what we have learned, we can expect that the loss of coronary protection in women after "complete" hysterectomy is accompanied by a rise in blood cholesterol. And this is the case. Dr. R. W. Stander of the Indiana University Medical Center tested twenty-eight women before and after surgical removal of the ovaries and found a distinct rise in blood cholesterol.

There are other studies involving women which will illustrate the harmful effects of high blood cholesterol.

One of these is the effects of diabetes. When young women are afflicted with diabetes their blood cholesterol rapidly rises. As a result diabetic women have the same rate of heart attack as diabetic men.

And, finally, we might note that among non-Western peoples, normally living on a low-saturated-fat diet, there is no significant difference between the rates of coronary heart disease in men and women *at any age*. The reason for this should now be obvious: the blood cholesterol is low in *both* sexes, and it *remains* low throughout their lives.

The variations in blood cholesterol in women correlated with their heart attack data before and after the menopause, both in health and in illness, has given scientists an invaluable set of clues to the understanding of one of the major links in the artery-blockage problem.

Even if all other known data were to be discarded, the evidence of the change in rate of coronary disease in women, which correlates with their cholesterol changes, is a powerful indictment of high blood cholesterol.

If we examine the non-diet factors as a group, they are found to have one "key" characteristic in common. They *all* react on the arteries through the fats and cholesterol in the blood. This "key" directly relates the effects of the *non-diet* factors to those of diet—the principal source of blood fats and cholesterol.

There is a second "key"—the fact that stress increases the blood coagulability, and lack of exercise decreases the normal ability of the blood to dissolve blood clots. Both of these effects are also a by product of our moderated, saturated fat diet.

These interrelationships form the "master key" to the understanding and the solution of the coronary epidemic.

The first of the "master key" relationships, the effects of diet on cholesterol in the blood, will be explained in the following chapters.

CHAPTER FIVE

The Deadly Cholesterol "Numbers Game"

Today you, like most Americans, are playing a "numbers game" against great odds, a game in which you stand to lose everything. For it's your life that's at stake.

And the "number" you're betting your life against is the amount of cholesterol in your blood: The greater the quantity of blood cholesterol, the greater your danger of a heart attack.

How high does the blood cholesterol usually rise before there is danger of serious atherosclerosis. The answer, unfortunately, is not a simple one. And before you can relate the answer to your own coronary health, you must know more about cholesterol, where it comes from, what it is, and how it behaves in the body.

Cholesterol, which in Greek means "bile solid," was discovered in the bile stones, which accumulate and grow in the diseased human gall bladder. As far back as 1769, the French scientist Poulletier de la Salle isolated the substance and described it.

Cholesterol is easy to identify, and it was soon found in other parts of the body; in 1834, in the brain and in 1883, in the blood. In 1846, another Frenchman, Lecanu, made a discovery that is assuming critical significance in the light of recent coronary researches: He found that a large amount of cholesterol is present in eggs.

Cholesterol is one of the sterols (solid alcohols) found in all living things. By the time the prehistoric mammal had evolved, nature had devised its last and most perfect sterol, *cholesterol*, found in almost every organ and every tissue of the human body, as well as in all animals. It is the only sterol never found in our diet vegetables.

Cholesterol has one unusual property; it is an excellent electrical insulator. It is used by the body to protect the delicate electrical network of the brain and nervous system. Without it, our entire thinking and reflex apparatus would be "short-circuited." Insulation of this type has to be tough, resistant, and hard to break down—and cholesterol has all these properties. It's extraordinarily stable, and it is in this quality, ironically, that its menace lies.

Cholesterol can act like sand in the lubrication system of your car; being insoluble in the oil, it falls out and clings to the inner walls of the system. In your arteries, cholesterol cannot be broken down or otherwise eliminated.

Although cholesterol is waxlike, it is also crystalline. Under a microscope one can see the long sharp points, the tiny deadly needles that can irritate the arterial tissue when they become embedded in it.

But is there absolute evidence that cholesterol *does* become embedded in the arteries?

In 1847, Dr. J. Vogel in his *Physiological Anatomy of the Human Body* stated that when atherosclerosis is present in the human coronary artery, so is cholesterol. Even before that, a more far-reaching connection was suggested by two Frenchmen, Becquerel and Rodier. At that time they observed that an abnormal rise in blood cholesterol might be caused by what they called "indigestion." The symptoms of angina are sometimes confused with those of "acute indigestion." And it is a known fact that angina can be induced by a high-fat meal.

What happened following the German and French discoveries? For the next century or more, investigators continued to regard cholesterol with increasing suspicion. Dr. N.N. Anichkov, the earliest research worker in the *prevention* of coronary disease, stated almost half a century ago that "without cholesterol there is no atherosclerosis." But since heart attacks were so rare that they were considered medical curiosities, no urgent need was felt for decisive research.

However, in the last few decades, with coronary disease soaring, the time for a decision concerning the role of cholesterol had arrived. The fate of millions now depended upon it.

Was high blood cholesterol a major cause of coronary heart attack?

Scientists devoted much research to this problem, but hesitated to make a final decision. Researchers demanded more data and insisted on more time to "put the pieces together," although the coronary "plague" was spreading, killing off our older citizens and attacking even the young at an increasing rate.

To Mrs. Mary Lasker, head of the National Health Education Committee, the mounting statistics on heart attack became a matter of urgent concern. The public had to be informed of the danger and of the known means of prevention. But where could she get the information to disseminate? She appealed to the American Society for the Study of Arteriosclerosis, requesting a brochure containing data on how to prevent heart attack. The society's reply was: "We're not yet ready." Theirs was the traditional reluctance of established medical groups to issue public statements concerning controversial scientific issues.

But Mrs. Lasker persisted. She possessed the necessary endurance and the requisite knack of persuasion. Finally, she prevailed upon the Society to prepare the document. The ASSA began the project in 1957, a few years before the historic AHA study of diet fats in relation to atherosclerosis already described in Chapter 4.

A committee of the nation's most distinguished heart specialists, most of them past-presidents of The American Heart Association, was appointed to study the evidence and prepare an authoritative public statement. The report is a milestone in the history of preventive medicine. The ASSA's *A Statement on Arteriosclerosis* announced that factors which predispose one to heart attack and stroke are: (1) overweight, (2) elevated blood pressure, (3) excessive cigarette smoking, (4) heredity, (5) ELEVATED BLOOD-CHOLESTEROL LEVEL.

There had always been a consensus of opinion among medical men that obesity, high blood pressure, and cigarette smoking were related to heart disease, but now the century old suspicion of the harmful role of cholesterol had been confirmed by a competent medical jury.

Supporting data for this latest finding came from hundreds of research reports on cholesterol and atherosclerosis. But one scientific mass-population survey, the Framingham experiment, supplied the most decisive evidence.

THE FAMOUS FRAMINGHAM EXPERIMENT

Let's go back to the 1940's and look in on Framingham, Massachusetts, the site of the most important mass-study of factors influencing coronary heart disease ever made.

At that time the controversy over cholesterol was already intense. One group of scientists asserted that blood cholesterol was a contributory cause to heart attack; another group opposed this concept. The argument became so intense that The National Heart Institute, the official government agency, undertook to help bring about a decision by a twenty-year *prospective* mass-study.

"Prospective," in this case meant that the people undergoing examination would start off being healthy, *not* sick. They would continue to live the way they had always lived. Everything would be "normal"; they'd eat and drink what they liked, behave as they pleased, and generally carry on as if no experiment were in progress. But from time to time they would be tested for factors known to be related to the onset of heart disease. And most important of all—a careful check would be kept on the level of each person's blood cholesterol.

A prospective mass study would require thousands of volunteers to return to the testing laboratory at intervals over a period of twenty years. Where could such people be found? The town of Framingham, Massachusetts was chosen as the ideal "test" town. Its inhabitants were accustomed to undergoing examinations of this type for other surveys. The public-spirited citizens of Framingham were willing, and when the call went out for adult volunteers, about 5,000 responded.

Between 1948 and 1950, without publicity or fanfare, the now-famous "Framingham Experiment" was begun. Its initiators were Dr. Thomas R. Dawber and Dr. Abraham Kagan. Periodically their "Heart-Study Unit" examined the volunteers, noted the cholesterol count and other statistics, and watched for the symptoms of coronary heart disease. If the experiment were to have any significance, the medical team had to match its clinical and laboratory findings against the incidence and development of coronary heart disease.

By July 1961 the "Framingham Experiment" was more than ten years old; and in the July issue of *Modern Concepts of Cardiovascular Disease,* Dr. Dawber was able to conclude that, "There is convincing evidence that [blood] cholesterol levels are definitely related, both to the presence . . . and the development . . . of coronary heart disease."

The "Framingham Experiment" did more than just generally establish the link between blood cholesterol and coronary heart disease. Dr. Dawber and his associates began to relate the *amounts* of blood cholesterol to the *numbers* of heart attacks in each blood cholesterol group.

Over a ten-year period, in the group with a cholesterol level below 200, the coronary disease count was *forty-five.* At the 200 to 220 blood-cholesterol level, the count of coronary cases was *sixty.* At the 220 to 240 level, the count was *eighty.* At the 240 to 260 level, it was *one hundred and forty.* And when the cholesterol level surged over 260, the number of coronary victims mounted to *two hundred.*

Even in 1958, enough valuable information from the Framingham study was made available to the ASSA committee. This data, added to the voluminous data from other sources, resolved all doubts. A *public* statement by the ASSA could now safely be made: *High blood cholesterol was a definite cause of coronary-artery disease.*

This was an announcement of historic importance. For the first time in medical history an official medical group had publicly taken the first step toward the establishment of a Coronary Prevention Program.

Measurement of blood cholesterol is a simple procedure: The basic method was formulated by two chemists, Liebermann and Burchard, in the 1880's. The cholesterol "solution" is treated with sulphuric acid. This results in brilliant color reactions, ranging from red through violet to green, depending upon the amount of cholesterol present.

Although new analytical techniques have been developed, the methods employed today are, fundamentally, variants of the Liebermann-Burchard color reaction. By comparing the shade of the color with known standards, the analyst can determine rapidly and with reasonable accuracy the quantity of cholesterol present in a blood sample. These tests are so easy to perform and so inexpensive that blood-cholesterol has been studied in connection with almost every disease known to man.

To identify a *high* blood-cholesterol level, we must understand what the *normal* cholesterol level is. Is it to be obtained by taking a national average of "healthy" Americans? Is the *average* figure necessarily the *normal* figure?

Although the statistical studies made in the United States vary, the average blood cholesterol index stands today somewhere between 230 and 260, depending on location. For instance, California has a high average blood cholesterol compared to the other states.

But we also know that the average American is not a coronary normal. So our average high blood cholesterol may simply be an indication of "hidden" coronary disease, and it would be useless for establishing a valid cholesterol norm.

How, then, can we determine the true index of a normal cholesterol level at which whole populations are free of coronary? What is this figure?

Dr. Bernard Amsterdam, in the *New York State Journal of Medicine*, considers a blood-cholesterol level of 180 as the maximum.

"120 to 180" is the optimal normal, says Dr. William Dock, Professor of Medicine at the State University of New York.

"200 or less" according to Dr. M. E. Groover, in the *Journal of the College of Physicians*.

"Below 200" said Dr. N. Jolliffe of New York City's Department of Health.

"150" according to Dr. Louis H. Nahum of the Yale School of Medicine.

"120 to 160" according to Dr. H. A. Schroeder, in his book, *Mechanisms of Hypertension*.

"170" suggested by Dr. A. G. Shaper of the Makerere College Medical School in Uganda.

"150 to 185" according to Dr. W. D. Wright of the University of Nebraska, College of Medicine.

Correlate these findings with those of the "Framingham Experiment" and we can establish a working norm, a *practical* "safety zone," within the blood-cholesterol range of 160 to 185.

But since the current "average" American blood cholesterol index is between 230 and 260, it probably has been increasing decade by decade, far beyond the original true physiological norm. If the blood-cholesterol theory is correct, it should be possible to demonstrate this rise through published statistical data.

In the United States such records are not available. No medical group exists that has been functioning here, say, for forty or fifty years, under the same leadership, using the same measurements, keeping uniform records.

But a study of this type was possible in Holland. Dr. J. Groen published a report of Dutch cholesterol values for the years in which they were studied—1912, 1920, 1934, 1937 and 1948. During this period the blood cholesterol count gradually rose from 182 in 1912, to its modern level of 245 in 1948.

According to Dr. Groen, the Dutch have climbed the path of civilized diet, mouthful by mouthful, for fifty years, right into the danger zone of heart attack.

Similar evidence comes from England. Although the average blood-cholesterol level is still below the United States level, it has been creeping up gradually during the past thirty years. There is some reliable data on cholesterol levels in England during the pre-coronary years, the low-fat years of 1920 to 1925. Fortunately, Sir Berkeley Moynihan kept careful records of blood cholesterol in his patients during this period. In 1925 he published this data in the *British Medical Journal*.

He found blood cholesterol ranging from 150 to 200 in the normals. Based on his findings in atherosclerotics, he considered those with 160 to be normal, 160 to 192 high normal, and 192 and over high.

Compare these low 1925 cholesterol levels found by Dr. Moynihan with the known higher British levels in 1940 and 1960, and a pattern of increase emerges, very similar to that observed by Dr. Groen in Holland. The validity of Dr. Moynihan's cholesterol measurements can be evaluated by the fact that they enabled him to predict a treatment thirty years ahead of his time. Patients with a cholesterol of 190 and over *were prohibited the use of fats, eggs, goose, duck, pork, cheese; and urged to use skim milk, lean meat and fish.*

Dr. Moynihan's list of prohibited foods is almost identical to that arrived at by our most modern medical-research groups. Was Dr. Moynihan thirty years ahead of his time, or are we lagging in the practical application of this data?

For the United States the situation was worse, for our country's "food" prosperity started long before 1925, as shown by our national diet statistics. By the time accurate cholesterol tests were made in 1935 by medical researchers in the United States, the cholesterol count had already reached an average exceeding 200.

From this point we have moved to our present national average of 250. And in our highest coronary-rate state, California, Dr. R. L. Searcy reports that the average cholesterol level for a group of over 800 unselected clinically "healthy" men in the thirty to sixty age range was over 270.

The data from Holland, England and the United States form the basis for a historical study. Using the data just extracted from the historical "laboratory" we can divide the world into three groups.

1. The non-coronary countries in Africa and Asia where the blood cholesterol was very low forty years ago and is still very low today.

2. Those like Holland and England, which had a low average cholesterol forty years ago but have "civilized" levels today.

3. The United States, where the blood cholesterol level was on its way up forty years ago and which today has the highest known average blood-cholesterol level in the world.

The non-coronary countries still have their low rate of heart attack.

In Holland and England, the heart attack rate is known to have followed the rise in blood cholesterol until both are in a high "civilized" range today.

In the United States the rise in blood cholesterol preceded that of the other countries as did its rise in heart-attack rate, and both are now the highest in the world.

The United States is generally credited with the honor of being the birthplace of the coronary epidemic. Clinical heart attack was first introduced to world medical science by an American, Dr. Herrick in 1912.

The data just presented is too meager to stand by itself as a fully valid indictment of high blood cholesterol. But its implications are very deep, and should be a cause of grave concern to every American male with a logical mind.

Taken together with the other data so far presented, and with much which will be described later on, it helps to justify a course of action against the dietary and other factors known to lead to increased blood cholesterol.

What may we conclude from all this data? The sad situation is that our national "average" is *not* normal. Heart specialists such as Amsterdam, Dock, Groover, Nahum, Schroeder, Wright, and many others are correct.

The normal blood cholesterol for human beings should be in the region of 160-170-180.

There is only one way to bring our national average of cholesterol back to its true normal, the adoption of (1) a low calorie (2) a low saturated fat and (3) a low cholesterol diet.

The next section is about the last member of this inseparable trio. It will be explained how for a time it was separated, and how the mistake was rectified.

WHAT MEDICAL RESEARCH FINALLY REVEALED ABOUT THE LOW-CHOLESTEROL DIET

By the early 1950's the low-cholesterol diet was coming to be accepted as a method of coronary prevention. Many doctors endorsed it. The public had become accustomed to hearing about it.

Both the experiences of World War II and the accumulated data on eating habits of non-coronary peoples all over the world indicated that a diet low in saturated (animal) fat *and cholesterol* might be of great importance in preventing coronary heart attack. In addition there were a vast number of animal experiments in which the animals were fed cholesterol either in a pure form, dissolved in oil, or naturally contained in the foods they ate. In either case the same pattern of results emerged: an increase in diet cholesterol was followed by an increase in blood cholesterol; and this, in turn, led to increased atherosclerosis. On the basis of *all* the evidence—which pointed to the need for a low-fat diet as well—many doctors began to prescribe a low-cholesterol, low-fat diet for their patients.

Then something happened that resulted in a temporary discrediting of the low-cholesterol diet. It was a setback which has handicapped the fight against coronary heart disease for many years.

How did it happen?

Experiments with *animals* had demonstrated the relationship of diet cholesterol to blood cholesterol, but few direct experiments had ever been made on *man*. Animal experiments are valuable as guide lines but a firm foundation for a prevention program can only result from experiments on human beings conducted under normal conditions. Around 1950 groups of investigators began cholesterol-feeding experiments on man. These tests were based on incorrect assumptions. But the errors were not discovered until years later, and so they led to the *false* conclusion that the amount of cholesterol in food does not lead to an increase in cholesterol in human blood.

The experimental conditions upon which the false conclusions were based were incorrect for many reasons. Among these were the following errors. The "human guinea pigs" were fed pure "crystalline" cholesterol "unnaturally" dissolved in vegetable oil. In one series of experiments, the cholesterol was an additive to fat-free diets; in another series, to so-called "normal" diets. At *all* times, the added cholesterol supplemented the subject's "normal" large cholesterol intake. And most important— the overall amount of time allowed for many of these experiments was far too short.

But at that time, the hidden errors in the tests which discredited the low cholesterol diet were not understood. The incorrect conclusions received immediate and unquestioning approval.

The experiments were conducted by some of the most eminent workers in the field, and the data had the appearance of being highly scientific. In addition there was an important psychological reason for the non-critical acceptance. As a nation, we were reluctant to accept the proposition that our highly esteemed diet might be harmful, and we snatched at the first seemingly scientific endorsement of the status quo.

Dietary habits can be changed, but the psychological resistance to change is formidable. When any evidence turns up pointing an accusing finger at a favorite item in our diet, a hue and cry goes up: *give us more evidence —we're not satisfied—recheck the evidence.* But let any evidence be introduced giving our diet a clean bill of health, and we accept it without many questions.

An even more distressing problem was the fact that the false conclusions about diet cholesterol indirectly cast doubt on the value of the low-saturated-fat diet. For during the years preceding the confusion the press, radio and television had familiarized many thousands of people with the low-cholesterol diet. To many who suffered from heart disease this diet held out hope for the future. Now, people were told that the low-cholesterol diet was worthless. Confidence in the expected protection against a coronary heart attack was undermined, and the low-cholesterol diet was on its way *out*. In the confusion that resulted, the low-saturated-fat diet was also discredited.

Now, with no need to avoid high-cholesterol foods, people who had removed them put eggs and dairy products, foods loaded with dangerous saturated fat, back on their daily menu. The misconception of the actual meaning of the low-cholesterol diet *plus* the prompt acceptance of the anti-diet-cholesterol experiments resulted in incalculable confusion.

Even today the misconceptions caused by the incorrectly managed diet-cholesterol experiments still persist. It is interesting to see just how seemingly minor mistakes in the experiments were able to cloud the truth for so long a time on such a vital issue.

Let us examine these errors in method.

1. *Pure crystalline cholesterol*

According to Drs. Cook, Edwards, and Riddell, summarizing their findings in *The Biochemical Journal*, crystalline cholesterol is poorly absorbed by the human body; absorption of egg-yolk cholesterol is *four* times as complete.

2. *Cholesterol added to a no-fat-diet*

Reports Dr. Ancel Keys in *The Journal of Nutrition:* Cholesterol absorption by the body *requires the presence of fat.* On a fat-free diet, the body does not absorb cholesterol. No matter how much cholesterol is fed, it will be eliminated in the digestive tract and none of it will show up in the blood. To *test blood-cholesterol changes on a fat-free diet is meaningless*.

3. *Cholesterol added to our "normal" high cholesterol diet*

The consensus of a number of investigators is that our normal diet is already so heavily laden with cholesterol that the body can hardly absorb any additional amounts. Cholesterol added to a habitually frugal diet, will increase blood cholesterol significantly. But if cholesterol is added to our habitually cholesterol-rich diet, the increase in our already high blood cholesterol is much less significant.

4. *Short-term experiments*

In order to see results similar to those on laboratory animals, which have a comparatively short life span, observations of human beings must be carried out over relatively long periods of time. The usual tests—which rarely exceeded a few weeks—were often meaningless.

In short, the experiments which delayed the medical and the public acceptance of the life-saving, low-cholesterol-diet for nearly a decade were made under the *wrong* conditions, with the *wrong* quantities, in combination with the *wrong* foods, over *wrong* periods of time. *The conclusions had to be and were wrong.*

That diet cholesterol *does* affect blood cholesterol was clearly demonstrated by the new and valid experimental studies conducted during the years 1960-1962. Of all this work, the most impressive is that of Dr. W. E. Connor and his associates at the Iowa State University College of Medicine.

The Connor experiments were conducted under rigorously controlled conditions. His volunteers were inmates of a prison, so the time element was no problem.

Dr. Connor set out to eliminate all variables in the diet except cholesterol. He accurately measured the total calories, the amounts of saturated and unsaturated fats, the carbohydrates, the proteins, the vitamins and the minerals, and he kept them all constant. He varied only the amount of diet-cholesterol, which was fed only in the form of natural food. If blood cholesterol varied, only the natural diet-cholesterol could be responsible.

Here was a tightly controlled experiment. No one could reasonably doubt the validity of *these* test conditions. Once and for all the results would decide whether or not diet cholesterol influences the levels of blood cholesterol. And the result? Here it is in Dr. Connor's own words: "Dietary cholesterol has a significant effect upon the [blood] cholesterol in human beings."

In a short while, Dr. Connor's evidence resulted in what is virtually official medical recognition of the role played by diet cholesterol in raising blood-cholesterol levels. It came from the leading medical periodical in the field, *Nutrition Reviews.*

In 1960 all the scientific data on the problem of diet cholesterol and its relation to blood cholesterol had not yet quite been resolved, according to *Nutrition Reviews'* experts, but by October 1961, with the publication of additional results by Dr. Connor's group, the official voice of medical nutritional science in the United States had the following to say: "From these studies, one must conclude that ingestion of dietary cholesterol does elevate the [blood] cholesterol in man, and probably should be considered as a potential factor influencing the [development] of atherosclerosis."

In 1962, Drs. Bruce Taylor and George E. Cox of Northwestern University presented separate reports showing that the amount of cholesterol the human body should absorb is only one-tenth that of the amount now considered safe. Their analysis was that, although some animals have the ability to handle large amounts of cholesterol, human beings are not as fortunate.

Dr. Taylor eliminated the pitfalls of previous, short-term experiments and fed his "human guinea pigs" cholesterol-rich egg yolks for eighteen months. His conclusion was that the maximum food cholesterol should be only two-tenths of a gram per day. This limit is reached after eating only one quarter of a pound of meat and a half an egg yolk. Dr. Connor's allowance of cholesterol was only half this amount.

Other reports, of tests using the latest techniques, on diet-cholesterol research have recently appeared, such as that of Dr. Alfred Steiner's group at the Goldwater Memorial Hospital. All have confirmed the harmful role of cholesterol in the diet.

The obstacle to understanding the coronary problem has been removed, and from the scientific point of view, the diet-cholesterol misunderstanding is at an end.

Are the harmful effects of this medical misunderstanding truly over? Vindication of the theory that diet cholesterol influences blood cholesterol has come so late—and official approval is still so recent—that the news hasn't quite filtered through.

The roadblock has been removed by our top medical research scientists. But it will take considerable time before the American public is back on the right road.

UNSATURATED FAT—KEY TO THE CHOLESTEROL MYSTERY

In its historic report of 1961 on "Dietary Fat and Its Relation to Heart Attacks and Strokes," the American Heart Association mentioned three methods of reducing the cholesterol in the blood: (1) reduce the total amount of food eaten (2) reduce the percentage of fat calories (3) change the type of fats eaten from the saturated animal type (which predominates in the American diet) to the unsaturated, vegetable type.

The first two principles had been known for decades. But the third, the unsaturated-fat method of reducing the blood cholesterol, had only been discovered and generally accepted during recent years. Until this discovery the second, or low-fat method of reducing blood cholesterol was not fully understood. This was due to lack of knowledge concerning the effects of saturated and unsaturated fats and to research which often uncovered "exceptions" to the low-fat rule.

But Dr. J. Groen, who in 1952 was working with his associates at the Wilhelmina Hospital in Amsterdam, was convinced that if these "exceptions" were scientifically studied, they could be integrated into a general rule. Basing his hypothesis on early studies, he thought the difference between saturated and unsaturated fat was the key to the problem. He began with this idea in planning the basic experiments. First, he worked with large groups of normal individuals. Second, he used not two, but three diets in order to get a more general answer to the question. And, third, he switched his groups back and forth from one diet to the other to make sure that the results were not due to exceptional individuals or other unusual factors.

Now it can be seen why Dr. Groen could report in the November 1952 issue of *Voeding* that there was statistically only one chance in ten thousand that his findings were incorrect. And to make sure that his answers would be meaningful as well as accurate, he used great forethought in the selection of the three specific diets. Each was a "duplicate" of a diet followed by the world's three main population groups.

First, his "vegetarian" diet was similar to that used by the majority of people in less industrialized "backward" areas.

Second, the "frugal" diet was similar to that of the lower economic groups of Europe.

Third, the "Average American" diet represented that of the most industrially advanced groups in the world.

And it should be noted that the amount of calories on all diets was the same.

Not only were these diets natural, but in addition their

The Three Basic Daily Diets

	VEGETARIAN	FRUGAL NETHERLAND DIET	"AVERAGE" AMERICAN DIET
Bread Vegetables Fruit	As desired	As desired	As desired
Meat and Fish	None	1½ oz.	8 oz.
Eggs	None	2 per week	14 per week
Cheese	None	1 oz.	1½ oz.
Milk	3½ oz.	¼ to ½ pint	As desired
Buttermilk	As desired	As desired	None
Butter Fat	No Butter No Cream	Margarine and Butter mixture as desired	Butter and Cream as desired
Nuts and Oils	As desired	Little	Little

use would clearly delineate the effects of different fats on blood cholesterol. In retrospect, it is easy to see how this historic report could clarify most of the scientific enigmas of the previous diet-fat experiments and to see why it was to become the cornerstone for the diet section of the coronary prevention program.

The vegetable diet was high in unsaturated oils and with almost no saturated fats; the frugal Netherland diet was intermediate in both types of fats; and in the average American diet fat was mostly of the saturated type. What was the effect on the blood cholesterol?

"In general," Dr. Groen concludes (1952), "the blood cholesterol fell on the vegetable diet and rose on the 'high' [saturated fat] diet."

When the change was made from the vegetable diet to the high-fat diet, the blood cholesterol rose. When the change was made from the American diet to the frugal Netherland diet, the blood cholesterol fell.

With the statistical chance of error reduced to one in 10,000 Dr. Groen had established this basic truth: *Increase the amount of unsaturated fats in the diet, and the blood cholesterol drops; increase the amount of saturated fats, and the blood cholesterol climbs.*

At this point it is important to realize the significance of the extreme care and forethought used in setting up the experiment. Dr. Groen himself states that "If we had used a smaller number of subjects or if the duration of our experiment had been shorter, e.g., if we had stopped it after the first period, the influence of the diet might have seemed different. We would then have concluded that only a pure vegetable diet had an influence and that there was no difference between the [frugal] and the [American] diet."

The first period was actually three months and the whole experiment went on for nine months. The number of subjects was sixty.

Dr. Groen's experiment was a scientific landmark in the history of coronary disease research. Never before or since has an experiment in this field been conducted for so long a period on such a large number of young, healthy people and given rise to such important conclusions.

Even so, Dr. Groen still was not completely satisfied that enough data had been collected. Dr. Groen checked the cholesterol content of the foods his volunteers were eating, and he found that the greater the amount of saturated fats in their diet, the greater the amount of *dietary* cholesterol.

Therefore, Dr. Groen tempered his conclusion: The high blood cholesterol which occurred as a result of the average American diet, could be due to either the high-saturated-fat diet, or cholesterol in the diet, or to a combination of both.

But whatever the explanation, one fact was certain; reduce the saturated fats which are the *main source* of cholesterol in the diet and the blood cholesterol will drop.

In 1952 Dr. Groen voiced his desire to extend his experiment in order to find out specifically the effects of diet cholesterol. Had the funds for this extension of research been available, there is no doubt but that the diet cholesterol setback described in the last chaper would have been avoided.

But this was not all. Dr. Groen had one more prophetic proposal. As he states: "A similar experiment however . . . in an older group extended over many years . . . would yield important results for the study of the connection between diet, high blood cholesterol and the development of atherosclerosis."

But, unfortunately, as in the case of Dr. Raab's similar request twenty years earlier, Groen's proposal was to go totally unheeded for a long time.

On the problem of unsaturated versus saturated fat, however, Dr. Groen's scientific influence was decisive. There was no possibility of doubt or controversy about his results. A new era was inaugurated. Almost simultaneously Dr. Lawrence Kinsell of the Highland Alameda Metabolic Institute published a confirming report that sparked an explosion of scientific activity in this field. A hundred similar experiments followed, extending the research of Dr. Groen and Dr. Kinsell in a number of ways, but all verifying the value of unsaturated fat in reducing blood cholesterol. During the following decade the virtually unanimous conclusion of medical science was that the major cause of high blood cholesterol was a high-calorie, high-saturated-fat diet.

It is apparent that the key to understanding blood cholesterol is to be found in the manner in which saturated and unsaturated fats react in the human body.

The *saturated* fats are animal fats. The *unsaturated* fats are vegetable fats. This is a general rule. But there are several *exceptions* to this rule.

Exceptio probat regulam is the original Latin for the

common expression, "The exception proves the rule." But as Dr. William Dock has frequently reminded the medical world the true meaning is: the exception *probes* the rule.

Let us *probe,* then, the animal fat "exception," the fish. The water in which fish live is frequently extremely cold. Had their fats been saturated fats, which solidify at low temperatures, they would have frozen stiff—and frozen out of the evolutionary struggle. Unsaturated fats are liquid even in Arctic temperatures. The fish remain limber; they can swim about easily without stiffening and losing mobility, no matter how cold the surrounding waters. By way of contrast we know that hogs fed to develop "solid" saturated fat sometimes freeze hard if exposed to severe weather. They actually "crack up."

During their evolutionary struggle for survival, fish have developed the ability to manufacture an especially soft type of unsaturated fat, which is even *more* unsaturated than vegetable oils.

What's true of fish is also true of Arctic mammals, seals, whales and polar bears, which have a more unsaturated body fat than the other mammals.

Let's continue to probe—this time by examining the vegetables. In general, *their* fat, which is usually contained in the seed, takes the form of predominantly unsaturated oil.

But there are also exceptions to this general vegetable fat rule. In tropical and semitropical regions certain fatty fruits, notably the coconuts, have evolved fats with a high melting point. These fats remain solid even in tropical temperatures. As hardness and saturation are inseparable, so coconut fat, the world's *hardest* natural fat, is the world's most saturated fat.

These exceptions make it necessary to formulate a *more basic general rule,* which is this: The saturated fat is *solid* at room temperature. The unsaturated fat is *liquid* even at fairly low temperatures.

THE CRITICAL DIFFERENCE BETWEEN "HARD" AND "SOFT" FATS IN OUR DIET

To understand the nature of these fats we must find the basic reason for the hard-soft, solid-liquid distinction of the general rule. We can do this by looking at the way the basic building blocks of the saturated fats, the carbon and the hydrogen atoms, are "attached" to each other. The compactness of these atoms tells why the saturated fat is hard . . . solid.

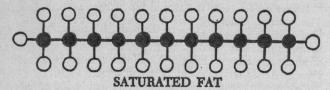

SATURATED FAT

You can see a layer of carbon atoms sandwiched between two layers of hydrogen atoms. It looks tight, hard, solid. The "longer" the saturated fat chain, the more solid the groups of these "sandwiches" will be.

Now what does unsaturated fat look like? Let's break the rigidity by removing two hydrogen atoms from the saturated fat. Now the diagram looks almost as if a hinge had been built into the structure:

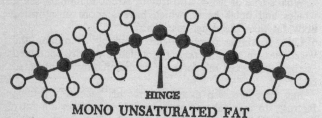

HINGE

MONO UNSATURATED FAT

The result is a more "flexible" unit. The unsaturated molecule now bends, softens. This shows the difference between hard saturated fat and the soft unsaturated oil. As the number of such "hinges" increases, the molecule becomes increasingly more "bendable"—the oil becomes more "liquid," more polyunsaturated.

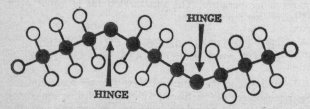

HINGE

HINGE

POLY UNSATURATED FAT

Possessing this basic knowledge of the structure of fats, it will be easier for us to understand how the two types of fat we eat react on the cholesterol in the body so that they change the level of cholesterol in the blood.

As we already know, cholesterol has important work to do in almost every tissue of the body. It's the insulating sheath for nerves. It's the raw material for hormones, the chemical agents that determine our growth, energy, and sexual characteristics. Cholesterol can handle these jobs by itself—it's then known as "free" cholesterol—but, *most often, cholesterol works in combination with a fat.*

Only a small percentage is in combination with the saturated fats. The unsaturated type of fat seems to have the best "shape" for this combination. Medical scientists have made many experiments which prove this conclusively. Unsaturated fats and cholesterol combine in a chemical "marriage," to form what chemists call an ester. It's in this ester, or "married," form that cholesterol carries out many of its functions.

But suppose the cholesterol has little or no choice. Suppose there is an excess of saturated fats in the blood and at the same time a shortage of unsaturated fats. Can the cholesterol "marry" a saturated fat? It can and does. But with this drawback: The saturated-fat-cholesterol ester is less efficient than the unsaturated-fat cholesterol ester. That means that *more* cholesterol is needed to do an equivalent job. As a result there has to be more cholesterol in the bloodstream.

But this "esterification process" isn't the only way in which saturated fats cause high blood cholesterol.

Bile is the chemical substance the body manufactures in the liver to digest fats. When fats enter the digestive system, the liver speeds into action and increases the output of bile. But the essential ingredient of bile is cholesterol. Therefore, as more bile is produced to digest the fats, less cholesterol is left over to be sent into the blood. And it has been definitely established that it is the unsaturated fats which stimulate the liver into high bile-production and that saturated fats only provide a *weak* stimulus.

Furthermore, we know how stable cholesterol is, how difficult it is for the body to break it down chemically and to dispose of it. But, a significant portion of the bile sent out by the liver into the intestines is eventually lost forever when the process of elimination is faster than the reabsorption of the bile by the intestine. This is the main method by which the body *can* dispose of cholesterol.

Additional evidence of the cholesterol-reducing effect of unsaturated fat through bile production was found by Dr. Barry Lewis of the University of Cape Town. Three of his patients were ill with a fistula in the bile sac, which enabled him to directly measure bile production. On an unsaturated sunflower-seed-oil diet there was a remarkable increase in the bile. But with the saturated coconut oil there was no bile increase.

In the large intestine, the useful lactic bacteria secrete enzymes which break down the bile. In 1957, Dr. M. N. Camien at the University of California found that saturated fats interfere with the growth of the beneficial lactic bacteria. But this can be corrected by unsaturated fats, stimulating the bacteria to speed up bile breakdown. Saturated fat not only interferes with the body's "normalizing system," via the excretion of cholesterol in the bile acids, but also causes the loss of beneficial intestinal bacteria.

In 1960 Dr. Grace A. Goldsmith studied bile levels after substituting unsaturated fats for saturated fats in the diet. Her research data included the combined effects measured by both Drs. Camien and Lewis. There was a 20% to 25% increase in the elimination of bile. And, naturally, eliminated from the body with the bile was the cholesterol that went into its manufacture.

Through these two important functions, the manufacture of esters and the elimination of bile, the type of fat in the diet determines the level of blood cholesterol. There are additional relationships between fats and cholesterol. But the sum total of all relationships is:

An unsaturated-fat diet results in low blood cholesterol; A saturated-fat diet results in high blood cholesterol.

Up to now we have learned that excess cholesterol in the blood is a major cause of artery blockage. In addition there is another basic cause of trouble, the fats which are the inseparable partners of cholesterol in the blood. The story of the "fatty globules" in which both cholesterol and fat "float" through the blood stream is the subject of the next chapter.

CHAPTER SIX

The Vital Fat Chemistry of Your Blood

THE LITTLE KNOWN "FAT-BLOOD-CELLS"

The red blood cells and the white blood cells, the oxygen carriers and the germ fighters, are known to almost everybody. But how many persons know about the *fat blood cells?*

There are three families of these fat "cells" in the blood. Actually these are not true cells but they are *"fatty globules,"* and their size—relative to the red blood cell—is shown below.

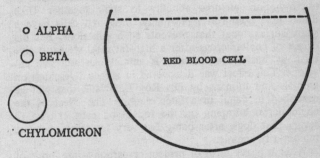

o ALPHA

○ BETA

CHYLOMICRON

RED BLOOD CELL

The red cell measures 3,000 to the inch, or, using microscopic measurement, 7 microns. The chylomicron is about one-seventh this size, which accounts for the "micron" part of the name. The "chylo" part comes from the fact that the digestive juice, chyle, is responsible for breaking down the fat.

For the names of the other two smaller globules the scientists use the simple Greek letters "Alpha" and "Beta."

The chylomicron, which in spite of its "giant" size is only a fat food particle and not a living cell, is one of the most unusual inhabitants of the blood. The amount of chylomicrons varies widely from hour to hour, meal to meal, unlike that of any of the other inhabitants of the blood, the number of which remains relatively constant.

The first key point relevant to the prevention of the present coronary epidemic is the fact that under normal conditions almost all of the chylomicrons from the evening meal are cleared out of the blood circulation before breakfast.

In the atherosclerotic, precoronary individual there is a gradual loss of this normal ability to eliminate the chylomicrons from the blood before the next fatty meal, and he therefore suffers from a chronic overload.

There are many ways in which an excess of chylomicrons causes trouble. The red blood cells already occupy about half the available space in the blood stream. The flexible, dish-shaped red cells with their remarkably smooth surfaces, slither closely past each other within the artery walls. Now into this traffic jam, after each fatty meal, rushes a horde of chylomicrons, as many as five for each red cell, and a type of "bumping" takes place.

After a high-fat meal, the red blood cells are seen in micro-motion pictures actually to stick together (like dimes in a coin roll). Normally, these red cells have a shiny surface coat that prevents such adhesions. But the excess of chylomicrons after a high-fat meal seems to give them a "buffy coat," which is actually an adhesive envelope. This effect was discovered in a recent research on animals and humans by Dr. Roy L. Swank that will be described in detail in a later chapter. The effect of the chylomicron bumping on the red blood cells can be so severe that dogs, after being fed very fat meals, become temporarily anemic.

After a heavy meal of protein or carbohydrate, none of these effects on the red blood cells has ever been seen. It is evident that there is sufficient reason for nature to have evolved a method of preventing any build-up of the fatty chylomicron globules in the blood. This method is twofold.

First, the special slowness of the fat digestive process. The fat "sticks to the ribs." This long period of digestion prevents the dumping of a full fat load into the blood at one time.

Second, as the chylomicrons enter the blood stream, a

special mechanism is brought into play to clear them out quickly.

When this mechanism is unimpaired, as among young women and non-Western people, the blood is cleared of chylomicrons in about five hours. This protective mechanism is known as the "clearing factor."

Until about fifteen years ago, most scientists had considered blood sugars to be the body's primary source of energy, but research in recent years has changed this concept. Weight for weight, fats have twice the energy of proteins and carbohydrates. The energy of the heart muscle is mostly dependent upon the fuel supplied by fats.

The recent discovery of the importance of fats for muscle energy should not lead to any concern regarding insufficient fat in the diet. A diet with 15% of fat calories is more than adequate to maintain optimum health. Moreover, the body manufactures fats out of the carbohydrates in the diet, and this process goes on, to some extent, regardless of whether the diet is high or low in fat.

The liquid part of the blood stream is almost all water, very little solids. The other nutrients, proteins and carbohydrates, are easily dissolved in water. But fats *cannot* dissolve in water. Then how can the blood carry such insoluble materials?

Not till 1950, when Dr. John W. Gofman published the results of his research in *Nature,* did science have the answer. Only then did detailed knowledge of the fatty particles in the blood, their composition and behavior, become a part of medical science.

One reason for this delay lies in the characteristic of fats mentioned previously—insolubility in water. Because of that, chemists had found these substances difficult to work with, and had devoted their energies to the more easily studied soluble compounds. As a result, fat chemistry, vitally important in heart attack, was ignored.

Only within the last decade have new techniques been devised for the study of the composition of the fats and other lipids and their behavior in the blood. From this recent work we can now piece together the story of the fatty globules.

This illustration shows the ingenious arrangement evolved in nature to handle the insoluble lipids.

Take the case of cholesterol, which is totally insoluble in blood liquid. The only substance in the body which is capable of dissolving cholesterol is fat. But the fat-cholesterol combination is still insoluble in blood. Obviously a special vehicle is needed to carry both these substances in the blood. This vehicle is the "fatty globule."

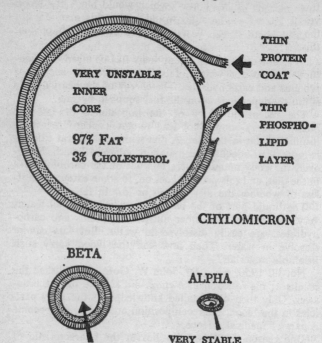

VERY UNSTABLE
INNER
CORE

97% FAT
3% CHOLESTEROL

THIN
PROTEIN
COAT

THIN
PHOSPHO-
LIPID
LAYER

CHYLOMICRON

BETA

ALPHA

INNER CORE OF
HALF FAT HALF
CHOLESTEROL

VERY STABLE
CORE OF FAT AND
CHOLESTEROL

THE THREE TYPES OF FATTY GLOBULES IN THE BLOOD

The fatty globule is actually a "spherical particle" which, like the red cell, simply floats in the blood.

You'll notice that the core material of the fatty globules is a mixture of fats and cholesterol. Covering the core is a layer of phospholipids. ("Lipid" is the general chemical name for fat-like substances; and "phospho" indicates that it contains phosphorous.) Serving as a coating for the entire globule is an extremely thin layer of protein.

The basic problem in nature is to prevent these microscopic "fatty globules" from sticking to each other and forming large fatty "lumps" which would block the blood vessel. Pure fatty globules would act in this manner. But the protective layers of phospholipid and protein prevent this "sticking."

The very existence of the globules of fats and cholesterol in the blood is the result of this four-way partnership. If the fats and cholesterol are to be carried by the blood to their destinations in the tissues, these four substances must always remain linked together. It is when the combination is unstable and the cholesterol and fats are deposited in the artery wall that the blockage starts.

The thicker the protective coat of phospholipid, the more stable the globule. The largest of the group, the chylomicron, has the thinnest protective coat, and is the least stable. The smallest of the fatty globules, the alpha, has the heaviest protective coat, and is the most stable of the whole group.

The following pages will show how the quantity of chylomicrons can become excessive, this being the first step down the path to "modern fatty blood."

THE "BLOOD POLICEMAN"
THAT CAN SAVE YOUR LIFE

Gardeners who make plants flourish by cooperating with nature are said to have a green thumb. There is no similar expression for the doctor who can make his patients flourish by cooperating with nature. But such doctors do exist, and among them is Dr. Hyman Engelberg of the Cedars of Lebanon Hospital in Los Angeles.

Dr. Engelberg had treated sixty-six victims of heart attack for an average of five years with amazing results, which he reported to the Annual Convention of the American Heart Association in 1960. According to normal statistical predictions, he should have lost at least six patients each year. But his annual loss had been *only two*. Of the fifty-six patients who were still alive, not one had again suffered a heart attack.

As a gardener restores worn-out soil to its original vitality by replacing an ingredient exhausted by misuse, so

Engelberg had added heparin, a "natural drug" occurring normally in the body itself. It was a true case of cooperation with nature; the restoration of the natural ingredient—artificially. Twice every week, large quantities of heparin flowed from Dr. Engelberg's hypodermic into the heparin-exhausted bodies of his patients. Twenty lives were actually saved, thanks to heparin, the "policeman of the blood!"

Later reports by Dr. Engelberg and others shows that even more impressive results can be had by this therapy.

Dr. Engelberg's treatment made use of the *combination* of both of heparin's "police functions." (1) to inhibit blood clots and (2) to regulate the fatty particles in the blood.

The natural heparin in the body helps break down and clear out chylomicron fatty globules in the blood. To understand this important natural process we will retrace the steps of a classic test made in England by Dr. D. W. Barrit.

Note: Details of this test may not be of interest to all. It can be omitted by skipping to page 115.

Dr. Barrit measured the large chylomicrons in the blood, not by counting them but by observing the amount of "cloudiness" they caused.

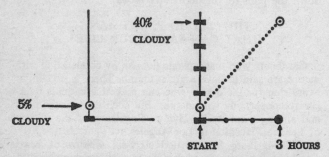

The blood serum is the liquid part of the blood, which remains after the blood cells have been removed. As the giant chylomicron fatty globules enter the blood, the serum becomes cloudy. The greater the accumulation of these large fatty globules, the more cloudy the serum becomes. Since the cloudiness obstructs light, Dr. Barrit simply measured the amount of light obstructed.

This is how the test was conducted. The persons being

tested were fed high-fat diets, and samples of their blood were taken three and seven hours after each meal.

What were the findings?

In the group with the lowest coronary rate, women before their menopause, just prior to the high-fat meal the blood serum was almost perfectly clear, the light-obstruction low. On the average it was about 5% of maximum cloudiness. On a graph it is represented like this:

After the meal, the chylomicron content began its rise. Within three hours, it reached its peak. At that time, the light-obstruction was about 40% of maximum.

During this time the natural response of the arterial walls is to secrete into the blood a special enzyme, a "clearing factor" which helps to break down and remove the chylomicrons. Heparin acts to "trigger" this process.

From this point on the "heparin-clearing factor" seemed to have the situation well in hand. The fatty cloudiness began to clear up, and at the end of seven hours, the light obstruction was down to about 10% of maximum.

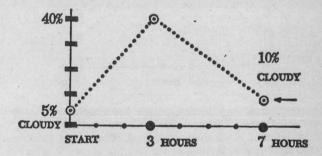

"Normal" men start with a higher light obstruction than women (10% as compared to 5%). The obstruction also reaches a higher peak (50% as compared to 40%) . . . and declines to a higher seventh-hour figure (15% as compared to 10%).

These are the approximate results reported by Dr. Barrit in the *British Medical Journal* September 15, 1956.

From Barrit's work one may assume that, since the male's blood is cloudier after a fatty meal and for a longer period than the female's, *the extended presence of fatty globules may contribute to his higher rate of cor-onary.*

If this were true, it would be of vital importance in the fight against coronary. Dr. Barrit decided to find the answer. He repeated his tests on a group of atherosclerotic men of the same age as the normals. Their blood serum was the most cloudy at the start, rose to the highest level of the three groups and declined slowly to a light-obstruc-tion value still higher than that of the "normal" male. In these atherosclerotics it took a good deal more than seven hours for the fatty particles to return to their pre-meal level.

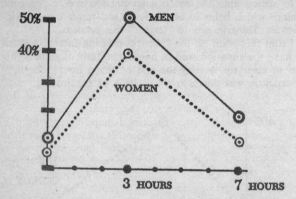

Here, then, is a picture of the heparin-clearing-factor system at work: it is most efficient in truly normal women, least efficient in atherosclerotic men. These facts indicate that there is a weakening of the clearing system in athero-sclerotics. Can this be proven by an experimental test?

Drs. Oliver and Boyd carried out an experiment to test this idea in 1953. They injected a small quantity of heparin into the blood of normal males, as well as into athero-sclerotics, three hours after a fatty meal.

In the normals, two thirds of the chylomicrons were cleared within a quarter of an hour after the injection. But in atherosclerotics, in that same quarter of an hour only one third of the chylomicrons were cleared, *just half of what was cleared in the normals.*

Since the same amount of heparin was injected in both cases we are left with the question as to what caused the

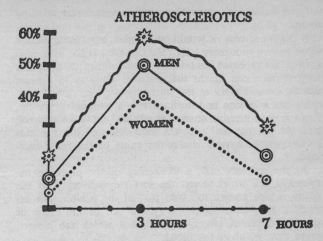

ATHEROSCLEROTICS

diminishing clearing effect in the atherosclerotic blood. Logically there must have been an "exhaustion" of the other half of the clearing team, the "clearing factor."

But what kind of fatty globules demand the most work from this team? By now considerable research has been done on this problem, and reports cited later in this book will show: The heparin-clearing factor combination exerted its effects on the *unsaturated* fatty globules far more quickly and efficiently than on the saturated fatty globules.

The data clearly shows that the combination of the heparin-clearing-factor plus *unsaturated* fats means less fatty globules in the blood. But something that is perhaps even more important; *unsaturated fats seemed to cut down the work load thereby reducing the possibility of "exhausting" the heparin-clearing-factor team.*

The "exhaustion" of the heparin-clearing-factor team has its parallels in other illnesses. Writes Dr. Engelberg:

"An analogy apparently may exist between insulin deficiency, elevated blood sugar levels and diabetes . . . on the one hand—and heparin and fat clearing deficiency . . . and atherosclerosis on the other . . ."

"However, it would appear that, whereas only a small part of the population cannot handle the average starch and sugar content of their diet, a much larger percentage is unable to metabolize properly the fat content of the average American diet."

Since Dr. Barrit's classic demonstration of the overloading of fatty globules in the blood of coronary-prone individuals that occurs after a fatty meal there have been innumerable other tests which have confirmed this fact. It has also been proven many times that this lack of ability to handle a fatty meal is one of the first steps on the way to a heart attack.

In any situation in which there is a temporary pile-up, there may be trouble at the delivery end or at the removal end. At the removal end, the exhaustion of the heparin-clearing-factor system is a major cause of the fatty overload.

At the delivery end, a weakening of the digestive enzymes which break down the fats for delivery into the blood is also known to cause part of the trouble. An exhausted fat-digestive enzyme system can be the cause of the formation of larger chylomicrons which are cleared more slowly out of the blood.

In an individual case it is not known to what extent either end of the "fat processing system" is responsible for the excess chylomicrons in the blood. But today it is a known fact that a lifetime of high calorie, high-saturated-fat meals is the basic cause for the increasing "exhaustion" of the natural enzymes required at both ends of the fat-processing system.

TESTS FOR DANGER
FROM THE CHOLESTEROL-FAT PARTNERSHIP

The three classes of fatty globules in the blood—the chylomicron, the beta and the alpha—are divided into countless sub-classes of large and smaller chylomicrons, larger and smaller beta globules, and larger and smaller alpha globules. There are, in fact, hundreds of sizes ranging from the largest chylomicron down to the smallest alpha globule. Each different-sized globule varies in regard to its relative content of cholesterol and fats. The larger globules contain proportionally more fat and the smaller globules more cholesterol. The chylomicrons can have a maximum of about 3% cholesterol, and their composition is almost identical to that of the food fats from which they were formed.

The largest beta globules contain about two parts of fat to each part of cholesterol, and as the beta globules get smaller, the relative cholesterol content increases. The smallest beta globules have about one part of fat to three parts of cholesterol.

Thus there are two major ways of describing the blood lipids (1) according to quantity of each specific size of globule, and (2) by total quantity of fats and cholesterol in all of the globules combined.

During what now seems the ancient history of atherosclerosis research, in the early 1950's, the group of scientists led by Dr. John Gofman of the Donner Laboratory at Berkeley insisted that it was best to know how many of each size of the fatty globules are present in the blood in order to recognize the coronary-prone individual and asserted that the cholesterol test told only part of the story.

But since the complete spectrum test was time consuming and expensive and required special apparatus, most heart specialists considered that the quick and inexpensive blood cholesterol test was most practical for general use.

Each group insisted that the overall weight of evidence was in its favor and that its method was best. A decision on this important question seemed urgent. A scientific medical group was appointed to evaluate both methods and to report back to the medical world.

In 1956 the report was published in *Circulation*. Which method was judged the best? Actually, the mechanical spectrum method seemed more accurate in its ability to indicate pre-coronary cases. But in order to achieve this accuracy, the Gofman group had introduced added refinements to their already complicated method.

The groups who were partial to the cholesterol-count method insisted that making improvements in the spectrum method during the evaluation trial was not a proper scientific procedure. The final result was a scientific stalemate.

A new practical solution to the detection problem came from research by Dr. Margaret J. Albrink during the past three years on the total amounts of cholesterol and triglycerides (fats) present in the blood. Dr. Albrink has shown enough data to make it clear that the total amount of fat in the blood is an even more accurate indication of the coronary-prone man than the blood-cholesterol test.

By measuring separately both the blood fats and the cholesterol it is now possible to obtain an approximation of the spectrum of fatty globules in the blood that can act as a low cost substitute for the more accurate but laborious Goffman method.

To understand the advantages of the cholesterol-plus-blood-fat test one should consider the three types of fatty globule disorders which afflict many American men. The first disorder is an excess of smaller beta globules. Since small beta globules contain twice as much cholesterol as fat, this condition may be diagnosed by the cholesterol test.

The second is the case of excess of larger beta globules, with a normal amount of small beta globules. The cholesterol test in this situation may show up as normal, since the large beta globules contain twice as much fat as cholesterol. This trouble, however, will be indicated by a high triglyceride (blood fat) test.

The third condition which is the most common problem in precoronary cases is an excess of both small and large beta globules. This is shown by a combined, test result of high cholesterol and high triglycerides.

These three examples show how the results of the cholesterol and blood-fat tests can roughly approximate the results of the Gofman spectrum test.

People known to be relatively free of coronary disease, such as young women and many non-Western men, have low amounts of both cholesterol and blood fats, and so all of their beta globules are low in number.

We now need to understand what causes the excessive build-up of the large or the small beta globules in the blood.

The excess of small beta globules is caused by too much saturated fats and cholesterol in the diet, contained in foods such as egg yolk, butter, etc. On the other hand, the excess of large beta globules is the result for the most part of a diet excessively rich in calories, especially refined carbohydrate calories.

Americans, whose diet is rich in saturated fats, cholesterol and refined carbohydrate calories, frequently have an excess amount of both bood fats and cholesterol.

Although the cholesterol-blood-fat tests give us much valuable information, they still don't tell the complete story.

Some of the blood fat may also be present in the form of excess chylomicrons which had not yet been cleared out of the blood from a previous meal.

The way in which our body handles these chylomicrons is also different in the normal and the atherosclerotic person. Dr. Barrit's work mentioned in the previous chapter showed that women, who are the least subject to coronary disease, are able to clear their fatty chylomicron globules out of the blood quicker and more efficiently than the more coronary-prone men. And, as mentioned before, atherosclerotics seem to have an "exhausted" system that permits too many chylomicrons to linger in the blood from meal to meal.

If Dr. Barrit's test, now called the Fat Tolerance Test, were applied to the non-coronary Bantu and Yemenite people, it should show that they can handle their chylomicrons better than Western people.

In 1960 a test was made by Dr. J. Metz at the South African Institute for Medical Research on three similar-aged groups, using Bantus, normal Europeans and coronary patients. The test was made following a usual hospital breakfast. The latest radioactive tracer techniques, which were used to follow the chylomicrons in the blood, showed that the Bantu had the lowest inrush of chylomicrons, the coronary patients the highest.

Similar tests were made in Israel by Dr. M. J. Schwartz at the Beilinson Hospital, comparing newly arrived Yemenite Jews to normals and coronary patients who had lived on a Western diet. The Yemenites—like the Bantus—also had superior ability to handle the chylomicrons, as was shown by the rapid clearing action.

From these important surveys, as well as dozens of others, comes indisputable evidence that individuals who can no longer handle a fatty meal without a large build-up of chylomicron fatty globules in the blood are well on the way to coronary disease. In other words they have a poor "fat tolerance."

Now we can understand what has happened to the fatty globules in the coronary-prone individual. He usually has an excess of every type of fatty globule—with only one exception. The coronary-prone has a relative deficiency of the alpha globules.

Later it will be shown that the chylomicron fatty globules and the beta fatty globules can—when they are in excess—become unstable and dangerous.

The alpha globule with its heavy protective coat *never* becomes unstable, and this is probably the reason why it does not cause any danger, no matter how great its quantity in the blood.

The spectrum of the large and small beta globules is not a fixed condition, and in general it will vary with changes in eating habits from season to season, being lowest in summer and highest in winter. It will also vary somewhat from week to week, and in some individuals, from day to day. Those with the greatest number of fatty globules will usually have a higher range of variations, and are usually the most coronary prone.

But no matter which tests are used, no matter which of the blood lipids are in excess, the best recommendation to bring them all back to the desired normal condition will still be a better understanding of and the proper adherence to the principles of the Prudent Diet.

CHAPTER SEVEN

How Today's Fat Became Harmful to Your Health

The past half century has witnessed the frightening rise in coronary disease. During the same period significant dietary changes took place which may in part explain this rise.

Dr. Paul Dudley White in his Convocation Address to the Twelfth Annual Meeting of the American College of Cardiology said: "The average American diet has been considerably enriched in animal fat in the last generation; this I have observed in my own lifetime, and it is during that period of 40 years or more that we have noted increasing numbers of increasingly younger patients with serious atherosclerosis."

Considerable evidence supports this statement. Let's go back as far as scientific evidence permits, say to about 1750, to Colonial America. One may assume that American dietary habits of this period generally resembled those prevailing in England. According to J. C. Drummond and A. Wilbraham (The Englishman's Food), the daily diet in England contained only about two ounces of fat, most of which came from unsaturated fish and seed oils.

By 1872 according to the statistics of Dr. C. Van Slyke, in *The Journal of the American Dietary Association*, the *fat* portion of a recommended diet for the American laborer and his family of four was a yearly 100-pound total of animal fat, including butter, milk, and lard as well as other meat fats.

This means a consumption of about 1¼ ounces of saturated animal fat per person per day. Add vegetable fats amounting at most to about one ounce, and the daily fat consumption was still barely over two ounces.

But from the post-Civil War period on, fat consumption was on the upswing. By 1909, according to the U.S. Department of Agriculture, the daily fat intake of the average American was up to four ounces, and by 1948 it had gone up to five ounces.

Our fat consumption has increased not only in total quantity but also in proportion to our total food intake. And that is not all. The diet of the average American of a century ago was not only comparatively low in fat, but what is more important the fat consumed was less saturated than today's fat, both in quantity and in quality.

In recent decades, we have gradually adopted a diet not only higher in total fats, but also higher in the fats most dangerous to the coronary arteries, the *saturated* fats. We always ate eggs, butter, meat, milk and other dairy products. But now we consume *more* of them.

In addition, the type of fats in these foods has been changing; not naturally, but artificially.

A NEW TYPE OF ANIMAL FAT

During these years our feed experts produced a new breed of animal, a supersaturated-fat animal, and a supersaturated-fat egg. Unwittingly, our food industry had transformed the old type of animal fats into a new type which turned out to be remarkably efficient in increasing the cholesterol in our blood. And, worst of all, our industrial chemists had actually changed the liquid, unsaturated vegetable oils into a new and most objectionable hard type, *artificially saturated vegetable fat.*

Remember the Western films in which you've seen great herds of cattle roaming over the limitless range? They healthfully ate grass and slowly grew into marketable animals. But greater profits could be made if the animals exercised less and were fed more efficiently on corn and other grain spiked with chemical stimulants. The result is swifter growth, heavier weight and a larger proportion of fat. Now a new kind of meat made its entrance into the American market, and the marbled steak was introduced to the American housewife.

Would the presence of too much *visible* fat in the beef cause the public to reject it? The answer lay in the power of publicity and advertising; this wasn't called "primed" beef but *prime beef*. It was not advertised as beef bred and fed for fast delivery and profits, but as the best beef. The U.S. Government obligingly labeled beef with the highest fat content *First Quality—Grade A*.

The harm didn't stop with the increase in fat. Unfortunately, the "priming" of cattle also changed the soft, yellow, partially unsaturated fat into a hard, white, *much* more saturated fat.

What about hogs? There was a time when scientists used lard as a source of *unsaturated* fats in laboratory experiments. In those days, hogs were fed "free range." They rooted for a good deal of their food. The old feeding methods produced lard which was soft and quite unsaturated.

But hog feeding, too, had to yield to the march of "production." By the middle thirties most hogs destined for America's larder were "scientifically" fed. This resulted in extremely heavy hogs whose fat was no longer soft and partially unsaturated, but hard and *much more saturated*.

We had transformed our major meat animals into producers of unusually dangerous saturated fats, fats of a type never before encountered in the course of evolution.

Now let us look at eggs and the problem they present, for what happened to cattle and hogs also happened to hens. Gone by the mid-1930's were the days of "free range" feeding of hens on worms, insects, seeds and grass that made up their natural diet. Substituted was "priming" for profit—at the expense of our national health.

Today's hens are compactly housed in cubicles in multistory structures. They have no freedom, no chance to exercise. They are fed on a "scientific" mixture designed to produce only one result—regardless of quality—the maximum number of eggs per day. The modern name for this is the "battery" system. The hen has become an egg-producing *machine*. And she *does* set production records. But at what a cost!

Without grass and worms, without exercise, without natural diet and activity she's lost the ability to produce a *normal* egg. The "machine" product is a *super-saturated-fat* egg, loaded with the type of fats *to be avoided at all costs* in an anti-coronary diet.

That a dangerous alteration has occurred in the composition of eggs is scientifically corroborated by Dr. J. Reiser. Writing in the *Journal of Nutrition* in 1951, he states: "The proportion of linoleic [a two-hinge unsaturated fat] in hens' eggs . . . a generation ago against today . . . has decreased sharply."

Today's mass-produced egg is a dual threat. To the super-saturated fats add cholesterol. The fact that this *new* type of egg yolk is more harmful can be proven by its effects on the chick for which nature intended it. As the chick develops and grows inside the shell, it feeds on the yolk. The cholesterol is used as insulating material for the chick's brain and spinal cord. From the report on "battery" egg chicks by Dr. C. W. Nichols at the University of California we learn, "these high lipid levels . . . in the newly-hatched chick are accompanied by a widespread deposition of lipids in the whole cardiovascular system . . ."

Based on experiments with chicks hatched from eggs laid by both free-range and "battery"-fed hens, Oxford University's Dr. Hugh Sinclair has reported that "mass produced" chicks hatched from eggs laid by hens living in "batteries" had more artery deposits than natural chicks hatched from eggs laid by free-range hens.

As regards milk the story is different. Cow's milk has always been and still is highly saturated. It is almost four times more saturated than human milk. Dr. H. H. Williams reports that the ratio of polyunsaturated (many-hinged) fats, compared to saturated fats, in cow's milk is less than one third as compared to human milk. We've long believed that cow's milk was practically "designed" by nature for direct human consumption. Today scientists, aware that cows milk is loaded with very highly saturated fat, are beginning to doubt the value of whole milk for adults.

How does the cow change the unsaturated fat in the grass it feeds on into the highly saturated milk fats?

The cow has several stomachs. Bacteria in these stomachs help carry out the digestive process. One particular species can even digest straw. These unusual bacteria can change the unsaturated vegetable fats in the grass into a very saturated type of animal fat. It is this very saturated type of fat which is transformed into the highly saturated fat in the milk.

FOOD SHELF LIFE VS. HUMAN LIFE

So, during the past forty years we have been changing the fats in our domestic food animals. Changing the *quantity* and also changing the *quality*. From a saturated, hard, animal type of fat that is already dangerous . . . to an extra-hard, extra-saturated fat, that is extremely dangerous.

The unfortunate changes in our animal fats is one of the reasons for this country having the highest blood-cholesterol level in the world.

But our food chemists' discovery of a "synthetic fat" in the laboratory made our already bad situation even worse.

Let us go back to 1912, to Stockholm, where the French chemist Paul Sabatier is receiving the Nobel Prize for discovering a way to make low-cost soap. His process involved the hydrogenation of inedible fish and vegetable oils, which changed these "waste products" into a hard white "soap fat" that could serve as a substitute for the more expensive lard. Later American food chemists used the same process for making a type of "food fat" which is another major cause of our present day coronary crisis.

The Lancet editorialized in 1956: "The hydrogenation plants of our modern food industry may turn out to have contributed to the causation of a major [coronary] disease."

By hydrogenation the food chemists could take a multi-hinged oil, force hydrogen under extereme heat and pressure into the "hinge joints" and harden the oil into a synthetic hard solid fat. By doing away with the "hinges," they now had a new unperishable food fat. Here was one answer to "short shelf life," the major profit problem of America's fast-growing, mass-production food industry. Food made with natural oils may turn rancid if left on the grocer's shelf too long. But foods made with oil sufficiently hydrogenated by Sabatier's process can keep "fresh" almost indefinitely.

One extra benefit for the food chemists was that the new process permitted them to manufacture fats of any consistency they desired. This "miracle" of modern science is good for the manufacturer, good for the distributor, good for the grocer—but a grave health risk for the consumer. It is dangerous not only because it changes unsaturated fat into saturated fat, but because in the hydrogenation process it is particularly the most beneficial *polyunsaturated* many-hinged fats that are destroyed most rapidly and in the greatest quantity.

When vegetable oil is hydrogenated, the most powerful natural safeguard against atherosclerosis is changed from nature's benign Dr. Jekyll into the food chemist's malign Mr. Hyde.

What has this artificial shelf-life lengthening process done to the food of the American people? According to the statistics of Dr. J. B. Brown, Director of the Nutrition Institute of Ohio State University, essential vegetable oils equivalent in food value to almost one-sixth of all our food calories are thrown into the hot vats of the chemists, there to be artificially transformed into an unnatural product containing the one property which food merchandisers prize above all else—stability.

For each person in this country the farmers can produce daily only about two-thirds of an ounce of the natural, *pure*, two-hinged oil. But after the chemicals in the hydrogenation tanks have completed their work, they have destroyed fully half the country's supply.

This bears repetition—*half* of all the vital, cholesterol-lowering oil produced in the United States is being stripped of its most essential value, for purely commercial reasons, to lengthen shelf life and thereby make food distribution more profitable.

It would be difficult to find in a modern supermarket a "manufactured" food product which contains fats that have *not* been hydrogenated.

Very few people have ever seen pure hydrogenated fat. It is white, and so unnaturally hard that it is brittle. It it almost identical to a "plastic." It is unchewable, unpalatable and—in its pure state—quite inedible.

This description also fits the natural saturated fats . . . when they are purified and separated from the unsaturated fats. Only in combination with the soft unsaturated fats are the natural saturated fats palatable, edible and digestible.

There is already so much dangerous hard, brittle saturated fat from the dairy and meat fats present in our diet that these new "plastic" hydrogenated fats are more than the human system can handle.

WHY THE MEAT GRADING STANDARDS WERE REVERSED

The quantity of animal fat we eat is our individual responsibility, but the quality of this fat is the responsibility of our Federal government and of the food industry.

How has each group met its responsibility? In the past the meat industry took the path that looked most profitable and championed the high-fat animal.

However, their scientists have studied the coronary disease problem in this country. They have read the handwriting on the wall. Their salesmen were bringing in reports from the butchers that a growing number of consumers had become aware of the danger in fat meat, and were demanding only the lean cuts.

Realizing that the high-fat animal they had created was becoming unprofitable, the meat producers belatedly went along with the tide of science. In 1963 the National Live Stock and Meat Board had an exhibit at the yearly convention of the American Medical Association. The lighted marquee over their exhibit reminded the twenty-four thousand doctors and others in attendance that "There Are More Low Fat Meat Cuts Than You Think." The meat industry, in many medical-journal advertisements, is claiming the development of new kinds of animals, modern *lean* cattle and modern *lean* hogs. They now make the unwarranted boast that "this development is our contribution to the fight against coronary heart attack." *The "old-fashioned" animal*—and in the illustrations in their medical ads they caricature its gross fatness—*the "old-fashioned" animal must go*, they insist. But, of course, their *modern* lean animal is the *real* old-fashioned animal.

Consider how fat cattle are "made." From the great ranches of the west roll freight cars full of lean young cattle to the feeding pens. Here they are efficiently stuffed with local corn and grain until their muscles have become degenerated by fatty infiltrations. This is called the marbling process. The theory is that the "veins" of fat tenderize the meat. When enough fat and meat have been added to bring them up to a profitable weight, they are shipped to the slaughter houses.

A few years ago the cattle cars coming to the slaughter houses of the big cities brought many fat and few lean cattle. Today, according to the meat industry advertisements, the reverse *should* be true. Not that this is a difficult problem. It is a well-known fact for instance that southern cattle, fed on orange rinds and other local surplus products, are much leaner than the northern corn-fed cattle.

With this "new" type of lean animal returning to the market, what now happens to the government standards which said "Grade A meat has a firm, white, well-marbled fat, etc."? Well, the old standards are being repudiated. According to the new, July 1962 standards set by the U.S. Department of Agriculture, the lowest-quality meat is now the fattest, and "Grade A" meat is the leanest. With this new grading, the meat industry will get higher prices for the leaner meats, and so will be motivated to produce even more lean animals.

The new 1962 meat grading standards were to be reviewed a year later before a final code was formulated. At present the new code has been finalized only for the Army. Here the code will be on a strict yield basis, i.e., the percentage of red meat which can be obtained from the carcass.

There is no doubt that this latest grading has been urged by the Army officials who want more red meat. The recommendation of the Army medical advisors—told in Chapter 3— are finally showing results.

And what about the egg industry? Has it, too, seen the handwriting on the wall? Regretfully, *no*. Unlike the meat industry, which is controlled by a few multi-million dollar concerns, the egg industry is in the hands of many thousands of small producers. The producer who attempts to take his chickens out of the mass-production batteries and restore them to the old, and more costly, free-range system is immediately priced out of competition.

But regardless of type, awareness of the coronary problem has grown, and *eggs* have become suspect. As a result the public isn't eating quite as many eggs as it did formerly.

The condition in the milk industry is the same. The American public is learning gradually about the coronary dangers in dairy fats, and consumption is falling off. The purchase of skim-milk dairy products has not declined but the sales volume of butter and other dairy products is declining annually.

The state of California, with the country's highest blood-cholesterol level and highest coronary rate, has been the first to try to remedy the danger caused by high saturated-fat milk. The state law was changed to permit the butter-fat content of milk to be reduced from 4% to 2%. The Eastern milk producers are now clamoring for a similar revision of the law which still requires the high 4% butter-fat content.

The change in food-buying habits of the past two years shows that a constantly growing informed section of the American public has already become aware of the coronary danger in the high-fat diet.

CHAPTER EIGHT

Your Defenses Against a Coronary Thrombosis

HOW YOUR BODY'S EMERGENCY REPAIR SYSTEM OPERATES

You are at the zenith of your career. You are a dynamic, driving, aggressive individual accomplishing the things you want to accomplish, getting them done the way you have planned. You have a wife, children, and the mortgage on your dream house has just been paid off. The future couldn't look brighter. Then—without warning—you're dead.

You've been killed by a bit of matter smaller than the head of a match. You've been destroyed by a blood clot in your coronary artery.

Who is to blame?

Has nature constructed our bodies with built-in booby traps? Or has nature tried to do everything possible to prevent this kind of death, only to be thwarted by us?

Let's go back a few years to the morning when Dr. M. Friedman and his team of medical researchers began a new investigation whose object was: *To study the choles-terol-level changes in business executives under stress.* No sooner had their project gotten under way when one of the men they were studying suffered a coronary thrombosis and died within two hours.

The investigators got to work immediately, and tried to uncover any incriminating evidence. The main clue came from a most unlikely source, the dead man's dentist. Only the day before, he had made a simple incision on the patient, whose blood had clotted, the dentist revealed, *with great rapidity.*

The coronary victim's blood clotted swiftly *on the outside,* just as it did the next day on the inside. Something had happened to the blood of this man that *predisposed* it to clotting.

Nature has developed a system for preventing these internal blood clots. It's a system of extraordinary ingenuity, a physical and chemical marvel that has taken billions of years to evolve. But in the past hundred years, through stress and poor diet, we have been breaking down the safeguards normally present in blood. How can the "balanced" clotting ability of blood be restored?

Let's begin by examining the *normal* blood-clotting mechanism, which is actually an automatic repair device. When a blood vessel is ruptured, severed, or injured in a way that causes a leakage of blood, the clotting mechanism swings into action, attempting to seal off or plug the vessel and stop the loss of blood.

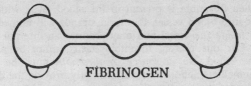

FIBRINOGEN

This is effected by an enormous protein molecule called fibrinogen, known to scientists for over a hundred years. But only recently have they fully understood what it does and what it looks like.

Let's look at the molecule in closeup through the eye of the electron microscope. In 1959, Dr. C. E. Hall saw for the first time the details of the basic building-block with which the blood repairs its vessels. This is what it looks like in an actual photo.

For a molecule, fibrinogen is tremendous. Seventy laid end to end are as long as a red blood cell. But even more astonishing is the unusual "dumbbell" shape and the built-in "hidden hooks" that can link the large knobs together.

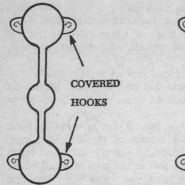
COVERED
HOOKS

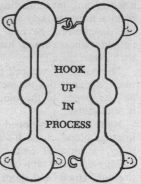
HOOK
UP
IN
PROCESS

When the hooks are linked, this interlocked chain is called *fibrin*. It is the skeletal network around which the blood clot forms.

How are the fibrinogen molecules activated to interlock?

Stepping into the picture now is another factor called *thrombin*. It's a giant molecule which forces the fibrinogen dumbbells to link up into the fibrin strand.

When thrombin is present in the blood, even without a break in a blood vessel, the fibrin strands will immediately form *inside* the vessel and may produce an internal blood clot. For this reason, thrombin itself cannot be present in the blood. But a *source of thrombin* must be ready for immediate action so it can promptly provide the thrombin needed to activate the fibrinogen when a break does occur. This dilemma is ingeniously resolved by nature.

We normally carry in our blood a substance that's "almost-thrombin"—scientists call it *pro-thrombin*. Like a sharp knife in its sheath it can't do any harm. It *cannot* activate the fibrinogen and cause a clot.

But after an injury, the wound releases a chemical that

combines with other chemicals already in the blood, to form a team which as a group can activate the "almost thrombin."

In the second stage, this chemical team removes the sheath from the "almost-thrombin," transforming it into the "sharp" and powerful chemical activator, thrombin.

In the third stage, the active thrombin immediately starts to cut off the protective covers from the fibrinogen dumbbells and the exposed "hooks" automatically link themselves into a neat thread of fibrin, as shown in the illustration.

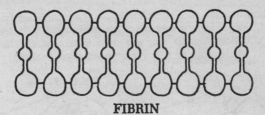

FIBRIN

When the wound occurs and the "almost-thrombin" is activated, what prevents the fibrin from clotting all the blood? Nature has provided a mechanism which localizes the clot. It's built around still another factor called the *blood platelet*, which is similar in shape and about one-third the size of a red blood cell. At the moment of injury the blood-vessel wall sends out a chemical messenger, that "attracts" some of the platelets to the wound. The medical blood clotting experts call the platlets which are attracted "sticky." These "sticky platelets" automatically fasten themselves to the edges of the broken blood vessel wall. Originally round and flat like coins, these platelets now have a scalloped form.

The localized fibrin continues to grow from the scalloped edges of the platelets until it bridges the gap.

Across the break in the blood vessel wall is a mesh of platelets and strong strands of fibrin. Blood can still leak through it, but as the blood flows, the web catches the red blood cells. It's the red blood cells trapped in the meshes of the fibrin that give the external blood clot its distinctive color.

With all the spaces between its strands now filled, the fibrin-repair network has done its temporary job. A patch has been formed over the wound that prevents blood leakage during the time it will take for the body to build new tissue in order to make the repair permanent.

This is only an outline of the very complicated system nature has evolved to prevent loss of blood from outside wounds. The mechanism of blood-clotting *inside* the body is similar, and it is a "normal" occurrence when during an internal hemorrhage the same fibrin is used to form a temporary patch.

PEOPLE WITH "THICK" BLOOD

When a person's blood-clotting ability is sufficiently reduced, the slightest injury can cause him to bleed to death. This affliction, hemophilia, was once a rare illness, heard of only in the case of a few European royal families.

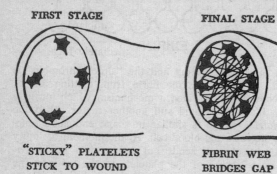

FIRST STAGE

FINAL STAGE

"STICKY" PLATELETS
STICK TO WOUND

FIBRIN WEB
BRIDGES GAP

Until recently it was popularly thought that this was an all-or-nothing disease: either the blood clotted or it didn't. But now, however, it is known that the disease exists in varying intensities, from slight loss of clottability to almost total loss. The amount of clotting factors found in hemophiliac blood is less than one-seventh the amount found in normal blood. As the quantity of clotting factors in the blood becomes reduced from its normal level, the bleeding tendency gradually increases.

Currently, there are over 10,000 cases of "real" hemophilia in the United States, according to recent reports and many more cases of bleeders of lesser severity.

How is this deficiency of the clotting mechanism repaired?

The first line of defense in arresting hemophilic bleeding, has been the use of natural clotting factors already present in the blood of a normal person—the blood transfusion. This usually raises the level of clotting factors in the hemophiliac to critical minimum.

The comparatively large number of cases demanding urgent medical attention has made it necessary for our doctors and researchers to study the defects in hemophiliac blood with painstaking effort through tests, analysis and clinical experiments. Out of this work has come knowledge of over a dozen major clotting factors present in normal blood, all necessary to prevent excessive bleeding.

But how much is known about the problem of *excess* clottability? Very little, because excess clottability is a *hidden* disease. The thickening of the blood is invisible. The victim *doesn't know* that it's happening to him and feels no ill effects. What's more, since there are no clinical symptoms, even the most skilled diagnostician can overlook this problem; that is, up to a certain point. *After* the heart attack, full attention is immediately focused on the *clinically evident* "thickening" of the blood.

It is understandable that a large amount of medical research has been devoted to hemophilia and other bleeding conditions because low blood clottability presents an obviously acute problem to both patient and physician.

It is ironic, however, that the opposite condition, high clottability—which afflicts tens of millions today—has begun to receive proper scientific attention only during the past few years.

What type of person has a high degree of clottability?

The answer comes from the well known Canadian researcher Dr. J. F. Mustard: " . . . subjects with clinical evidence of atherosclerosis have hypercoagulability of the blood . . ."

The presence of atheroma is associated with some thickening of the blood. However, it is among more advanced cases of atherosclerosis that the more serious blood-thickening is most frequently found.

The *clinical* atherosclerotic's blood is already relatively thicker, slower moving, more sludgy, fatty, and sticky. It is blood on its way to becoming thrombotic, with a tendency to form the final blood clot. But it may take special tests to measure these conditions.

Much of the important research which established the

connection between thick blood and clinical atherosclerosis was conducted in England by Dr. Lawson McDonald
at London Hospital. As a result of his pioneering work,
published in many British medical journals, the *American
Journal of Cardiology* invited Dr. McDonald to summarize his work for medical men in this country. He did
so in an article in the March, 1962 issue.

Dr. McDonald had concentrated his studies on three
groups of patients: (1) patients with angina (2) patients
after heart attacks and (3) a control group of "normal"
patients. He kept track of three of the important factors
contributing to the clottability of the blood.

One of these factors is the amount of fibrinogen circulating in the blood. It was higher in the angina group
than in the normal group, and highest in the heart-attack
group.

Another factor is the amount of "stickiness" of the
platelets. Remember, platelets become "sticky" before they
become attached to the wall of an "injured" blood vessel.
The platelets were most "sticky" in those who had a heart
attack. Stickiness in the angina group was greater than in
the normal group.

A third factor tested by McDonald was the amount of
thromboplastin in the blood. Thromboplastin is the scientific name given to the whole group of blood-clotting
factors that stimulate the weaving of fibrinogen into its
web of fibrin. The increase in the amount of thromboplastin follows the same pattern as the increase of the
other two factors.

It was with this type of research, meticulously conducted
and scientifically analyzed by the most modern statistical
methods, that Dr. McDonald " . . . clearly demonstrated
. . . for the first time . . . hypercoagulability of the blood
in [atherosclerotic] heart disease."

THE FATAL BLOOD CLOT

Now it is easier to understand why many doctors after
a heart attack will often use a drug known as an anticoagulant, a substance that has the ability to reduce excess
coagulability of the blood.

One of the drugs used is *heparin,* which is actually one
of the natural anticoagulants already present in the blood.
Heparin is a giant molecule that is capable of perform-

ing many "miracles" of control. One of these is the activation of the clearing-factor which removes chylomicrons after a fatty meal.

Heparin also has the ability to prevent abnormal thrombotic clotting of the blood. Since an excess of a variety of clotting factors must be present to form an unnatural blood clot, it is necessary that heparin have a special type of ability to react on many of them. This special power lies in the fact that heparin is an "electrical" molecule, and its large size permits it to have many negative electrical charges on its surface. It is with these electric charges that heparin is able to accomplish many of its functions in controlling both blood lipids and blood-coagulating factors.

Heparin is not only present in the blood, but also in various organs of the body, especially the lungs, where there is most danger from harmful blood clots.

It is the lungs (the transformers of "blue" unoxygenated blood into red blood) that constitutes the end of the line for the whole blue-blood vein system. This is the place where any blood clots which may have formed anywhere in the entire venous system must end up.

Actually, it was in the lungs, not the blood, that this anticlotting factor was first discovered, although not isolated, by the celebrated Russian, I. P. Pavlov, in 1887. And it was from the liver, again not the blood, that Dr. Mclean isolated heparin, in 1918. The lungs of cattle are the principal source of the heparin used by doctors today.

We have known about heparin for a long time and have had a chance to study its functions. It can be viewed, as was said, as the "policeman" of the blood. Consider the clotting factors as a dangerous mob; when they gang together, it's the policeman's job to "break it up." The doctor injects heparin because the patient put many of his heparin policemen out of action. By the time the heart attack occurs, the clotting mob had grown so strong that the doctor has to send in not one squad of policemen but a whole platoon. In other words, his dosage of heparin is greater than that found in normal blood, where it is present in very small quantities.

Now you can see why, when the doctor's hypo sends heparin rushing into the blood stream, an attempt is made to rescue the patient not on just one important front, but two. With the heparin, counterattacks are launched against the high-clottability—due to excess of thrombotic factors

—and against the dangerous excess of fatty particles as well.

Is the injection of heparin a case of locking the stable door after the horse has been stolen? The answer is yes and *no*. Yes, because we have been careless and permitted the horse to be stolen, permitted the heparin in our blood to be exhausted by our "civilized" diet. *No,* because there are plenty of horses left. By changing our diet (as part of a total anti-coronary program) we *can* restore the natural heparin production.

But if proper preventive measures are not taken, the blood can continue to grow more and more thrombotic and finally produce that clump of matter no bigger than a match head that can snuff out a life. How is that final clot formed?

The patient is atherosclerotic. The coronaries supplying his heart with vital food and oxygen have been dangerously narrowed. A small clot can now end his life.

The low supply of normal heparin in the blood has permitted many clotting factors to accumulate and to create a dangerous condition. In addition the artery blockage has not only reduced the blood supply to a mere trickle, but it has also slowed it down to a point where even a very small clot can get a foothold. This time the clot may be too solid for the exhausted fibrin-dissolving enzymes to dissolve it quickly.

The clot sticks—and grows large enough to block the narrowed coronary artery. This is a *coronary thrombosis*.

But there must be some final event that produces the thrombosis. How about stress?

Yes, stress is a factor. Stress *can* provide that final stimulus that precipitates the match-head-size deadly pellet. *But* this is the exception rather than the rule. Here is a percentage analysis compiled from several reports showing just what the patient was doing when the heart attack occurred.

ACTIVITY	PERCENTAGE
Sleep	*15*
At rest	*15*
Everyday activities	*45*
Mild exercise	*10*
Emotional stress	*10*
Heavy physical effort	*5*

Is there a *last* precipitating event that is the true cause of a thrombosis?

The facts show that, in most cases, the answer is *no*. It's not the last moment that counts, but the long succession of preceding moments, the lifetime of gradual artery blockage, of increasing blood clottability until the final event that stops the heart. *You don't prevent a heart attack by avoiding the final damaging moment; you prevent it by avoiding a lifetime of damaging moments.*

UNCLOTTING THE BLOOD CLOT

But suppose a blood clot (a thrombosis) were now to form in your coronary artery. Has your doctor any means of reversing this calamity, of dissolving the blood clot? The answer is yes. Dr. M. S. Mazel, Medical Director of Chicago's Edgewater Hospital, has been able to save many patients who came within six hours, when the clot was still "soft like Jello," by a drug which prevents the final hardening of the clot.

This drug is identical to a substance found in the human body, "invented" in the evolutionary process to protect our body's narrow channels from becoming blocked. That is why urine, milk, tears and seminal fluids, which, like blood, flow in narrow tubes, are rich in anti-clotting elements. In the blood the clot-dissolving substance is an enzyme (chemical activator) called *fibrinolysin.* "Lysin" means to dissolve; fibrinolysin is a "fibrin dissolver." Of all the clot dissolving substances, fibrinolysin is the most important.

With the help of this newly discovered clot dissolver, many doctors have reported significant improvement in many patients having blood clots in veins, lungs, and leg arteries.

The best way to combat the threat of coronary thrombosis is not after the blood has clotted, but in the early stages before its actual formation, by means of prevention.

The web-forming element has already been mentioned. This is the fibrinogen in the blood, those dumbbell-shaped molecules that link with one another to form the characteristic web of fibrin. Fibrinogen is very active, always on the alert, not unlike a fireman ready to leap into action the moment the alarm sounds. That is why some of the fibrinogen molecules are constantly being activated into fibrin in the blood stream. So sensitive is the fibrinogen molecule that its normal life span is only a few days. But if not used up in "repairs," it becomes linked up with other molecules of its kind to form potentially harmful strands of fibrin.

At the moment fibrin is formed, a clean-up gang gets to work and dissolves it. Actually these dissolving substances exist in the blood stream as *almost*-fibrinolysin which changes into active fibrinolysin at the first hint of fibrin formation. (The reaction is similar to almost-thrombin changing into thrombin.)

What happens if nature's ingenious system of fibrin-dissolving substances becomes inefficient and cannot do its work properly? This is precisely the situation in the blood of atherosclerotics.

In May, 1960, a research team headed by Dr. Hershel Sandberg of the Philadelphia General Hospital, examined the blood of fifty-eight heart-attack victims, compared it to the blood of "normals," and came to this conclusion: in heart attack patients, there is a definite interference with the fibrinolysin mechanism. In other words, the atherosclerotic has a poor clot-dissolving system.

To this data Dr. Nirmal Sarkar in the British publication, *Nature,* (March, 1961) added that almost all normals studied by him had the natural ability to dissolve 95% of a "clot" in their blood within twenty-four hours; but the atherosclerotics were unable to dissolve more than sixty-four per cent of the "clot" in the same amount of time.

In actual practice it has been found that the weakest fibrin-dissolving systems are found in the blood of patients with severe atherosclerosis of the legs. The Australian researcher, Dr. P. J. Nestel, experimenting in 1959 with blood from thirty such patients, found that test-tube clots took a long time to dissolve, but his data in *The Lancet* showed that normal "control" blood in the same test tubes dissolved clots in less than one-third the time.

It would seem, then, that in the blood of atherosclerotics something slows up the production of fibrinolysin or interferes with its action.

Research into causes of fibrinolysin inhibition started some years ago. Dr. H. B. W. Greig, pathologist at the South African Institute for Medical Research, published an account of his pioneering experiments on this problem in the July, 1956 issue of *The Lancet.*

Here's what Dr. Greig did. He took samples of blood and allowed them to clot in test tubes. Then by a special test he measured the reduction in the clot caused by the natural clot-dissolving enzymes within a given period of time. Here was a scientific way of determining the effectiveness of the clot-dissolving fibrinolysin already in the blood.

His patients were normal men and women. The samples of their blood were taken first following a non-fat meal, later following a meal rich in butter, eggs and cream.

Dr. Greig's results: *After the heavy fat meal there was a decided decrease in fibrinolysin activity.* However, when vegetable (unsaturated) fats were substituted for the saturated fats in the fat-heavy meal, *there was no interference with the clot-dissolving process.*

After a year of new and intensive experimentation he again reported in 1957 that diets high in butter, fat and eggs always slowed the clot-dissolving system. Vegetable oils, on the other hand, made the system more efficient.

Dr. Greig further improved fibrinolysin action by removing some of the fatty globules from the blood. It is the beta fatty globules, according to his research, that retard the efficiency of clot-dissolving enzymes.

Yet Dr. Greig recorded that when saturated fats in the beta globules were replaced with unsaturated fats via a long-term change in diet, there was no adverse effect.

The work of Dr. Greig was widely accepted by medical scientists as an important contribution to the prevention of blood clotting. But scientists seldom accept a series of experiments until others have been able to repeat them and get the same results. Dr. Merigan and his associates at the University of California School of Medicine used the Greig technique of alternating fatty and non-fatty meals but based their results on the chylomicrons that swarm into the blood stream after a fatty meal. Merigan's conclusion ". . . chylomicrons appearing in the [blood] plasma after a fatty meal are responsible for the inhibition of fibrinolytic activity."

Dr. Nestel at the University of Melbourne set himself the task of checking Dr. Greig's work another way. The technique he used was based on measuring the total time it took for a clot to dissolve in a test tube. Then he compared the dissolving time to the amount of beta fatty globules already in the blood of the subject. The interference with the clot-dissolving system was proportional to the amount of excess fatty beta globules.

Dr. Monamy Buckell of London's Charing Cross Hospital provided accurate evidence by checking the clot-dissolving tests at exactly the same time each day; and found that fatty meals definitely interfered with the normal clot-dissolving ability of blood.

Dr. J. Gajewski of Warsaw used all the technical controls previously employed by the other medical investigators and added a new safeguard against error by eliminating effects due to exercise. His answer was the same: Fatty meals slowed down the blood's ability to dissolve blood clots.

In 1961 additional proof of the value of vegetable oils came from Dr. Eugene E. Clifton at the Clotting Mechanisms Section of the Sloan-Kettering Institute. He observed that volunteers on a diet supplemented with highly unsaturated safflower oil showed increased anti-clotting activity over the control group.

But Clifton's work, like that of the others, wa a test-tube experiment. The earliest anti-clotting experiments on animals were performed by Dr. H. C. Kwann of the Queen Mary Hospital in Hong Kong, a few years ago. His report appeared in *Nature,* (February 2, 1957.) Dr. Kwann used rabbits and formed visible clots in their almost transparent ears by the injection of thrombin. He divided his rabbits into two groups: the first, fed on a "normal" diet; the second, fed on a high cholesterol diet.

In the "normal" diet group, Kwann saw the clots dissolve perfectly. Of the rabbits in the high-cholesterol group, only one showed partial clot-dissolution. In the others, the clot went on to form a substance that, under Kwann's microscope, resembled *atheroma.*

Dr. Kwann's rabbit experiments were extended a few years later in the United States by Dr. W. A. Thomas and his associates at the Albany Medical College. They studied the effects of diets rich in sugar and vegetable oil and compared them with butter and margarine diet effects on the clots they injected into the rabbits' veins.

Both butter and margarine severely interfered with the natural clot-dissolving process. After both sugar and corn oil meals, twice as many of the clots which had been injected were dissolved, in comparison to the butter tests.

Dr. Clifton extended the blood-clot tests to laboratory dogs. He found that in the normally fed dogs, the clots "all disappeared completely [in] 5 hours . . ." But in the fat-fed dogs, autopsy at 5 hours showed "large coherent bulging masses of clot . . . in all the veins."

Dr. Clifton has summed up the results of his several years of research in this field as follows:

"We have shown in our laboratory that if you give animals diets rich in fat, the clots that are formed in these animals are more difficult to lyse [dissolve] than those formed in normal animals. Furthermore, these clots tend to remain and become embedded in the wall in a manner similar to what has been described in human pathological specimens."

In Japan in 1962, Dr. S. Furuta of the Shinshu University repeated Dr. Clifton's research. In the dogs fed non-fat meals the blood clots which were artificially injected into their veins were found to be completely dissolved. After a butter-fat meal almost all of the clots remained undissolved. But after a vegetable-oil meal the natural clot-dissolving system was also able to dissolve almost all the injected clots.

The many confirmations by well-controlled research have resulted in a general medical acceptance of the fact that fatty meals are a source of danger owing to their interference with the natural clot-dissolving process.

Later it will be shown that fatty meals are also responsible in many ways for the condition of higher coagulability in blood which causes the formation of thrombotic clots in the first place.

The next chapter will show how artery blockage starts and how it finally succeeds in clogging the arteries with its dangerous deposits.

But before this, it will be of interest to list the three main ways in which high fat meals contribute to dangerous artery blockage. They are responsible for:

1. The excess fatty globules which in turn cause deposits of cholesterol and fat in the artery wall.
2. The hypercoagulability which results in small clots that add fibrous material.
3. The interference with the natural fibrin-dissolving mechanism which increases the rate of atheroma deposits.

CHAPTER NINE

Life and Death in Your Arteries

HOW ARTERY BLOCKAGE BEGINS

The prevention of additional artery blockage is a matter of life or death for the middle-aged adult male. The goal of prevention is reached by maintaining the proper balance and stability of the contents of the blood. It is the improper nutrition of the microscopically thin innermost layer of the artery which starts the artery-blockage formation.

For many decades scientists have been analyzing bits of this innermost layer, the intima, taken from normal sections of coronary arteries and comparing it under the microscope with sections taken from blocked coronary arteries of heart attack victims.

But Dr. David Rutstein, who was working on tissue culture research at Harvard University, wanted to see, through the microscope, just how artery blockage grew in *living* artery tissue. He had been watching the effects of "steroid" drugs on "living" artery-wall specimens, growing in his test-tube cultures, for a possible relationship to atherosclerosis. Since cholesterol is chemically related to this group of drugs, it was also used as part of the test.

To Rutstein's surprise, when cholesterol was tested, it seemed to be entering the cell walls!

Here was a reaction too interesting to be ignored. Dr. Rutstein decided to follow it up with a complete series of tests. Because of this fortunate accident, it is now possible to see from Dr. Rutstein's unusually clear photomicrographs, exactly what happens to the inner (intima) walls of the arteries under conditions closely approximating those existing in atherosclerotic blood.

Dr. Rutstein tested every major factor which was suspected of being related to artery blockage: cholesterol, beta fatty globules and saturated and unsaturated fats. Using living intima tissue cells in his test tubes, he increased the concentration of fatty globules (lipoproteins) in the nutrient solution. He could then observe in his microscope the cholesterol deposits increasing in the intima tissue. Rutstein had actually created the beginnings of an atherosclerotic culture in living arterial tissue.

Having induced the start of atherosclerosis in artery tissue, could he reverse the process?

Dr. Rutstein removed the cholesterol-laden tissue from the beta-lipoprotein-rich solution and dropped it back into a bath of normal blood; he then waited and watched. On the fifth day the intima tissue was back to normal. The excess cholesterol had departed from the intima. In a test tube at least, the beginning stages of artery blockage could be reversed.

But for Rutstein this was only the beginning. He now treated the living intima with a nutrient fluid high in beta globules, to which fluid he added a quantity of saturated fats. Not only did cholesterol again deposit in the intima, but now it did so at a quicker rate. *The saturated fats had aggravated the atherosclerotic condition.*

What happened with the addition of unsaturated fats? Using a pure polyunsaturated fat (linoleic, or two-hinged), Dr. Rutstein observed its reaction in more concentrated nutrient solution of beta globules. Though there was a high enough concentration of fatty beta globules to have produced a cholesterol deposit, under the microscope there was no evidence of it. Unsaturated fats, in quantities normally used by the body, seemed to have stopped the atherosclerotic process.

Confirmation of this work first came from Dr. Ancel U. Blaustein at the annual convention of the American Heart Association in 1960.

Dr. Blaustein, working in the laboratories of the New York Medical College, went further than Rutstein in simulating physiological conditions. To feed his intima culture, he used actual blood serum of patients whose high-cholesterol levels were in the range of 350 to 550.

When Blaustein added unsaturated fats, as Rutstein had done, deposits of cholesterol were inhibited. The addition of saturated fats, however, increased the infiltration of cholesterol deposits into the cell walls.

Further confirmation soon followed from Dr. Lazzarini-Robertson. In 1960, at the International Conference of Drugs Affecting Lipid Metabolism, he announced results of experiments that supported the original Rutstein research.

In 1961 Dr. Lazzarini-Robertson reported further data based on his electron-microscope studies. He could almost "see" that the inner intima had microscopic fingers (villi), which seemed to guide fatty globules right into the cell walls.

However, all these test-tube experiments could only suggest how atheroma starts. For the complete understanding of this problem studies had to be made on the intima of living human beings.

The story begins, as before, with the lipids in the blood.

"The normal intima," state Drs. E. F. Hirsch and F. Weinhouse (*Physiological Reviews*, 1943), "has a lipid [fat, cholesterol and phospholipid] distribution almost identical with that of the blood lipids."

This was to be expected, since fatty globules in the blood are part of the nutrients needed by the intima. It is only when these fatty globules are present in excess in the blood that things begin to go wrong and that their cholesterol contents are deposited as artery blockage in the artery wall.

That cholesterol deposits in the atheroma had been known for a hundred years. Much research has been completed which shows that individuals with a high blood cholesterol have more than four times as much cholesterol deposits as those with average blood cholesterol. But how about the *fats* in artery blockage?

One fairly conclusive way to prove that the fatty lipids in artery blockage do come from those in the blood, is to "fingerprint" the complete spectrum of all the many different types of saturated and unsaturated fats, both in the blood and in the artery blockage. If it is true that the fatty components of artery blockage come from the blood, then the chemical spectrums of the fat from both places should be identical.

A team of medical "detectives," Drs. N. Tuna, L. Reckers and I. D. Frantz Jr., used the latest scientific techniques in obtaining chemical "fingerprints" at the Cardiovascular Research Laboratory of the University of Minnesota. The fat-spectrum fingerprints matched. Summing up their research in the August 1958 *Journal of Clinical Investigation,* they reported as follows: "The data were interpreted as support for the concept that [the artery blockage] is formed by infiltration and indiscriminate deposition of blood lipids in the artery wall."

For many years pathologists, who at first were almost the sole research workers in the field of artery blockage, had been seeking the origin of a strange layer of cells, which always appeared in "foam like" formations within the intima layer of the artery in the first stages of atheroma. But only after Dr. W. J. S. Still of the Royal Free Hospital in London combined his electron-microscope technique with the atherosclerotic research experience of Dr. R. M. O'Neal of the Washington University Medical School was the mystery of the fatty layers of foam cells in artery blockage finally solved.

To begin with, there is a wandering cell which passes freely through the cell walls, in and out of the blood stream. This cell is called the *macrophage,* and scientists have long suspected that it might be the origin of the foam cell. This macrophage cell is a scavenger and it has the ability to envelop and destroy, by digesting, foreign bodies and germs, the harmful elements in the blood and within the tissues of the body.

With normal, low content of lipids in the blood, very few macrophages are seen. As the quantity of blood lipids doubles and triples, so does the number of macrophages.

An increase in the macrophage count is not solely dependent on the quality of the fatty globules. The quality of the blood fat is also influential. One of Dr. O'Neal's students found three times as many wandering foam cells (macrophages) when the blood fat came from a butter meal as compared with the lesser number after a corn-oil meal.

The electron-microscope photographs of Dr. O'Neal and Dr. Still clearly show these fat-laden macrophages actually creeping, half in and half out, into the lining of the artery wall. But once inside the artery wall, and full of fatty globules, the wandering cells stop their wandering, and remain stuck inside the intima.

These macrophages continue to enter the intima, and pile up in thin layers. The electron photographs show them to be identical to the foam cells. At last the mystery of a half century has been solved. Nature has been tricked.

The protective germ-eating macrophage had been turned into a destructive agent by the excess fatty globules of the blood.

Among other medical scientists who have been studying this problem is Dr. Enos, who was one of the group that discovered the high rate of artery blockage in the young American soldiers killed in Korea.

Dr. Enos was also interested in the relation between excessive artery blockage and the high-calorie fatty diet of our soldiers. He correlated these two conditions with the newest knowledge on macrophages and foam cells, and made this significant comment in the March 1962 issue of the *American Journal of Cardiology:* "It can be stated without reservation but with some chagrin that the young American male subject has the best-fed coronary lipophages [macrophages] in the world."

In the past, some skeptical scientists have refused to accept the data that blood cholesterol was responsible, and they formulated the theory that the artery wall was responsible for chemically manufacturing the cholesterol found in artery blockage. However, within the past few years new scientific developments have provided additional overwhelming proof that it is the excess blood lipids which cause the damage.

For instance, there is the radioactive-tracer research performed by Dr. C. W. Adams at the Guys Hospital Medical School in London in 1962. Atomic research enabled him to feed radioactive cholesterol to animals, then to watch the step-by-step journey of this "tagged" cholesterol from the blood to the inner layers of the intima lining, and finally to photograph—via electron emission—its deposit through the entire intima.

One of the marvels of surgical science is the woven plastic artery, used to replace atherosclerotic arteries. In experiments it has furnished the "final" proof demanded by skeptical scientists. Since plastic is lifeless and can't manufacture anything, if the artery wall is responsible for blockage, the woven plastic insert should remain atheroma-free.

A research team headed by Dr. Richard A. Tarizzo, of the Laboratories of Surgical Research, Presbyterian St. Luke's Hospital, made such plastic artery grafts on laboratory animals as well as on patients. Did the new shiny nylon arteries stay clear and clean? They did *not*.

According to Dr. Tarizzo, "The general impression that synthetic vascular grafts do not develop atherosclerosis has not been substantiated by our experiments."

The truth was that the plastic tubes began to accumulate atheroma *as if they were alive*. It was not the action of the artificial artery wall but the *blood* that supplied the building material for the growth of atheroma.

So concerned was Dr. Tarizzo with the effects of a high-fat diet, which might again clog up the clear, clean artificial arteries and ruin his painstaking operations, that he wrote, "an important practical clinical advantage may be gained by keeping patients with [plastic arterial] grafts on a low-cholesterol diet . . ."

Among the many investigations supporting Dr. Tarizzo were those at the Royal Victoria Infirmary in London, where autopsies on patients with nylon-artery-graft operations showed that, "development of atherosclerosis need not be dependent on any process inherent in the wall of an artery."

It is now beyond question that the start of artery blockage comes from the fatty globules in the blood. But we should not lose sight of the fact that local conditions in the artery wall can encourage this invasion. This conclusion is based on the data from three authorities. Dr. W. H. Hauss of Germany, after studying the peculiarities in the arterial wall *before* atheroma growth, states that the early *spotty weakness* in the artery was precipitated by a high-fat diet. Dr. T. Shimamoto of Japan, whose microscope showed a *spotty* inflammation of the artery before atheroma started, could produce this inflammation either by drugs or by a high-fat diet. Dr. Sandler from Emory University traced an enzyme deficiency to the actual *spot* the atheroma was to form on and blamed the enzyme weakness on a lack of polyunsaturated fats at the spot.

Local conditions may determine the sites on which artery blockage is to form; but it is an atherosclerotic diet and atherosclerotic blood lipids which are often both the inciting factor, as well as the growth factor, in artery blockage.

In conclusion: Many types of artery blockage can affect the intima of the coronary artery, caused by blood which is excessively rich in cholesterol and in large fatty globules.

This has been proven by many types of research, among which are: (1) Intima tissue culture analyses (2) Cholesterol deposit measurements (3) Fatty "fingerprint" correlations (4) Growth of fatty foam cells (5) Radioactive cholesterol tracers (6) Artery blockage in artificial arteries (7) Local conditions in the artery wall.

But fat and cholesterol deposits are only the beginning of artery blockage. The next section will tell how other factors in the blood become involved during the final stages of artery blockage.

THE SIX COMPONENTS OF ATHEROSCLEROSIS

Which is the most dangerous factor in artery blockage—is it the deposits of cholesterol and fat, or is it fibrin? Until a few years ago this question divided the medical world into two camps.

On this side of the Atlantic the American school held that fats and cholesterol, depositing from the fatty globuless of the blood, were the primary and critical cause of atheroma.

On the other side of the ocean a group of researchers in England, led by Dr. John B. Duguid, revived the century-old observation of Dr. Von Rokitansky who in his book *Manual of Pathological Anatomy says:* "The deposit is [a] product derived from the blood, and for the most part from the fibrin of the arterial blood." Now over a hundred years later modern scientists have discovered that this neglected report contained the final important clue needed for the complete understanding of all the stages of artery blockage.

The British scientists placed the emphasis on the thrombotic tendencies of the blood. According to their analysis, the principal cause of atherosclerosis is thrombotic clotting and on the subsequent partial dissolving of these blood clots with a final undissolved fibrous residue of artery blockage.

So far as this international medical controversy over atherosclerosis is concerned, there is truth in both the American and the British contentions. As a matter of fact, during the last few years, the two theories have been combined and now, together, present a more accurate picture of the artery blockage process.

Drs. N. Woolf and T. Crawford of the St. George Hospital Medical School in London, using a new fluorescent-light technique, directed their microscopes on atheroma deposits and observed that *atheroma-forming fibrin was accumulated mostly in and around the fatty deposits* on the artery walls. Something in the fats was causing fibrinogen in the blood to deposit as fibrin. It was not a case of one *or* the other; it was the combination of both one *and* the other.

The unified theory made its formal bow at the American Heart Association Convention when it was presented by Drs. W. A. Thomas, R. M. O'Neill and W. S. Hartroft. *The Thrombolipid Theory* is the name coined by this group after their six years of experimentation with high-fat diets on laboratory animals.

This group had made many research studies which indicated that not only do the lipids in blood and in artery blockage attract fibrin, but in addition, fibrin in the blood clots also attracts the fatty globules.

From Canada's Dr. Mustard came further evidence welding the British and American theories into one. It is Dr. Mustard's conclusion that lipids from platelets and fatty globules in the blood are trapped between the sticky platelets and the fibrin on the blood-vessel wall.

This newly discovered action of the platelets, writes Dr. Mustard in the *Journal of the Canadian Medical Association* (September, 1961), permits combining "the encrustation and the lipid theories of atherogenesis [start of atheroma] . . . commonly regarded as rivals."

Although the unification of the opposing schools removes the need for further debate, actually from a purely practical point of view it did not matter which of the two schools had the most correct explanation since the prevention program will *still act to inhibit artery blockage*. This program works on both fronts: (1) On fats and cholesterol and (2) on fibrin formation and thrombotic blood. And the way through which the atheroma inhibition is effected is the same, by means of the Prudent Diet which reduces both the excess blood lipids and the high coagulability of the blood.

We already have a clear picture of how the atheroma *begins*. But how does it *grow*?

Scientists can follow the atheroma growth by making autopsy studies on groups of progressively advanced age, such as was done in the study reported in 1961 in the *British Medical Journal* by a research team under the direction of Dr. Kenneth Hill, Professor of Pathology at the University of London.

The life history of artery blockage begins in childhood. Even then, along the walls of the artery, fatty streaks are observed. Slowly, year by year, these streaks grow.

At about the age of fifteen a new phase develops. The fibrin, which in the early years had for the most part been removed by the relatively healthy clot-dissolving mechanism, now increases in quantity, piling up in the form of fatty fibrous growths. The artery blockage is now beginning to reduce the flow of blood slightly.

Artery blockage does not grow in an even and uniform manner. It occurs in layers and patches. Some layers contain more fats and cholesterol, others are more fibrous. Later in life there appear layers which seem to be the residue of blood clots which were only partially dissolved.

How thick can the layers become before they cause a critical blockage? The amount varies with each individual, and the only test of specific critical blockage is the actual heart attack.

In 1960 an analysis of this problem was performed by a group of researchers led by Dr. William G. Beadenkopf of the New York State Department of Health. Their purpose was to determine whether there was an actual relation "between atherosclerosis in the coronary arteries and infarction in the [heart muscle]."

Dr. Beadenkopf's results settled all doubts concerning this relationship. He performed autopsies on 300 patients who had died of a variety of diseases, measured the thickness of the coronary wall, and correlated it with the incidence of infarction. He found:

1. In the group with atheroma thick enough to block off only about half of the inner artery pathway, 30% had infarctions;
2. When the artery blockage was only allowing less than one-fifth of the original blood pathway, myocardial infarctions were found in 60% of the patients.
3. When the arterial flow was reduced to a mere trickle (nine-tenths of the artery being blocked) only one out of four escaped infarction.

The infarction rate in general was proportional to the amount of artery blockage, but this did not hold true for each individual case. There are several reasons why some individuals had an infarction with *less* blockage. One is that artery blockage deposits are not uniform. Thus there exists an element of chance which may determine just where spots of sufficient thickness will fall opposite each other and narrow the channel to lethal proportions.

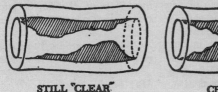

STILL "CLEAR" CRITICAL

The Beadenkopf survey supplies the background data for understanding some of the basic facts in heart attack. The first fact is that the coronary artery need not be completely blocked to cause damage to the heart. The second is that every heart and each heart muscle, depending upon its individual efficiency and state of health, has a critical requirement for oxygen. Reduction in the blood flow or an increased need for blood, or both, can cause the disaster.

The thrombosis, on the other hand, always stops the blood flow completely. But a thrombosis could never occur in a "clean" artery. As the progressive atherosclerosis makes the channel even more narrow the probability of thrombosis increases.

A significant survey of this problem was made in 1961 by Dr. T. Crawford, of St. George's Medical Hospital in London. The conclusion was that:

" . . . thrombosis was observed only when pre-existing atherosclerosis had narrowed the [coronary artery] to one-third or less of . . . normal . . ."

At this point it may be of use to summarize some of the essential facts concerning artery blockage.

What we do know about the contents of Artery Blockage

1. Fats and Cholesterol   *Deposited by the unstable fatty globules*

2. Foam Cell Layers   *Fatty contents brought in by the macrophages from the blood*

3. Platelets and Red Blood Cell Debris	*Actually the lipid and fibrous debris left over from undissolved blood clots*
4. Fibrin and Fibrous Tissue	*Both (3) and (4) are due to inhibition of the fibrinolytic system by excess blood lipids*
5. Hyaline Connective Tissues	*Actually a result of the degeneration of fibrous deposits*
6. Calcium Deposits	*May be due partly to excess calcium in the blood, or to imbalances, or both*

At this point it is important to reiterate that all the contents of the artery blockage may come under the influence of and be prevented by the Prudent Diet.

Must artery blockage inevitably cause infarction if the growth has reached the critical stage?

"All the evidence available," commented Dr. J. B. Taylor in 1961 in the *Illinois Medical Journal* "is contrary to this defeatist concept that atherosclerosis is a 'one-way' or irreversible process."

In 1916 this reversibility had already been demonstrated by the pioneer investigator, Dr. Krylow. Dr. N. Anitschkow, in 1928, also reported the disease "reversed" in rabbits after 18 to 24 months.

During the early 1950's, Dr. Wilens showed, in his reports based on autopsies performed on the arteries of patients who died from wasting diseases, that the artery blockage was often "resorbed." Where the diet was near starvation levels, as in the Nazi concentration camps, the arteries examined at autopsy were usually clear of atheroma.

Today pathologists often see arteries in which there are "hollows" where previously there was atherosclerotic blockage. These pathologists have no doubt about reversibility.

Consequently, three phases should be considered in a prevention program.

1. REVERSAL: Dissolving part of the fatty fibrous growths already blocking our arteries.
2. STATUS QUO: Prevention of any further extension of deposits of blockage.

3. PREVENTION of Coronary Thrombosis: By preventing the excess blockage usually required for this disaster, and by reducing excess blood lipids which increase the thrombotic factors in blood.

Luckily the same prevention program is effective in all three phases. Even if you cannot be sure that your artery blockage is being dissolved via the prevention program, it is certain that the goal of status quo and the prevention of coronary thrombosis can be achieved.

Up to this point excess amounts of blood lipids were considered as the primary cause of our present high incidence of artery blockage and heart attack.

Now we come to a *second major condition* which acts in combination with the blood lipids to further increase artery blockage. This is High Blood Pressure.

CHAPTER TEN

To Salt or Not to Salt

WHAT HIGH BLOOD PRESSURE DOES TO YOUR ARTERIES

"A Japanese farmer who lives to a ripe old age, and eats about two ounces of salt each day during his life, filters through his kidneys 277,000 pounds, or 138 tons, of salt!"

This believe-it-or-not statement was made in 1961 at a medical meeting on salt and high blood pressure by Dr. George Meneely of Vanderbilt University.

The Japanese, according to medical statistics, suffer from the highest blood pressure in the world, and they also are known to be the world's highest salt consumers. What is the connection between salt and high blood pressure?

The first fact to be considered is that high blood pressure, although *secondary* to high blood lipids, is a major cause of heart attack. The combined effects of *both* causes will produce the *greatest* amount of artery blockage in the *shortest* time. In women, whose blood lipids are normally low during early adult life, the comparatively few cases of early coronary disease almost invariably have high blood pressure.

The same holds true for both men and women in China and Japan, where, again, the rare cases of heart attack are usually accompanied by high blood pressure.

Blood pressure which is higher than normal will cause excess stretching, vibration, elongation, bending and other stress that exhausts and injures the muscles and other cells in the blood-vessel walls. The total effect of these small injuries is to make the blood vessel more susceptible to artery blockage.

That high blood pressure accelerates the rate of growth of artery blockage has been an accepted fact for many years. But it was the Framingham Experiment which provided the most valid statistical confirmation of this knowledge. At Framingham, Dr. Dawber and his associates measured not only cholesterol levels but also blood-pressure levels. And they compared them with the incidence of heart attacks in their volunteer group over a period of ten years.

We already have seen the data from Framingham on how the step-by-step increase in cholesterol was matched by a corresponding step-by-step increase in heart attack. Now, let's see what happened in groups where everyone had the *same* cholesterol level but different blood-pressure levels.

Five cholesterol groups, ranging from "low" to "high," were studied. In each group, as blood-pressure levels varied from low normal to abnormally high, the heart-attack rate rose correspondingly, reaching a top rate of 500% over base. The *base* rate, of course, varied depending on the average cholesterol level of the group.

Whether the cholesterol grouping was a low 180 or a high 300, those in each grouping with the highest blood pressure had a heart attack rate five times as great as those with low blood pressure.

Other experts have reported even more drastic figures. One authoritative study comes from the eminent blood-lipid specialist, Dr. John W. Goffman. In his book, *Coronary Heart Disease,* published in 1959, Goffman estimated the risk of myocardial infarction at various diastolic pressures. Diastolic pressure is the *low* figure on a blood-pressure report.

As the pressure goes from 60 to 70, the risk doubles. From 70 to 85, it doubles again. And from 85 to 100, it doubles for the third time. Simple arithmetic shows that as the diastolic pressure rises from a normal of 60 to a high of 110, *the risk of myocardial infarction goes up 800%!*

Similar statistics were obtained in England by Dr. R. G. Brown and his associates from a large study of systolic pressures. These are the *high* figures on your blood-pressure reports. Dr. Brown found that as the systolic pressure rises from a norm of 120 to a high of 200, the risk of heart attack increases uniformly. The increase in risk from low to high was the same as Gofman's—800%!

These and many other similar studies indicate that one thing is certain: to reduce heart-attack risk, the blood pressure must be lowered.

The Metropolitan Life Insurance Company experts have stated that, " . . . even a relatively modest elevation of blood pressure has long-range effects on longevity."

WHAT SALT DOES
TO YOUR BLOOD PRESSURE

What causes high blood pressure? Medical science knows of many causes: stress, toxic substances such as cigarettes and gasoline fumes, etc., food additives, insecticide sprays, the side effects of drugs, and industrialization are suspect. Regarding the elimination of these caustive agents, it's difficult to give advice; for most of us they are inseparable from our way of life.

However, there is one cause of high blood pressure which can be remedied. Sodium chloride (common table salt) is a major cause of high blood pressure.

It would seem, therefore, that if salt intake were restricted, blood pressure would drop. But according to *Science News Letter* (August 12, 1961), "only about one-fourth to one-third of patients with high blood pressure respond to salt restriction." Because in many cases blood pressure does not fall, it was thought that excessive salt intake was not a basic cause of hypertension. Nevertheless experiments indicate that the *initial* cause can still be excess salt even when salt reduction does not effect a cure.

In 1954, Drs. L. K. Dahl and R. A. Love, who had devoted much research to the relation of diet-salt and hypertension, decided to make a survey study of the problem. They checked a large number of men for both salt intake and blood pressure.

The first group among those studied alleged that they never salted their food. The investigators estimated the average daily salt intake of this group at about two or three grams. This was the low-salt group. The second group stated that they salted their food, even before tasting it. Their daily salt consumption, according to the Dahl-Love estimate, was twelve to eighteen grams. This was the high-salt group. The third group was the "normal," or "medium" salt group. They used salt according to taste and consumed an estimated four to ten grams daily. Statements on salt intake were verified by means of urine analysis.

Drs. Dahl and Love examined each group for hypertensives. They found: (1) In the high-salt group 10% were hypertensive (2) In the medium-salt group 7% were hypertensive and (3) *In the low-salt group there wasn't a single case of hypertension.*

Dr. Norman Fallis made a test in 1962, the object being to see if victims of high blood pressure might be high-salt eaters due to poor salt-tasting ability. Twenty high-blood-pressure patients were matched with twenty normals. Each of the forty were given a series of drinks to test how sensitive their taste buds were.

Their ability to taste sugar in these drinks was almost the same. However, Dr. Fallis found that the high-blood-pressure group required two to sixteen times the amount of salt in the drink before they could taste it.

A direct experiment on the role of salt in hypertension was performed by Dr. Meneely, who gave us the astonishing statistics on the salt intake of Japanese farmers. Groups of rats were placed on a high-salt diet, and other groups on a low-salt diet. The low-salt group *did* show lower blood pressures than the high-salt group. When he increased the intake of salt in various groups he found that after a period of time the blood pressure in these groups went up proportionally to the increases of salt in the diet.

Now for still another type of experiment from which we can draw "reasonable inferences," as the scientists say. If excess salt in the diet causes high blood pressure, then in subjects with *high* blood pressure, we should find *more* salt in the body than in those with *low* blood pressure.

This experiment was harmless and could easily be performed on human beings. Dr. E. J. Ross matched individuals for age and other relevant characteristics, and separated them into a high-blood-pressure group and a normal-blood-pressure group. The results appeared in *Clinical Science*. On the average, the normal-blood-pressure group had less body salt than that found in the high-blood-pressure group.

After a thorough search of the medical literature, I have been able to find only one other research report in which accurate measurements of the amount of salt found in hypertensives was compared with that found in normals. In this research it was the quantity of salt in the blood (as sodium and as chlorides) which was measured. The results, obtained from residents of the Central Asian City of Tashkent, fully corroborated those of Dr. Ross.

Dr. S. N. Babadzhanov of the Tashkent Medical Institute reported in 1963 that the significant range of sodium in the blood of normals was 290 to 300 milligrams. In those with high blood pressure the significant range was 308 to 334. The chlorides in the blood showed similar results.

And even more important was Dr. Babadzhanov's statement that, "High levels of these substances in the blood were encountered thrice as often in patients with stage two diseases as in patients with stage one . . . In the course of treatment, as the patients' general condition improved and the level of their arterial pressure fell, a definite decrease in blood sodium and chloride levels was observed."

The influence of salt on blood pressure usually operates very slowly. Many years go by before the increase in blood pressure is noticed. But research can't wait this long, and so Dr. J. McDonough of the St. Louis City Hospital persuaded ten young adults to use an average of one ounce of salt a day for three weeks. This is the approximate daily amount used by Northern Japanese farmers. As a result of this high salt intake, according to Dr. McDonough, "There was a gradual, progressive, highly significant increase in systolic and diastolic pressures."

Up to now we have been talking about salt causing high blood pressure in the "normal" person. But how about the effects of salt on those millions suffering from our country's most prevalent ailment, overweight?

Here is a sensitive area for research because overweight is *known* to be very frequently accompanied by high blood pressure. Is there a link between the obese individual's high blood pressure and his salt intake?

No experimental tests have yet been made by placing groups of people on a high-salt, overweight-producing diet. But the fact that a weight-reducing diet will lower blood pressure only if salt is *also* restricted was reported in 1958 in the *New England Journal of Medicine*. Obese, hypertensive patients *did* respond to weight-reducing, salt-free diets with a significant drop in their blood pressure. But in only one case out of twelve was there a drop in blood pressure on a "normal" high-salt reducing diet.

And now one more piece of most convincing evidence. In 1952, Drs. L. Tobian, Jr. and J. Binion had compared the amounts of sodium in the arterial walls of hypertensives and normals, and reported their results in *Circulation:* "The arterial walls of hypertensive individuals proved to contain abnormally large quantities of sodium."

Of all the blood vessels, the capillaries are most accessible to direct examination. Dr. C. D. De Langen, in his laboratory in Utrecht in the Netherlands, has noticed by direct microscope observation that capillaries under the fingernail can be affected within two weeks by as little as one half ounce of extra salt per day.

Reporting the after effects on the nail capillaries, Dr. DeLangen wrote: "Lively contractions were observed. The capillaries, checked in the fingernail and the skin, had become coarse and thick . . ."

Moreover, the group, acting as its own control, was switched back and forth from low-salt to high-salt diets. The high-salt diet always induced damage. As Dr. DeLangen concludes: "When taken in too large quantities [salt] may act as a capillary poison."

Is the effect of salt on atherosclerosis manifested only through an increase in blood pressure?

Dr. Douglas Talbot of the American Medical Research Foundation made a startling discovery. First he studied the rise of blood fats after an experimental "fat load" had been fed to twenty young men. Then he added extra salt —twenty grams (two-thirds of an ounce) a day—to their diet and repeated the fat-load experiment. *On the high-salt ration, the rise in blood fats was much greater.* Dr. Talbot says of his findings (*Annals of Internal Medicine,* February, 1961) that they " . . . would certainly suggest that early limitation of salt might offer a means of controlling atherosclerosis."

There have been other medical investigators to note these effects. In the *Journal of Experimental Medicine* (October, 1960) Dr. L. K. Dahl reported an experiment on *The Effects of Excess Salt Feeding on the Elevation of Cholesterol in Rats and Dogs:* "Among female rats and dogs, which were fed excess salt for periods of about one and four years, respectively, elevations in [blood] cholesterol . . . were frequent . . . and, in some cases, quite marked."

Dr. Meneely fed a 7% salt diet to rats for two months, and observed the "disturbed lipid metabolism . . . deposition of lipids in arterioles [small arteries] throughout the body . . ."

And Dr. DeLangen, in 1959 in *Nutritia and Dieta* states that, " . . . the fat content of the blood stream may increase markedly under the influence of much extra salt in the diet."

DeLangen had previously discovered a direct effect of common table salt on the arterial wall. He experimented with many animals, particularly the rabbit, and reported at a Symposium on Arteriosclerosis at Basel in 1956: "[Although] relatively large quantities of cholesterol and fat are needed to cause atheromatous changes in the experimental animal . . . when an extra quantity of sodium chloride is added to the food, much smaller quantities of cholesterol and fat are required . . ."

Although the specific method by which salt causes the increase in fatty globules is not yet known, the data from many laboratories presents very convincing evidence of the harmful reaction caused by salt. In addition, as will be shown later in the book, a high-fat diet also has an effect on the salt in the body.

"SALT LICKS" WITHOUT SALT

Is a low-salt diet a *deficient* diet? Don't we need plenty of salt in our diet to keep us fit? This is a popular notion —but is it true? For instance, everybody "knows" that animals need salt for their health, crave salt, even go miles out of their way to visit "salt licks." But has any scientist ever proven this—or is it just a myth?

The May 1953 *Nutrition Reviews* reported the findings of A. R. Patton, of the Chemistry Department of the Colorado Agricultural College. Patton denies the possibility of wild animals getting any salt out of the so-called "salt licks." He states: "I arranged with forest rangers to send me samples of the mud from the many localized spots where the wild forest animals congregated from far and wide to lick the soil. Although all of these sites were known as 'salt licks' the one chemical property they all had in common was complete absence of sodium chloride [salt]."

Although this was printed in *Nutrition Reviews* about ten years ago, no refutation of Patton's important survey has yet appeared in any scientific journal.

There is a "licking disease" in Europe among wild animals known in Germany as *Lechsucht* and in other countries as "Pica." Such animals usually have an iron and copper deficiency due to local soil deficiencies and the "licks" supply the needed minerals. This disease has been largely eliminated by now with mineral supplements. In large areas of Florida, animals have an anemia disease known as "salt sick," and outcroppings of iron-bearing rock have been used by wild animals as "licks." But the sodium-chloride level in these rocks is extremely low.

In 1958, also in *Nutrition Reviews,* a letter appeared from G.L. McClymont, Professor of Rural Sciences at the University of New England, Australia, concerning the need for salt of domesticated animals. He writes, "despite an ancient and continuing belief in the practice, there is, as far as we are aware, a complete lack of critical evidence that grazing sheep have ever responded to salt supplements; and many negative experiments have been recorded in *this* country."

It is true that farmers in the United States do use supplementary salt for their cows, but the result is that a quart of milk contains the extremely high content of 1½ grams of salt per quart. For a five-month-old infant, this is equivalent to ½ ounce of salt to an adult.

ARE SALT TABLETS NECESSARY

There is a common belief that salt lost in sweating must be immediately replaced. In many of our factories, the management supplies salt tablets to keep the workers in "proper health." But, are these salt tablets necessary?

Rommel's *Afrika Corps* swept across the Sahara to the gates of Egypt, fought and lost a bitter battle before El Alamein, and retreated over hundreds of miles of blazing desert; yet, when the campaign was over, the English found the captured troops in good physical condition even though the Nazi soldiers were *not* supplied with salt tablets.

The story of the *Afrika Corps* supports the findings of many experiments performed with low-salt diets on human beings under desert conditions. What happens, according to the scientific studies, is this: After the first few days of acclimatization, the subjects cease to lose salt through perspiration. Apparently, there's a normalizing body mechanism at work that conserves salt. Dr. Frederick M. Allen, pioneer investigator of the low-salt diet, put the case clearly in his report in *Nutrition Reviews,* of September, 1949: "The comfortable endurance of all ordinary weather conditions by thousands of patients on rigid salt-poor diets shows that this need [for added salt in hot weather] has been exaggerated."

There is actually enough *natural* salt in vegetables, meats and other foods, even though they have not been processed with salt in any way, to supply the salt required by our body. Proof of this fact is found in the known past history of many peoples throughout the world who have never used salt.

The Kirghiz of Turkestan never added salt to their food, nor did the Bedouins of Arabia. The American Indians, when the first explorers arrived, knew nothing about the use of salt and called it "white magic." Vilhjalmur Stefansson the great Arctic explorer states that "In pre-Columbian times salt was unknown, or the taste of it disliked, and the use of it avoided through much of North and South America." It was during Stefansson's Arctic explorations among the salt-abstaining Eskimos that his desire for salt disappeared within three months.

The world-renowned Dr. Albert Schweitzer offers corroboration with his statement that "the natives two hundred miles from the coast . . . (on my arrival in Gabon in 1918) . . . consumed no salt."

Other non-users of salt include Greenland and Arctic Eskimos, Australian Aborigines and Chinese in the mountainous western Szechwan region. The Siriono Indians of

Eastern Bolivia, ignorant of salt until traders introduced it, first found it distasteful, as is the usual case when any group has its first contact with salt, though later they become fond of it.

Regarding the amount of salt used, Dr. Dahl states: "Some of the primitive groups probably were averaging about one gram per day."

When primitive groups have low blood pressure, it causes no surprise. Since they live far from the stress of modern civilization, it is as most scientists expect it to be. But when such groups are found with high blood pressure, the reasons must be investigated. One such group was found in rural Nigeria.

Studies in 1960 by Dr. D. G. Abrahams have shown that in general, a comparison of blood pressures in similar-age groups of rural Nigerians and Europeans showed both groups to have similar high values.

The Lancet, in an editorial comment on Dr. Abrahams researches, finds it "interesting to note that, although the Nigerians studied by Abrahams et al., were illiterate and uncivilized, they partook freely of the rock salt which is plentiful in the district . . ." and the editor goes on to " . . . wonder whether the baneful effect of 'civilization' on blood pressure is not perhaps, after all, simply a matter of salt intake."

When groups living far from civilization reveal high blood pressure, they have almost always been found to use an abnormal amount of salt in their diet.

Dr. F. W. Lowenstein, a medical officer in the World Health Organization, made use of a nutrition survey to study the blood pressures of two tribes of Indians, the Carajas and the Mundurucus, living in Northern Brazil.

The Carajas have consistently low blood pressure. The Mundurucus, living not far away, have a high blood pressure similar to, but somewhat lower than, that found in Europeans.

Dr. Lowenstein studied both groups to find reasons which might account for this difference. The way of life of the Carajas was the same as that of their ancestors, but that of the Mundurucus had been changed after the advent of the missionaries. One significant change was the use of tobacco, and the other was the regular use of table salt, which previously was unknown to both groups.

What is the human requirement for *food salt?* The

opinions vary from one half gram up to one gram a day. The average American actually consumes ten to twenty times his salt requirement each day.

Suppose this average American tried actively to avoid all salt except that which occurs "naturally" in his food—how low could he reduce his salt intake? According to Dr. A. Grollman of the Southwestern Medical School, the very lowest figure he could obtain is three grams. This unfortunately high figure is due to the excessive amount of "hidden salt" in almost all commercially prepared foods.

Dr. Dahl and his associates at the Brookhaven National Laboratory have been very active in the study of the effects of salt on high blood pressure among many groups throughout the world. Since those with the highest blood pressure in the United States are the Southern Negroes, it was only natural for Dr. Dahl to study this situation. His conclusions were reported in the April 19, 1958 issue of *Science News Letter:* "My interviews with Negroes from that region indicate that, for most of them . . . a prominent article in the diet . . . in one form or another . . . from early childhood . . . has been . . . *salted* pork."

So interesting did Dahl find this discovery that he traveled to Japan to continue his salt studies. While the incidence of high blood pressure is generally high throughout Japan, it is higher in the North than in the South. It gradually diminishes as one travels south through the islands, where the rate of high blood pressure is only half of what it is in the North. Dr. Dahl looked for a relationship between the drop in blood pressure and salt intake and he found it. In the South of Japan, salt intake, although high, was about half of what it was in the North.

Another one of Dr. Dahl's international studies was reported by him at the International Symposium on Hypertension in 1960. Five groups of different peoples were studied and their salt intake carefully checked by daily urine analysis. The daily salt intake ranged from four grams by the Alaskan Eskimos to twenty-six grams by the Northern Japanese. The Eskimos had no high blood pressure, but the incidence in the other groups rose gradually, parallelling their salt intake. It seems incredible, but almost half of the Japanese people living in the areas with the highest salt intake are victims of high blood pressure. But what protects the other half of the Northern

Japanese who also eat their ounce of salt daily, but don't succumb to high blood pressure?

The possibility that heredity may be involved in high blood pressure was not overlooked in Dr. Dahl's studies. By breeding rats and watching their high-blood-pressure reaction to salt feeding, he was finally able to isolate a strain in which excessive amounts of salt did not induce high blood pressure. These rats obviously were born with kidneys which could quickly and easily eliminate salt.

Another strain was isolated which was born with a tendency to high blood pressure. Of this later group Dr. Dahl says, "However strong the genetic tendency to hypertension may be in this strain, the addition of a high salt diet seems necessary to unmask the trait."

Dr. Dahl's final conclusion is, "Thus far, however, we have not encountered *groups* which customarily consume high salt intakes that had a low prevalence of hypertension or *groups* in which low salt intakes were the rule, associated with high prevalence of hypertension."

Dr. J. H. Weller of the University of Michigan Medical School puts it another way. He says that on the basis of the known researches concerning salt, "It may be stated unequivocally that sodium plays a prominent role as a *permissive* factor in the development and persistence of hypertension."

The question must be asked: If the possibility of a significant reduction in high blood pressure is as simple as the withholding of the salt shaker from the table, and the removal of the box from the shelf of the cook, canner and baker, then why is it not more widely recommended by the doctor?

The answer is that without sufficient motivation the low salt diet is unpopular with both the patient and the doctor. Although the taste for salt is acquired, and is not physiological, it has become so strong that strong motivation is required before a change is made.

"DE-SALTING DRUGS"
THAT REDUCE BLOOD PRESSURE

Now that the relationship of salt, high blood pressure and coronary heart attack has finally become clear enough to provide the incentive to make a change in our saltshaker habit, the chemists have come up with a new wonder drug.

This wonder drug is called Thiazide, and it is the chemist's answer for those who want to eat their salt and get rid of it the same day. Already a dozen different chemicals similar to Thiazide are being prescribed by doctors.

Since the effects of the Thiazide drugs are due to their ability to *force* the kidney to excrete salt, the next logical step should be a controlled clinical trial to see which is better—drugs or diet. This test has not yet been officially made, but the opinions of the medical experts at a discussion during the second Hahnemann Symposium on Hypertensive Disease may be of interest. Drs. Brest, Grollman and Freis were each of the opinion that the pressure-reducing effect of a low-salt diet was just as good as that of the drugs. Only one participant, Dr. Hollander, held the opinion that in his practice the drugs were slightly more effective than the low-salt diet.

The frequent objection to a low-salt diet on the part of many doctors, which has been mentioned in several medical reports, is "poor patient acceptance." Many doctors have said that they found it impractical in most cases to make a patient adhere to a diet restricted in salt.

As one doctor recently put it: "It is so easy to write a prescription for a tablet that a patient will take, so gratifying to observe a fall in blood pressure after the drug has been taken. It is more difficult to educate the patient about low-sodium diets; it is more time consuming."

Since less than half the patients on a low-salt diet show a reduction in blood pressure, the doctor is at a loss to know if the patient is still allowing salt in his diet or if the patient is one who may not immediately benefit from a low-salt diet. Dr. A. C. Corcoran has reported that with the use of the powerful salt-losing drugs, it was no longer necessary to check the urine for salt, to see if the patient was "cheating."

But since high blood pressure, according to Dr. James Conway of the University of Michigan Medical School, is "a disease in which drug therapy once started, will be maintained for life," let us see what the possible effects of the Thiazide drugs over such a long period might be.

The first problem is that of the "low salt syndrome."

This illness is never a result of a natural low-salt diet, but it has occurred after use of the salt-eliminating drugs.

The drug substitutes for the low-salt diet have other dangers. Like all potent drugs they have "side effects." In *Post Graduate Medicine,* Dr. M. D. Phelps states in January, 1963, that due to Thiazide drugs, "Latent diabetes may be transformed into clinical disease, and clinical diabetes may be accentuated to the point where previously effective doses of insulin . . . no longer provide adequate control." Dr. Morton Fuchs of the Hahnemann Medical College says regarding Thiazide drugs, "Increased blood uric acid levels may be produced frequently to pathologic levels . . . Clinical acute gouty arthritis may be produced . . ."

It is an accepted fact that malignant (extremely serious) hypertension seems to have almost disappeared. According to Dr. A. M. Fishberg, the Director of Medicine in the Beth Israel Hospital, this is probably due to the fact that today all patients with elevated blood pressure are put on a restricted salt diet.

Says Dr. Fishberg: "I believe firmly, much more firmly than I did a few years ago, in the value of sodium [salt] restriction. For a long time I was skeptical about it, but in the last few years I have come to think it is of tremendous importance . . ."

"I now also believe that lesser degrees of sodium restriction may slow the progress of hypertensive disease."

CHAPTER ELEVEN

Anti-Heart-Attack Drugs

HOW DRUGS CAN HELP—AND HARM—YOU

With so many modern "miracle drugs" devised in our chemical laboratories and produced by our pharmaceutical factories and with so many millions of dollars expended annually on research, why has chemistry not produced the needed miracle drugs, one drug to lower blood cholesterol, for example, another to lower the beta fatty globules and a third to clear the blood of chylomicrons after a fatty meal?

These drugs do exist. They're on the market. Hundreds of thousands of coronary-heart-disease victims are using them right now. And they seem to work . . . but at what price?

One advantage of a drug is easy patient acceptance. Diet change requires indoctrination of the patient, and what busy doctor is able to take the time for that? For the patient, dieting is a change in habit; it requires will and effort.

But the drug, the pill, the rapid, painless remedy that requires no change in our daily habits—why, that's just the thing to satisfy both the doctor and the patient.

But are today's anti-coronary drugs harmless?

Let's discuss one somewhat familiar drug, the anti-blood-fat drug, the female sex hormone.

Dr. Jeremiah Stammler, Director of the Heart Disease Control Program of the Chicago Board of Health, headed a team of research workers on a five-year study of 275 men who had recovered from heart attacks. Each had been treated with "estrogens," female sex hormones. The treatment, the *New York Times* reported on April 19, 1962, "appears to cut in half the death rate."

How? Because "the male pattern of blood-fat levels can be altered to a female pattern [of low blood fats]." From it, Stammler concludes: "The positive results of our investigation . . . lead us to recommend . . . estrogens to the medical profession for use in the long-term management of myocardial infarction."

But "side effects of the estrogen treatment include breast enlargement," the *Times* reported, "and decrease in libido and potency [sex urge and sex ability]." The estrogens, therefore, won't be suitable for all until all demasculinizing effects are eliminated. Drug companies are busy working on that problem, but until they come up with a solution, the estrogens remain a last-ditch measure.

So we must turn to another type of drug. Why not look for one that will directly inhibit blood cholesterol? The pharmaceutical houses put their finest research teams on the job, tested hundreds of chemical compounds on laboratory animals, and came up with *Triparanol*.

The trade name is MER/29, and it is a "cholesterol-inhibiting" drug, introduced to the medical world in 1959. Here was a drug that, *if* it worked, might be the anti-coronary wonder weapon.

Immediately upon its introduction, innumerable clinical trials were instituted, and scores of reports appeared in the medical press. Yes, MER/29 *did* reduce blood cholesterol. It looked, now, as if medical men had the drug needed to combat coronary disease. But, once again, the question arose: were there any harmful side effects?

Dr. W. P. Achor and his team of researchers at Rochester, Minnesota, put eighteen patients on MER/29 and took blood cholesterol samples for three months. At the end of that period, blood cholesterol was down 13%. But of the eighteen patients, six suffered a considerable loss of hair, and one was afflicted with a serious skin disease with a fish-like, scaly appearance.

These side effects were obvious. But side effects can also be *hidden*. Dr. Hyman Engelberg reported that he had treated thirty-nine patients with MER/29, but had to discontinue treating four of them because of toxic effects. These were still "open" side effects, but he also put his finger on a *hidden* side effect. Sixteen of his patients showed a drop in blood cholesterol. But in eight of the sixteen who exhibited this drop and in three who didn't, what occurred as a result of the MER/29 pill was far more harmful than high cholesterol: a large increase in blood fats.

There was also the possibility of another side effect that made some medical men uneasy. To understand their fear, let's see how this cholesterol "inhibitor" worked. The body in manufacturing its cholesterol starts with a simple chemical called an acetate, and builds step by step, through more than a dozen different chemicals to the final body-usable cholesterol. The next-to-last link in the chemical chain is called desmosterol. What MER/29 did was to inhibit its transformation into cholesterol.

And here's why medical men were concerned when the chemical synthesis is stopped at the desmosterol stage. Instead of cholesterol accumulating in the blood, desmosterol piles up. According to Drs. M. M. Best and C. H. Duncan (*American Cardiology Congress*, 1961), it is possible that desmosterol was even more dangerous to coronary health than cholesterol. Cataract of the eye is a condition caused by deposits of blood lipids and cholesterol. Now certain side effects of MER/29 made doctors worry that the accumulation of desmosterol could be responsible for even more cataracts than cholesterol.

Action was needed to prevent this possibly blinding side effect. The Food and Drug Administration now put pressure on the manufacturer, and early in 1962 the drug was quietly removed from the medical market.

In addition to the drugs analyzed so far—the estrogens and Triparanol—more than a hundred others have been developed. Most of them are laboratory curiosities, but one, nicotinic acid, is well known and widely used.

Doses of nicotinic acid *will* cut down the blood lipids, lower the concentration of beta-fatty particles and cholesterol, but again, not without harmful side effects. "At the onset of the treatment," according to Dr. K. G. Birge (*Geriatrics*, August, 1961), ". . . flushing . . . is experienced . . ."

The problem of biochemists was to produce a nicotinic acid variant *with* anti-blood-fat, anti-cholesterol action but *without* the side effect of flushing. But the new compound produced a different kind of side effect: gastric distress leading to ulcers. The search was on again, and a new variant was found which did eliminate the gastric problem. But still there were side effects such as liver damage and jaundice in some patients and high levels of gout-producing uric acid in others.

Birge's report isn't the end of the nicotinic acid side-effect story. Dr. William B. Parsons, Jr. in *Archives of Internal Medicine* also has reported many complaints after nicotinic-acid treatment: dryness of skin, localized roughness and pigmentation, and during the second year of treatment, increased uric-acid level and test results similar to those caused by liver damage. Dr. Parsons further discovered that in some patients nicotinic-acid therapy induces diabetes!

Dr. Herbert Pollack, in the *Journal of Diabetes*, warns doctors who see high-blood-sugar patients "to inquire . . . whether or not they have been taking nicotinic acid . . ." Of three cases referred to him, Pollack was able to identify the diabetic cause as nicotinic acid.

Dr. Birge's summation: "Because of these side effects and their possible long-term implications, the use of large doses of nicotinic acid must still be regarded as an investigational treatment . . ."

The search for *the* anti-coronary drug continues. As Dr. David Steinberg of the National Heart Institute points out, since 1956 there has been a tremendous intensification of activity, centered around the blood lipids as the main target.

Most anti-coronary drugs are aimed at, and their usefulness is measured by, the reduction of blood cholesterol, blood fat, lipoproteins (beta fatty particles) and the chylomicrons.

This type of research more than any other shows that the medical scientists today are almost all fully convinced that the solution to the heart attack problem lies in the reduction of our abnormally high content of fatty globules in the blood.

One cause of high blood fats is the exhaustion of heparin, which as we have seen is the activator of the "clearing factor." If heparin is exhausted, why not replenish the supply? But heparin is quickly destroyed by the digestive juices so it cannot be taken as a pill. It is very effective when injected, but this requires the careful supervision of a skilled physician.

It is possible that in the future, if the situation is not brought under control by the prevention program, that just as hundreds of thousands of diabetics have had to resort to daily injections of insulin, so perhaps millions of atherosclerotics may have to resort to injections of heparin.

Just as the exhaustion of heparin in the blood causes trouble in the last stages of the enzyme handling of fatty globules, so the exhaustion of the fat digestive enzymes in the digestive system may be the cause of trouble in the early stages.

DRUGS OR DIET
WHAT MEDICAL SCIENTISTS SAY

Medical scientists have been seeking drugs to remedy the deficiency of fat-digestion enzymes. However, since the lack of enzymes is due to a lifetime of high-saturated-fat diet, the logical question to be asked is: Which shall we rely on—drugs or diet?

Let the experts answer.

The National Heart Institute is the official heart-research

agency of the federal government. Dr. David Steinberg, on the staff of the Institute, states: "Since it is prophylactic [preventive] in nature and would presumably entail the administration of drugs to healthy individuals, and since the treatment would probably be administered over a very long period of time (essentially a lifetime treatment)—any drug proposed must be remarkably free of short-term or long-term effects . . ."

But Dr. Steinberg says further: "Will it be possible to find an agent sufficiently specific to interfere with one particular biosynthetic pathway without altering body metabolism in a deleterious fashion?"

Dr. Jeremiah Stammler, in charge of the Chicago Board of Health Heart-Disease-Control Program, is an accepted leader in this field. In summing up a panel discussion at the Annual American Heart Association Convention in October 1961, he said in part: "Methods of prevention must be safe, and no one is sure of the long-term effect of drugs. Prevention cannot be based on drugs. If the coronary disease is a product of a way of life of which diet is one factor, then use of drugs is irrational. Diet is better than drugs."

The Emeritus Professor of Medicine at Athens University, Dr. A. P. Cawadias, stated in 1962 that, "The usual egg and bacon breakfast is responsible for many coronaries —and could be replaced with a fish breakfast."

"The role of medicines in the prevention of the ischaemic [coronary] and thrombotic episodes of atherosclerosis is, in the present condition of our science, secondary."

Dr. Irvine H. Page, addressing a Symposium of the American Heart Association in January, 1961, reminded the cardiologists present that, "People don't like virtue, unfortunately . . . and they think it's easier to buy pills . . . I am inclined not to go along with people who want to take pills to accomplish something that should be accomplished by virtue."

In an editorial on the dangers of drugs which lower cholesterol in the blood, Drs. B. Lown, O. W. Portman and F. J. Stare of the Harvard School of Public Health made it clear that, "It is our view that at this stage of knowledge, drug therapy should be employed only by the investigator and conducted under careful clinical and laboratory supervision." And in the same report, in August, 1962, this group gave their conclusion: "Reduction of caloric intake, moderate restriction of fat consumption and a reasonable substitution of polyunsaturated fat comprise at the present time a reasonable and safe approach."

The consensus of medical opinion in one important group was shown in a poll taken on June 28, 1961 at a convention of the American Medical Association. At a session attended by physicians interested in atherosclerotic research, this author listened with interest when the Chairman, Dr. Edward H. Ahrens, of the Rockefeller Institute, said: "Cholesterol seems to be one of the main problems in coronary heart disease. I think at this stage of our knowledge of atherosclerosis, it wouldn't be a bad idea if we took a poll of the members present to get a picture of the latest thinking. What methods do you favor to lower blood cholesterol? Let's do it by a show of hands."

Dr. Ahrens then asked, "To lower blood cholesterol, how many of you are now in favor of the nutritional method, the low-saturated-fat diet?" Almost every voting hand went up.

"And now how many of you are in favor of the combination of the nutritional method plus some drugs?" Only three hands went up.

Dr. Ahrens paused. He was ready now for the final question. "And how many," asked Ahrens, "how many of you are in favor of drugs alone?" The doctors present looked about them.

Not a single hand was raised!

Diet is safer and more practical than drugs in the coronary prevention program. Yet diet is not the entire story. A dozen or more factors are involved.

The next chapter will deal with all the factors comprising the complete prevention program.

CHAPTER TWELVE

A Practical Heart-Attack Prevention Program

TWENTY FACTORS
INVOLVED IN CORONARY DISEASE

The researches of medical scientists during the past ten years have revealed the causes for the alarming increase in coronary-artery disease. At the same time they have laid the groundwork for a unified program designed to halt the increase in artery blockage, as well as to neutralize and reverse the conditions in the blood which cause it.

With so many factors relating to atherosclerosis, it would seem difficult to design a practical, unified anti-coronary program. But if we arrange all the factors under three basic headings, the practical simplicity of the anti-coronary program becomes evident.

Group 1 **The Uncontrollables**	*Age* *Sex* *Heredity* *Geography* *Climate* *Body Build*
Group 2 **The Semi-Controllables**	*Stress* *Occupation* *Location* *Endocrine Disorders*
Group 3 **The Controllables**	*Poor Tissue Tone* *Vitamin Deficiencies* *Infectious Disease* *Toxic Factors* *Smoking* *Constipation* *Exercise* *Obesity* *High Blood Pressure* *Nutrition*

The characteristic common to all the factors in Group One—the uncontrollables—is that we can't do anything about them. Understandably, research scientists study these factors, but for our direct anti-coronary program such researches have not yet proven to be of practical use.

Fortunately, the control which is possible over the factors in groups two and three can be of decisive importance in preventing heart attack or postponing its occurrence for many years.

In Group Two—the semicontrollables—are the factors of external and internal stress, both products of our social, economic and political environment. The cold war, the high cost of living, and dozens of other stress-producing situations face us at every turn, and few of us are lucky enough to escape any of them. It might be possible, for instance, to reduce the coronary danger by moving from a city to a rural area. There is a two-to-one ratio of coronary disease between highly industrialized parts of the country like California, New York and the New England states and the less densely-populated, less urbanized states of Arizona, North Dakota and New Mexico. But, of course, few of us are in a position economically to undertake such a move.

We might also change our place of work and seek out a situation with more compatible associates and a more understanding management, even if thereby our earning power is reduced. But our national psychology makes us fear such a change as a mark of failure, for it is contrary to the accepted social pattern of "upward mobility." Most of us, in changing jobs, seek to move to a "better" one, offering more responsibility and more money—and also more stress and a greater coronary probability.

In addition, the socially imposed goals set by television, the movies and the press, intensify the drive toward a "high level of happiness." It is when we are frustrated in reaching the success goals with which we equate happiness that the major effects of stress make themselves felt.

We can see that coping with the semicontrollables is largely a matter of individual initiative. A person can conceivably alter his individual coronary-stress profile by resisting the national mania for setting his goal too far beyond his actual capacity. This is a problem that each individual has to try to solve for himself.

HOW YOU CAN PROTECT YOURSELF

Now we come to the third set of factors—coronary-influencing factors over which we have considerable control. These fall into two general groups: Those which affect the artery wall and those which influence the fatty composition of the arterial blood.

The main factor affecting the artery wall is poor *tissue tone*. Weak tissue, unhealthy and easily inflamed, is most prone to lipid damage. A major cause of weak tissue tone is a deficiency of essential vitamins and minerals.

Another cause of poor artery-tissue tone is infection. Infectious and virus disease may produce weakening inflammation of the artery lining and predispose it to the growth of artery blockage.

High blood pressure in combination with high blood lipids and poor tissue tone are the basis for artery blockage. With all three factors low, the arteries will remain clean. But the combined effects of all three can bring on a heart attack at an early age.

There are three main non-drug methods of keeping blood pressure normal: The low-salt diet; elimination of toxins in food and environment; and the avoidance of stress situations. All three are part of the prevention program.

Toxins present in our food also disturb the lipid metabolism, thus causing excessive blood fats. Currently there are over 700 chemical food additives in use. Of these only about half have been tested for toxicity by the Food and Drug Administration and even these have not been subjected to thorough, long term tests. How can we eliminate the possibly toxic substances in our foods? We can do it by strengthening the powers and increasing the facilities of the Food and Drug Administration so that it may properly test all food additives and forbid the use of those found even slightly toxic. In the meantime it would be wise to avoid as many of the packaged foods containing food additives and preservatives as possible.

Poisons in the air such as smog, smoke fumes, etc., also help trigger the "lipid mobilizing" hormone, but these poisons are more difficult to avoid.

And in addition to atomic fallout, there is insecticide and pesticide fallout which clings—invisibly—to our food.

The insidious presence of these factors is revealed only by the clinical medical report of the physician. The only effective method of getting rid of any of these coronary-promoting toxic factors is through social legislation.

Among the toxic factors one can control and eliminate are cigarettes, which impressive statistics now also prove to be a powerful factor in promoting coronary disease.

Another little-known cause of increased blood cholesterol that is directly under our control is constipation. It is the slowing down of the intestinal motion by constipation which causes excessive reabsorption and reutilization of bile and a consequent piling up of cholesterol in the blood. In the Prudent Diet "empty calories" are replaced by fruit and vegetables, and the extra fiber content naturally speeds up the elimination process.

Now we come to exercise, the easiest and yet the most difficult of all the controllable anti-coronary factors.

Exercise is easy because it costs nothing and is available to almost everybody. One obstacle to it is our modern pushbutton civilization, which almost eliminates the need of physical effort. Another difficulty is time. In this hurried life exercise has been crowded out of our daily program. A half-hour a day should be given over to exercise for the full value of the anti-coronary program to be realized. Exercise is also the second key to the overweight problem. In controlling obesity, a low-calorie diet is essential, but it must be combined with a proper exercise program.

If we re-examine the multifaceted causes of atherosclerosis—the uncontrollables, the semi-controllables and the controllables—we see that almost all of them exert their effects by acting directly and indirectly on the blood-lipid metabolism. This knowledge points the way to the final and most important phase of the whole coronary-prevention plan—the lowering, normalizing and stabilizing of the blood lipids by means of proper diet. This phase of the coronary-prevention program is so important that the next four sections are devoted exclusively to the Prudent Diet.

DR. JOLLIFFE'S ANTI-CORONARY CLUB AND THE PRUDENT DIET

The evidence is in. The rich American Diet stands convicted as the major cause of the current coronary epidemic. There is now no doubt, even in the minds of the most skeptical scientific specialists, that changes must be made in our customary fare.

But what changes? And how many? What must we give up, and what are the expected gains in terms of added years of life?

As yet, the answer is incomplete. Though there isn't enough data for an exact estimate, the Anti-Coronary Club has supplied evidence on which to base a rough guess. By cutting down on several simple foods, such as butter, eggs and dairy products, for example, and following a few simple Prevention Program rules, we may be able to reduce our heart-attack rate to one fifth the present expectancy.

Whether this will add two years or ten years to a specific life span, no one can prophesy. But this is certain: the adherence to an anti-coronary diet will not only add years to our life, but more important, it can add vitality to our years.

The effectiveness of the anti-coronary diet has been proven by the final research project of the late Dr. Norman Jolliffe.

Aware of the low rates of coronary among other peoples of the world, he felt that the high rate among Americans was inexcusable. Dr. Jolliffe was certain that something could be done. What's more, his clinical knowledge and background in nutritional research, combined with his experience in preventive medicine, uniquely qualified him to undertake a project destined to make medical history.

Dr. Jolliffe decided to make a public trial on an anti-coronary diet designed to be part of a complete anti-coronary program. As Director of the New York City Bureau of Nutrition, he was in a position to influence Dr. Leona Baumgartner, who was then the Commissioner of Health, to sign the executive order creating the New York City Anti-Coronary Club.

The nucleus of the Anti-Coronary Club was a group of four hundred volunteers, most of whom joined as a result of a single small newspaper advertisement. The volunteers were permitted to live in their own homes, carry on their work and social life exactly as before, and to continue all normal activities, with these exceptions: (1) change in diet, (2) restricted smoking, and (3) increased exercise by daily walking.

The other scientists associated with the study were Dr.

Seymour Rinzler and Morton Archer, a medical statistician. Archer carefully analyzed the data on coronary-heart disease from the Framingham Study. From these figures he could predict the normal incidence rates of each member in the Coronary Club if no changes in living habits were made.

But the Anti-Coronary Club was not to be an inactive group. This was its essential difference from the Framingham Study. The Massachusetts group was merely observed for the purpose of compiling medical statistics. There was no attempt during the experiment to induce them to make the slightest change in their way of life. In effect, the Framingham Study was to serve as the "control group" for the Anti-Coronary Club Study.

The 400 "human guinea pigs" were to be *active* participants. They were to learn just what caused heart attack and to understand the theory behind the course of action they were to take. They were to accomplish their life-saving feat by the simplest but most effective weapon—education. They were taught the principles of the Prudent Diet, the diet low in saturated fats but supplemented by adequate unsaturated fats.

The 400 volunteers lived on this diet, and Dr. Jolliffe studied their reactions to it. He took blood samples, recorded weight, and kept an eye on the members' general health.

It was primarily a reduction in the consumption of fat meat, eggs, fat cheese, butter, milk, ordinary margarines, and hydrogenated shortening. The volunteers were warned that many commercially manufactured, baked, canned and processed foods contain these forbidden ingredients and were to be avoided.

For the banned foods, there were adequate substitutes: vegetable oils, fish, lean meats, whole grains, skim milk, non-fat cheese, vegetables and fruits.

And one more very important rule was enforced; the club members were to reduce their weight and exercise more. So important was weight-reduction that members who failed in this respect were "suspended."

It was expected at first that about half of the group would become discouraged and drop out. These drop-outs were to have served as a control group. But contrary to expectations, almost all the members remained in the club.

The most important method of weight reduction, according to the Prudent Diet was the elimination of "empty calories." It is interesting to note that both of these important descriptive terms, the Prudent Diet and "empty calories" were originated by Dr. Jolliffe and have now gained world-wide acceptance.

"Empty calories" is an expression used to describe foods denatured by the commercial food manufacturers. In many cases, commercial processing of foods robs them of vitamins, minerals, enzymes, and other vital ingredients they naturally contain.

The most glaring example is sugar, which Dr. Jolliffe held up as the "pure" example of "empty calories." Other "empty-calorie" foods are (1) highly refined white flour (2) most saturated fats and (3) foods made by combining sugar with highly refined flour and saturated fats, such as most commercial baked goods.

The simple elimination of most of the "empty calories" was considered an important step in the Prudent Diet. Cereals, whole grains and vegetables were to replace the "empty calories."

After four years of the Prudent Diet, Morton Archer had compiled all the statistics on coronary disease in the Anti-Coronary Club. How did they compare with the predictions based on the Framingham Experiment? In 1962 the New York State Medical Society heard the official results. Dr. Rinzler reported: In the group of 400 "human guinea pigs," 25 "coronary events" might have been expected, but only 4 had occurred. The Prudent Diet had reduced the coronary rate by 500%!

This was front-page news. A method that could effectively combat the coronary epidemic had been scientifically demonstrated.

Anti-Coronary Clubs have spread to other American cities. Dr. Connor, rediscoverer of the harmful effects of diet cholesterol, is the head of a "Cardiovascular Clinic" in Dayton, Ohio. The Chicago Club is led by the eminent cardiac authority and head of that city's Board of Health, Dr. Jeremiah Stamler. Other clubs are operating in Los Angeles, Newark, Albany, Milwaukee and other cities.

In all these clubs the program followed is much like Dr. Jolliffe's. Emphasis is placed on the elimination of harmful foods in the diet and the substitution of proper natural foods.

There are minor variations in emphasis among the various groups. For instance, in Dayton, where Dr. Connor made his historic experiments on diet cholesterol, charts are used showing how to cut down on the high-cholesterol-containing foods. In Chicago, Dr. Stamler has placed added emphasis on the elimination of "empty calories."

The Prudent Diet, weight reduction, and exercise program recommended by the Anti-Coronary Clubs is producing anti-coronary results. But have any *harmful* side effects been noted? The doctors, researchers, statisticians, technicians, and nurses from New York to Los Angeles who have participated in the program answer "No."

Some of the additional advantages to be gained by the use of the Prudent Diet are listed below:

- The effects of the Prudent Diet on the blood lipids is (1) to reduce those which are in excess (2) to normalize the alpha to beta ratio and (3) to increase the stability of the globules.
- The Prudent Diet is medically recognized as the best type of reducing diet.
- The Prudent Diet is now becoming adopted by Diabetes Clinics as the standard diet.
- There are other metabolic ailments (as will be shown later) which are normalized by the Prudent Diet.
- There is no illness (known or hidden) which can be aggravated by the Prudent Diet.
- The Prudent Diet is PRUDENT.

THE FOODS
MOST DIFFICULT TO GIVE UP

How much discipline, motivation and self-control is required of those on the Prudent Diet?

In answering the question, which foods are the hardest to give up, Dr. Rinzler of the New York Anti-Coronary Club listed Danish pastry, coffee cake, plain cake, cookies and pies. For those who could not abstain from these favorite foods, his solution was home-baking using vegetable oils instead of butter, cream and other ingredients containing saturated fat and cholesterol.

This will not impose a lifelong burden on the harassed housewife. It will probably not take very long for the small as well as the large bakers to feel the economic pinch, and within a few years there should appear countless advertisements proclaiming the virtues of cake made wtih pure, unsaturated vegetable oil.

Dr. George James, the present New York City Commissioner of Health, has predicted that "during the next ten years . . . industry will have provided a large selection of low saturated—high polyunsaturated fat foods."

Another deprivation which caused "unhappiness," according to Dr. Rinzler, was the prohibition of ice cream, although the number of people favoring it was considerably less than those who had the Danish-pastry "habit." In Canada, Dr. Horlick, in his anti-coronary group, devised a permissible corn-oil ice cream.

Dr. Rinzler's next effort was to make the club members aware of the importance of reducing the size of the portions they ate, especially that of meat, which often contains deceptively large amounts of "invisible" fat. A major problem of our affluent society is the economic ease with which three-quarter-pound meat portions appear on our dinner plates. Says Dr. Rinzler, "in a balanced diet containing adequate calories, no normal subject need more than three or four ounces of animal flesh daily."

Surprisingly enough, the prohibition of butter and whole milk presented no difficulties to Dr. Rinzler's charges. For those who would not throw away their butter knives, various kinds of substitute spreads were devised. Among them was non-fat cottage cheese mixed with vegetable oil. Skim milk, fortified with added dry skim milk powder, was a satistfactory milk substitute when required.

All these recommendations are easy enough to carry out at home. Those who eat in restaurants may meet with difficulties at first. But, says Dr. Rinzler, "If a person can afford to eat in restaurants where the food is prepared to order, no problem exists."

However, for those who can only afford to eat in cafeterias, where the food is mass produced, some care is required. Here the recommended entree is fish or poultry, which preferably should be broiled, baked or boiled. Restaurant desserts are easy to decide on. They should be limited to fruits.

But can we rely upon the verbal reports of the club members as proof of their diet's palatability? What if they did not adhere to the Prudent Diet? Dr. Rinzler had two methods of checking. One was the blood-cholesterol index, the other was the actual drop in coronary rate over the years.

But Dr. Dayton in Los Angeles, who did not have the early start of the New York group, used a more rapid check-up method to see just what his people were eating. Actual "needle" biopsies of the stored fat on the club members' hips were chemically analyzed to measure the change from the hard, saturated body-fat accumulated on the usual American diet to the softer, unsaturated, multi-hinged type which, little by little, had replaced the old fat. This gradual change was the proof that the club members were adhering to the proper prevention diet.

Though having a biopsy taken is painful, so anxious were Dr. Dayton's charges to reduce their coronary-attack rates, that those who were inadvertently omitted were quick to complain about being overlooked.

One way to estimate how difficult it is to adhere to the Prudent Diet is by the number of people who continue to stay with it.

In the New York Anti-Coronary Club, at least, the difficulties cannot have been excessive, judging by the relatively small number of drop-outs.

Dr. Rinzler and Dr. Dayton were not the only ones who reported how easy it was for their coronary-club members to stay with the new program.

In the experience of Dr. Leon Swell at the School of Medicine of the George Washington University:

". . . This dietary regimen . . . was readily accepted by the family and required no adjustment or marked change in the family dietary habits."

An important factor in the attitude toward the Prudent Diet is the conviction concerning its *safety* as well as its other values. Dr. Ancel Keys recently stated: "I have no hesitation in my choice. Because the required dietary change is perfectly safe, is not expensive and can be made with *little or no sacrifice in longtime eating pleasure,* I conclude that it is wise to accept it."

NINE ELEMENTS OF AN ANTI-CORONARY DIET

The Western nations, with only one-third of the world's population, have three-quarters of the world's food supply. According to Rodger Dajoz' UNESCO report, there are about six pounds of food per person available in the United

States for every pound available to an Asian or African.

With this superabundance of food, we are eating our way into heart attack.

But in order to lower our high rate of heart attack, it is not necessary to adopt a Spartan diet. There are more pleasant ways to achieve the same result. Our magnificent variety of foods is unparalleled in history. Even the Roman emperors at their sumptuous banquets did not have the choice of foods available to the American housewife today.

The anti-coronary program starts in the local super-market. The problem is one of selection. To choose the foods that will combine good coronary health, good general health and enjoyable eating does not demand too much extra time or money; just a bit more knowledge of the nature of our foods.

Milk

One doesn't ordinarily regard this as a high-fat food, but it is. By calorie count, it contains 30% carbohydrates and 25% proteins, but its fat-calorie content is almost as great as that of the carbohydrates and protein combined—45 per cent. In addition, the fat of milk is of an extremely saturated type which should be almost entirely eliminated from the diet.

Since most cheese is made from whole milk, its average high-saturated-fat content is the same as in milk.

It is difficult to obtain non-fat cottage cheese or others made entirely from skim milk or whey, such as "Jack," "Sapsago" and "Slim Cheez." But this is the only type permitted on the Prudent Diet.

Meat

Under the old meat-grading system, the marbled, highest-fat meat was labeled Grade "A." But the meat industry, informed by its merchandising experts that the public was turning away from the fat meats, is now producing animals of the old-fashioned lean type. In accordance with the meat-industry's change the government has newly relabeled the leanest meat as First Grade.

But although the meat industry is advertising "modern *lean* animals" in the medical journals, and the U. S. government has reversed its grading procedures accordingly, this does not automatically assure you of lean meat in the butcher shop.

Getting the butcher to trim the fat off the *not-yet* "modern lean animals" is a complex psychological-economic battle. But since more fat on the butcher's block will mean less fat and cholesterol in your family's blood, a defeat in the butcher shop must be corrected in the kitchen.

Meat should be limited to small portions served only three to five times a week.

Gravy and meat soups should be prepared for use by first removing their very high-saturated-fat content. The usual procedure is to chill the gravy or soup in the refrigerator and remove the top cake of hard grease. The non-fat portion is permissible.

Poultry

Chicken and turkey fat is less saturated than beef or lamb fat and also contains a fair amount of polyunsaturated fats. For this reason the anti-coronary program recommends serving less beef and lamb and comparatively more chicken and turkey.

However, these meats contain enough saturated fats to make restrictions necessary. The skin and other parts should be discarded if they are fatty.

Duck and goose are exceptionally high in both saturated fat and cholesterol and have no place in the program.

Fish

The Prudent Diet recommends a general reduction in meat and an increase in the consumption of fish for the following reasons:

1. Fish contain much less cholesterol than does meat.
2. Lean fish have a very low fat content.
3. Fat fish—as well as lean—contain a type of fat which is very high in polyunsaturates which are highly recommended for the Prudent Diet.
4. Fish tends to decrease blood cholesterol while meat tends to increase it due to differences in the type of fat content.
5. Fish contain much less calories per serving than meat.
6. Fish proteins are equal in quality to those of meat.

Salad Dressings

The best way to introduce the ounce or more per day of vegetable oil into the diet is to use salad dressings.

Choose only those commercial salad dressings made with corn, safflower or cottonseed oil.

Usually, they run a bit high in salt content. There are two ways to overcome this. First learn to make your own salad dressing, second, extend the commercial salad dressing with added safflower or corn oil.

Margarine

Why is margarine not allowed? First: many margarines contain an excessive amount of hydrogenated fat—which is the worst type of super-saturated fat. Second: even the *best* of todays so called "pure oil" margarines still contain too much hydrogenated oil and so even the *best* is still *harmful*.

To make the general knowledge of the saturated and polyunsaturated fats of practical value, a chart is provided which shows the average amounts of these substances found in some of the popular foods in our diet.

Eggs and Cholesterol

Until our egg farmers make up their minds that the public is demanding an anti-coronary diet, they will not make the necessary changes and try to market a "natural," old-fashioned egg. This can only be obtained from hens let out of their mass-production "battery" cages and permitted the free-range foods—grass, insects and worms— enriched with vegetable-oil supplements.

However, even natural eggs will still remain a highly concentrated source of cholesterol. The chick naturally requires the 250 milligrams of cholesterol found in the yolk, and there is no research to show how to eliminate this product of evolution.

Since the 25 milligrams is double the daily maximum allowed by Dr. Connor (who did the pioneer research on diet and blood cholesterol), even "natural" eggs will have to be severely restricted.

A chart on dietary cholesterol content of the principal cholesterol containing foods follows. By properly choosing the amount of each of the animal protein foods, it will be possible to prevent our diet cholesterol from going out of bounds.

FATS AND OILS			• POLY UNSATURATED %	
			• SATURATED %	
PREDOMINANTLY	CORN	OIL	10	55
POLY	SAFFLOWER	OIL	8	72
UNSATURATED	SOY BEAN	OIL	15	52
MULTI-HINGED	SESAME	OIL	14	44
TYPE OF FAT	COTTONSEED	OIL	25	50
FOUND IN	ALL THIN	OIL	Low	High
SEEDS	WALNUT	NUTS	7	70
NUTS	ALMOND	NUTS	5	20
AND FISH.	PECAN	NUTS	6	22
THESE	WHEAT	GERM	15	54
OILS	OAT	MEAL	22	42
REDUCE	SUNFLOWER	SEEDS	12	63
BLOOD	ALL	SEEDS	Low	High
CHOLESTEROL.	ALL FISH FAT		Low	High
	CHICKEN	FAT	23	24
INTERMEDIATE	OLIVE	OIL	11	7
	PEANUT	OIL	20	26
HARD	BUTTER	FAT	55	3
SATURATED	DAIRY	FAT	55	3
ANIMAL	BEEF	FAT.	48	2
FATS	EGG	YOLK	32	7
INCREASE	LAMB	FAT	56	3
BLOOD	COCONUT	FAT	86	0
CHOLESTEROL.	HYDROGENATED	FAT	High	0

Food Cholesterol Chart
milligrams per 100 grams (3½ ounces)

Brains	2,000	Lobster	200
Egg Yolk	1,500	Shrimp	150
Duck	760	Crab	150
Liver (beef)	600	Cheese	150
Pork-Spareribs	600	Beef	110
Kidney	400	Veal	80
Oyster	325	Breast of chicken	80
Butter	300	Most fish	50
Calf Liver	300	Vegetables (all)	0

AN ANTI-CORONARY FOOD SHOPPING GUIDE

The problems involved in the double hazard of saturated fats and cholesterol in the diet make food selection a bit more complicated. To solve this problem, there are the guides to the food departments.

These guides are based on Dr. Jolliffe's Prudent Diet as well as diets from other Anti-Coronary groups in operation throughout the country. At first some of these recommendations may seem excessively restrictive. For those who are not yet fully convinced of the necessity for making the changes, further reading of the latest scientific findings on the causes and prevention of coronary heart disease may provide an added incentive.

Guide to the Meat and Poultry Department

The prudent purchaser should avoid all meats with thick or fine veins of fat and remember that even when well-trimmed, "marbled meats" still have a high fat content. Instruct your butcher to closely trim off all visible fats. Do your own grinding of lean meat.

Especially avoid meat in which the fat is inextricably bound such as tongue, bacon, rib cuts and others.

It is of almost no use to separate the good meat cuts from the bad by a simple list. The fat content of every cut varies widely depending upon how each particular animal was fed. Today all meat selection must be made by eye in order to be sure that it is fat free.

DON'T use:	DO use:
All Fatty Cuts	All Lean Cuts
All Rib Cuts	Such As:
Tongue: invisible fat	Lamb-Lean
Duck: high both in fat and cholesterol	Veal—Lean
	Beef—Red Only

Use organ meat in strict moderation. Consult cholesterol chart.

Guide to the Fish Department

Fish is high in poly-unsaturated fats and low in cholesterol and is therefore an excellent food which should be served more often.

DON'T use:	DO use:
Salted fish, such as herring	All fresh and frozen fish.
Do use: in strict moderation: smoked fish	Canned fish packed in corn oil and cottonseed oil to be preferred to those packed in olive oil.
Because of the relatively high cholesterol content, be moderate in the use of shell fish. (Consult the cholesterol chart.)	

Guide to the Fat and Oil Department

Almost all seed oils are high in the beneficial poly-unsaturated fats.

DON'T use:	DO use:
Animal fats	Corn oil
Butter	Safflower oil
Cream	Other *thin* vegetable oils. (See oil list.)
All margarines	
Hydrogenated fats, in any form or quantity	Salad dressings made with corn and safflower oil
Mayonnaise	Nuts which are high in poly-unsaturated fats: Almonds, Walnuts
Nuts high in saturated fats: Cashew and Brazil	
Daily maximum of saturated fats to be *one ounce*, and preferably much less.	Sunflower seeds
	Daily maximum of vegetable and fish oils and fats to be *two* ounces.

Note: The combined amounts of ALL types of fats in the diet to be 2¼ ounces—or 20% of the total calories—whichever is less.

Guide to the Dairy Food Department

All fatty dairy foods must be eliminated or severely curtailed, with the exception of skim milk and non-fat cheese.

DON'T use:	DO use:
	(in moderation only)
Butter	Non-fat dry milk
Whole milk	Skim milk
Cheese (except those made from skim milk)	Buttermilk and yogurt made from skim milk
Sweet or sour cream	Uncreamed cottage cheese
Whipped cream	Other cheeses made from skim milk
Eggs (a *maximum* of two or three yolks a week, including those in prepared foods).	

Guide to the Delicatessen Department

It is hard to decide which are more potentially harmful, the dairy or the delicatessen foods. The saturated-fat calories in many delicatessen items average about seventy per cent of the total.

Delicatessen foods also contain harmful ingredients other than high-saturated fat. They are high in salt, used in pickling and preserving, and have a high content of toxic chemicals used to prevent decomposition.

DON'T use:	DO use:
Corned beef	The only foods which are permitted for use (if necessary) from the Delicatessen Department are the home-style prepared foods, such as:
Sausage	
Liverwurst	
Bologna	
Frankfurters	
Salami	
Pastrami	Roast Beef
Luncheon meats	Roast Turkey
Canned meats	Roast Chicken

Guide to the Dessert Department

Don't use any desserts or baked foods made with saturated fats and eggs. These fats, combined with sugar, generate an extra cholesterol-promoting effect.

DON'T use:	Permissible:
Custards and rich desserts	Fruit
Commercial Pies and Pastries, etc.	Home-made "frozen desserts" based on vegetable oils and honey.
Commercial baked cakes of any type, including: PLAIN CAKE POUND CAKE DANISH PASTRY COOKIES etc.	Home prepared gelatin desserts flavored with fruit and honey. Use in moderation: Home-baked cakes, pies, cookies, made without saturated fats, based instead on corn or safflower oil and honey.
Whipped Cream Cakes	
Frozen Creams	
Ice Cream	
Candy, chocolate	
Sweet food in general	

Guide to the Fruit and Vegetable Department

Vegetables and fruits may be used in any amount and variety, limited only by your weight scale.

DON'T use:	DO use:
Canned vegetables packed with salt.	All fruits and vegetables— preferably fresh.
Canned fruits with added sugar.	Whole grains, legumes and root vegetables.
Frozen fruits or juices with added sugar.	Use in moderation only: Canned or frozen fruits or juices with no sugar added. Canned or frozen vegetables.

Snack Foods for Social Gatherings

Snack foods are neatly intertwined with television and socializing. Their harmful effects show up on the weight scale and in the cholesterol count. With planning and ingenuity, many delicious anti-coronary snacks can be made.

DON'T use:	DO use:
Package crackers (usually made with hydrogenated oils and heavily salted)	Whole-grain crackers
	Fruit (fresh, dry)
Cheese and cheese crackers	Nuts (walnuts, almonds, pecans, peanuts, sunflower seeds)
Commercial Potato Chips	
Commercial "Dips"	Carrot and Celery sticks
Delicatessen Foods	Fish, meat and vegetable tid-bits
Candy, Chocolate	
Cookies, Cakes	Other foods on the Do Use Lists
Ice Cream	

Bread

Most commercial breads contain varying amounts of saturated fats such as hydrogenated fats, milk, egg yolks, and sometimes butter. Also, most white breads are "hollow foods," owing to the ultra-refining of the white flour.

Today, in every sizeable city, stores can be found that sell good home-style, whole-wheat loaves with labels clearly stating that none of the saturated fats have been used. Also examine the label for additives and any type of "preservative," which should be avoided.

. . . and Potatoes

Few foods are the cause of more misinformation than the potato. Although usually classed as a food to avoid in a reducing diet, it contains no more calories than an apple or orange. The same is true of the other starchy vegetables: beans, peas, rice, barley, buckwheat, etc.

As to quantity, this is another matter. The daily conference with the scale will be the deciding factor here.

ANTI-CORONARY RECIPE IDEAS FOR PEOPLE WHO ENJOY TASTY FOODS

Is the price we must pay for a longer life on the Prudent Diet the loss of gourmet pleasures? Must we not throw away all our treasured recipes and give up all tasty food? Far from it.

Pick up a good French cook book, and nearly half the recipes in it can be used, almost unchanged.

This is also true of recipes from Chinese and Japanese cook books. Other cook books, such as Greek and Armenian, also contain many usable recipes. This is to be expected. These nations are noted for their low coronary rate and the very low amounts of saturated fat in their diet.

But French cooking is generally regarded as the richest in the world. How then can so many French recipes be incorporated in the Prudent Diet?

In part the "richness" of French cooking is a myth. The richness in taste lies mostly in flavors imparted by onions, garlic, mushrooms, herbs, and spices, rather than in the fat content of the basic foods.

Take a mouth-watering steak prepared by a good French cook. It actually conforms quite satisfactorily to the requirements of the anti-coronary diet. The French butcher has already trimmed away most of the excess fat (which was not a great deal, since the grass-fed French cow is leaner than its "corn fed" American counterpart). Then the good French cook gets to work and completes the trimming job with her sharp little knife.

True, a little butter may be spread on the meat, but this is not essential, for it is the herbs, garlic and mushroom flavors that the French cook depends on to give it its incomparable taste. Compare this to an American-style sirloin steak, which depends mainly on the brown fat for flavor.

A French dish internationally known as a gastronomic triumph is bouillabaise, which knowing gourmets speak of with reverence. And yet it fits in quite well with the Prudent Diet. The usual recipe for bouillabaise is based almost entirely on varieties of fish expertly seasoned and served as a thick soup. The only caution is to go easy on the use of shellfish.

So we see that many favorite cook-book recipes with a few minor substitutions can be included in the Prudent Diet. All that is needed is to exercise an awareness of the ingredients in order to make the proper selections.

It might help to circle in red the recipes in favorite cookbooks that do *not* lean on eggs, butter, milk, cream, cheese and other saturated fats. These recipes are probably suitable for inclusion in the Prudent Diet. For those with international food tastes, the anti-coronary diet will present no problem.

But individuals who favor good, old-fashioned American food are in trouble because traditional American cooking is rich in all types of saturated fats. The utmost caution and knowledge will have to be used in trying to salvage the American cook book. But again, by means of a few simple substitutions, many recipes can be kept in our diet.

Substitution Number One is vegetable oil for butter, margarine and other hydrogenated shortenings. The conventional American cook book does not stint on butter. So we must find a substitute which, even if it doesn't have the distinctive taste of butter, will be just as pleasant in its own way. Flavored vegetable oils can be perfect taste substitutes. Herbs, spices, garlic, onions and other ingredients will impart an exciting and distinctive taste and aroma.

Here are a few simple oil flavors: *Onions fried in corn oil*. The oil acquires a flavor resembling that of rendered chicken fat; and the well-fried onion rings are also very tasty. *Salad dressing flavors*. The simple, practical way is to mix, in equal portions, any Italian style salad dressing with additional plain corn oil. This can be used successfully as a substitute for butter in garnishing cooked vegetables or for seasoning mashed potatoes.

In most cases no special preparation is required and a vegetable oil can be substituted for butter in many cook book recipes.

Subsitution Number Two is skim milk for the usual whole-fat milk. Sometimes reinforcement with skim-milk powder is advisable to maintain a creamy quality. In other recipes an extra bit of oil may be added when necessary. The omission of the butter-fat portion of the milk will generally go unnoticed.

Substitution Number Three is a replacement for the fatty cheeses. This is not easy to find. The use of non-fat cheeses such as uncreamed cottage cheese with a bit of flavored oil will often do as a substitute. But since there is no substitute for some of the more distinctive cheeses, it may be best to get used to doing without these flavors.

Substitution Number Four is a replacement for eggs. This is going to call for much ingenuity. It is just an unfortunate fact of life that the egg is one of the main troublemakers in coronary disease. It is difficult and often impossible to find an acceptable substitute to replace the mixing, thickening, sticking, hardening and other mechanical-chemical virtues of the egg.

Since the coronary-promoting components of the egg reside mostly in the yolk, it is often suggested that egg white alone be used as a substitute. This may be satisfactory now and then, but the continual throwing out of yolks is too wasteful for the average person. There is a dry, eggwhite powder on the market, but this is rarely used except by commercial firms.

Where the egg seems indispensable the recipe must be abandoned or used only within the limited weekly egg quota. But, fortunately, this is not always the case. In most recipes the eggs were added as an afterthought, to make the dish richer. Here the omission of the eggs will not damage the recipe.

Substitution Number Five is spices and herbs for salt. The replacement of salt with spices in recipes is both difficult and easy. It is difficult because at first the absence of salt is very obvious and has to be artfully compensated for by extra herbs, spices, and other food flavors. Later on, however, it is easy because experience has proven that after six months on a "no-salt" diet, the craving for salt usually disappears—and no substitution is required.

By now, interest in the anti-coronary diet has grown and there are many anti-coronary cook books. They have been published mostly during the past few years, and the popularity of this type of cooking is growing. The expert cook can create her own anti-coronary cook book out of the old ones with the use of the five substitutions just mentioned.

However, the anti-coronary cook books already in the book stores can save much time and energy. A list of such books will be found in the appendix.

CHAPTER THIRTEEN

Medical Facts
About Reducing Weight

EXPOSING THE "CALORIES DON'T COUNT" DIET

The problem of overweight has bedeviled this country for many years. In 1922, Dr. E. P. Joslin, founder of the Boston Joslin Diabetes Clinic, ranked the use of the bathroom scale in degenerative disease comparable in value to that of the thermometer in acute illness. Today it is generally accepted that overweight predisposes a person not only to diabetes, but also to high blood pressure and high blood lipids and eventually to heart attack.

There is nothing in preventive medicine that has been the subject of as much myth and misinformation as that of weight reduction.

One of the reasons for this is the fact that clinical weight reduction has such low prestige value in the medical profession. By now there have been so many machines, gadgets and "methods" introduced by non-medical "experts" that everything in this field has been labeled *charlatanism*.

In addition the overweight person is too often in the grip of an overwhelming psychological compulsion originating in the powerful and primitive hunger instinct.

Simple admonitions, usually followed in other illnesses, are of no use. Unless the physician can indicate some immediate possible disaster, there is often little hope of change. So failure, in the eyes of the practitioner, seems inevitable and treatment only a waste of time. As a result of these and other reasons, research in weight reduction has lagged.

With the whole field of weight reduction relatively abandoned by the research scientists, faddists and pseudo scientists have rushed in. There is no need for surprise therefore when year after year new panaceas are first proclaimed and then dropped in favor of the latest seven-day wonder. So the regrettable lack of medical criticism of the most recent "Calories Don't Count" method is easily explained, although not condoned.

Weight reduction is usually treated merely as a matter of "burning up" more calories than we eat. But since not all weight loss takes place through oxidation or "burning," this is an oversimplification. We must find the specific answer to the question of *what* substances are being reduced and *how* they are being reduced.

Three main body substances are involved in weight changes: fat, protein and—most puzzling of all—water. Until the mystery of water retention was cleared up a few years ago, it was difficult to explain the failures in weight-reducing programs.

But once we have the answer to the weight reducing failures induced by water retention, we will also have the secret of the incredibly foolish "Calories Don't Count" myth which has caused untold confusion and possibly serious damage to countless numbers of its innocent victims.

We can get rid of excess protein and fat in the body only by "burning up" this excess. But one pound of pure body fat contains about 3,500 calories, which even if no food were eaten, is more than can be used up in a hard day's work. Weight changes due to reduction in body fat take place very slowly.

The number of calories in a pound of pure fat is almost the same as that in two pounds of dry protein. But protein in the form of muscle tissues is combined with a great deal of water. The fact is that a pound of fat has the same caloric value as eight pounds of muscle, which consists of two pounds of protein and six pounds of water.

The most dramatic and rapid means of losing weight is through loss of body water, a method which has nothing at all to do with "burning up" of calories. Body weight is sixty percent water, a large part of which is not "locked" in chemical combinations. By losing or gaining water, we can alter our weight—up or down—by a dozen pounds.

Doctors frequently prescribe drugs, when it is medically necessary, whose chemical action causes large weight reductions through loss of water from the tissues which is then eliminated in the urine. Here, then, is what appears to be an easy and painless method of weight reduction. But the water-removing drug can only be taken for a limited time, and when the drugs are discontinued, the lost water is quickly regained.

Now we can begin to understand the reasons for apparent failures in many weight-reduction programs.

The quick changes in weight due to shifts in water content can mask the slow changes in weight caused by the intake and combustion of calories.

For instance, we can put on a pound of solid fat and simultaneously lose five pounds of water and be under the illusion that we are on a "reducing diet."

THE FALSE "SUCCESS" WHICH DECEIVES THE CALORIES-DON'T-COUNT "REDUCER"

The water-loss reaction is the reason for the popularity of many "trick" diets, especially the well-known "Calories Don't Count" Diet, which urges the obese individual to eat a very high fat diet, luring him with the unattainable promise of continuous and safe weight reduction.

This is not a safe method of weight reduction, nor will it "melt away" fat as claimed, unless the food calories are just as low as on any other weight-reducing diet; in fact,

the whole "Calories Don't Count" diet is scientifically incorrect from every possible point of view.

But it does bring about the seemingly amazing quick loss
of weight, and even though it is temporary, this effect often
leads the trusting individual into the belief that here at last
is the "eating way" to reduce. It took the combination of
two recent research projects on both sides of the Atlantic
to demonstrate the scientific reason for the temporary loss
of water weight at the start of a high-fat diet.

The first one came from the St. Georges Hospital in London, where Dr. T. R. E. Pilkington and his associates did
extensive work on weight reduction.

With two groups of patients on sparse 1,000 calories a
day diets, one of which was a normal mixed diet and the
other mostly fat, Dr. Pilkington and his collaborators observed the expected, steady, daily loss in weight on both
diets.

Now a third diet was tried consisting of exactly the
same 1,000 calories, but mostly carbohydrates. Immediately the weight loss stopped. In fact weight began to increase, and remained up for almost two weeks, before it
started down again.

Why was there a temporary gain in weight? Dr. Pilkington gives the answer. The weight increase on the low-
calorie, carbohydrate diet was caused by retained water.
But after two weeks the body had absorbed its quota of
water, and the weight again started to decrease at the expected rate.

Actually the body had been losing fat even during the
temporary "weight gaining" period at the start of the
carbohydrate diet, but this was masked by the retention of
water. Here then is the explanation of the plaintive cry
of many overweights, "I can't even lose weight on a few
slices of bread a day; there must be something wrong with
my glands."

But what causes this water retention which is the nemesis
of millions of would-be weight reducers?

The answer was supplied by Dr. W. L. Bloom, Director
of Medical Education and Research at the Piedmont Hospital in Atlanta. He measured the amount of salt lost
through the urine of his low-calorie, weight-reducing
patients. On a low-calorie, but high carbohydrate diet,
almost no salt was eliminated.

The salt in the diet was retained in the tissues of the

body. However, since there is an automatic regulating system which prevents the "saltiness" of the body from becoming excessive, extra water is retained, causing the temporary increase in weight.

When the major content of the diet was changed back to fat and protein, the diet salt was again eliminated and as a result the copious flow of urine registered as weight reduction.

The mystery of the often dramatic—but inevitably only temporary—success attending the *beginning* of the high-fat, high-protein "Calories Don't Count" diet was now solved.

The relation between salt and water in the body has been known for many years. Doctors have long used a low-salt diet to correct excess water retention, as in dropsy and heart failure.

The quick loss of weight on a high-fat diet had been shown in 1898 through the long-forgotten experiments of Dr. N. Zuntz.

Twenty-five years later Dr. F. G. Benedict in searching for an explanation of the temporary quick weight loss on high-fat diets reported that "all the experiments showed a loss of salt and water into the urine at the beginning of a high-fat diet." However Benedict did not follow up this observation and searched for other causes.

In 1921 Dr. G. Lusk insisted that the true explanation of the high-fat diet weight loss was to be found in the shift in water balance. But this explanation still seemed too simple, and it was buried for thirty years, until Dr. Bloom's research showed *why* Dr. Lusk's explanation was correct.

The next question is: how does the high-fat diet cause the elimination of salt from the body? Unfortunately this is still a mystery since there is no medical research data available to answer this question.

But there is no doubt in the minds of the medical researchers of the validity of the data which shows that a high-fat, high-protein diet will cause reduction of weight only by elimination of salt and water, and only at the beginning of this diet.

However the main problem is not the mystery of the biological cause and effect, but the mystery of why it frequently takes so long to transmit important medical knowledge to the public before unscientific theories can cause so much confusion.

The modern American is not only over-fat, but also frequently water logged due to excessive salt retention in the body. These two conditions must be handled by *different* methods. Dr. S. K. Fineberg, in his weight reduction clinic at the Harlem Hospital in New York, was well aware of the problem of water logging when he stated that, "Prolonged salt and water retention during weight reduction was the greatest single cause of failure in the treatment of obesity." Dr. Fineberg's work indicates that from ten to twenty pounds of water may be retained in the body due to excess salt even though the body-fat stores are being eliminated on a low-calorie reducing diet.

Dr. G.G. Duncan of the Philadelphia Hospital told the A.M.A. Convention in 1963 that potato chips, pretzels and salty ham can raise body weight three pounds in one day.

The natural method of preventing water logging due to salt retention is the direct approach—the elimination of salt from the diet. In this way the violent fluctuations in weight caused by water changes will be minimized and the true reduction in excess body fat will be seen by a daily reading of the bathroom scale.

The proper reducing diet for excess fat as well as excess water in the body should be based on the low-salt Prudent Diet, which contains adequate protein, a low-saturated-fat intake and a complete avoidance of "empty calories."

FAT PEOPLE WHO DON'T OVEREAT AND THIN PEOPLE WHO "EAT LIKE A HORSE"

It would seem that everything else being the same, fat people on the average would be eating more than slim people. But the facts have been checked and rechecked by almost a dozen medical surveys and the answer is always the same: there is frequently little difference between the amount of food eaten by many obese individuals compared to similar normal individuals.

Obviously the answer must be that the overweights who eat "normally" use up less "energy calories," and many surveys have shown this to be true. The best yardstick of activity is walking, and the pedometers used in innumerable tests almost always indicate that overweight people walk about half the number of miles covered by similar individuals of normal weight.

Another reason for the apparently greater "efficiency" of the metabolism of a fat person compared to a thin one is, according to Thannhauser's *Metabolism and Metabolic Disorders*, that "after a high-calorie meal, the skin temperature of a normal individual rises *more* than that of an obese individual. The fat envelope acts as a heat conserving shield."

The puzzle of the overweight who doesn't seem to overeat is matched by the equally puzzling case of the thin person who "eats like a horse." This exception to the "calories do count" rule is a source of confusion to the unsuccessful reducer. Discouraged, the overweight person reasons that there must be some built-in biological factor which keeps the thin man thin in spite of his overeating. Next they apply this theory to themselves but in reverse. They claim to have a "glandular condition" which keeps them plump even though they don't overeat very much.

In some cases there may be a hormonal imbalance. The thyroid is the "energy" gland, and when it is overactive, the body does burn up fuel faster. The under-active thyroid personality on the other hand is slow moving. His body uses up fuel more slowly, and the excess piles up as fat.

But the *average* thin man we are talking about and his obese opposite are not true glandular cases. They are *physically* normal. What controls the rate at which their food is burned up is an often easily evident tense or placid attitude toward life and physical activity.

For background data on this we must go to the recent research of Drs. G.A. Rose and R.T. Williams in the *British Journal of Nutrition*. They tested a group of small eaters (2,400 calories) and compared them with a similar weight group of big eaters (4,600 calories) and found that the basal metabolism didn't provide the answer. In both groups, on the average, it was the same.

But they did find that the first fifteen seconds of activity is a wasteful "start up" period, using up twice the usual calories. Another very wasteful activity was tense "fidgeting" which can double the body's calorie consumption.

The paradox of the thin-man-who-eats-like-a-horse-and-never-gains-an-ounce now yields to a simple solution: It's the thin man's stop-and-go psychology that stimulates him to short but energy-wasteful bursts of activity . . . numerous "starts" that burn up excess calories. The fat man may accomplish the same amount of useful work by the end of the day as the thin man, but the fat man's energy expenditure is smooth, his habits are easygoing, his activity proceeds at a steady level. Excess food calories are not burned up as they are in the start-stop way of life.

For the sedentary man who doesn't exercise enough or who, by nature, does not use the start-stop method of burning up his excess calories, a very low calorie intake is one solution to his overweight problem. But this incurs the risk of poor nutrition from lack of vital proteins, vitamins, enzymes and minerals.

The sedentary man with a low-calorie intake must make every calorie count. His diet allows room only for the most essential foods, the proteins, the unsaturated fats, the vitamin and mineral bearing vegetables and whole grains. For him the elimination of "empty calories" is of crucial importance.

There are other known ways, and perhaps many still undiscovered, by which the food calories of the thin heavy eater can be directly turned into wasted energy and heat.

One heat-dissipation system which helps to keep our body temperature normal is evaporation of water from the lungs in breathing and by the visible and invisible evaporation of sweat from the skin.

Another little-known heat-dissipation method is by an unfelt and invisible vibration of the skin muscles which aids in the direct transfer of heat from body to air. This microscopic tremor was only discovered recently by Dr. H. Rohracher of the University of Vienna. Sleep decreases the amount of these tremors and under stress the amount of the heat-wasting vibration almost doubles.

According to Dr. R. S. Gubner of the Equitable Life Assurance Society, the "average" American carries a load of *pure fat* which is over twenty percent of his true fat-free weight.

One of the most dangerous problems is that of the individual whose "weight" condition is hidden. He may seem normal or even underweight, but he is "over fat." This condition was discovered by Dr. Kenneth Sanders when he compared the weights of coronary patients at the Middlesex Hospital in London with healthy controls matched for age, sex, nationality, and other factors.

The weight of the coronary patients was the same as that of the controls, but the fat content of the two groups was quite different. Measurements showed that the pinched skin (a method of fat measurement) of the coronary patients was very much thicker than that of the healthy group.

This means that the coronary group was not overweight as far as the scale could show—but they were overweight in their body-fat content.

None will disagree with the statement that Americans are under-active and over-fed and that over-eating by so many people is only possible in an economy of abundance such as is found in this country.

The only way out of America's modern dilemma according to Dr. Charlotte M. Young of Cornell University is (1) Better mental health facilities to correct compulsive eating, (2) Education in the use of leisure time to reduce boredom eating (3) Re-education to reduce our excess social eating.

There is no doubt (and many surveys have shown this) that a large number of overweight Americans are using food as a tranquilizer to overcome feelings of insecurity, anxiety and depression. These individuals need the greatest amount of motivation before they can be won over to the Prudent Diet program.

From a practical point of view the first step in any weight reduction plan is the purchase of an accurate bath-room scale. The second is the establishment of a daily weighing-in routine, preferably just before dressing every morning. The third step is to establish a program of eating and exercise which will transform the body from its present fatty water-logged state into the lean and solid condition seen in groups who have clear arteries and a low rate of heart attack.

CHAPTER FOURTEEN

New Ideas on
Coronary Prevention

WHY SATURATED BODY FAT IS DANGEROUS

It is now known that the use of the Prudent Diet has reduced the liability to coronary disease. The Anti-Coronary Clubs and other groups have established the Prudent Diet as decisive in the prevention program. Some, however, still demand more tests before they concede that we should all abandon the present "luxury" diet. They are willing to wait eight more years until the results of a proposed *new* "Nation-wide Anti-Coronary Club" are in. But why wait? If they need additional proof, there is another type of test which can serve as a conclusive confirmation of the findings of the Anti-Coronary Clubs.

The principle of this test is the chemical analysis of body fat. It is used to trace the hidden history of a person's past diet. Let us examine the body fat of those who have changed from the Western diet to a Prudent Diet: Thousands of tests have established that their body fat gradually changes from a predominantly saturated type to a more unsaturated type. This gradual change is now used by the medical staffs of the Coronary Clubs as a means of checking on continued adherence to the Prudent Diet.

To understand the significance of this change clearly, it is necessary to follow the step-by-step course of diet fat as it is transformed into body fat. First, the diet fat enters the blood in the form of fatty globules, with little change in chemical composition. These fatty globules are, in turn transformed, again with little change in chemical composition, into body fat.

Individuals living on a typical high-calorie, high-saturated-fat, American diet, have blood fats which are higher in quantity than normal and mostly of the same saturated variety as in the diet; and their body fat also has the same composition. On the low-calorie Prudent Diet, the quantity of fats in the blood declines to a low-normal, and is of a predominantly unsaturated variety. The body fats gradually become identical with those in the blood. In other words, the type of fat we eat, the type of fat in our blood and our body fat will eventually all match.

With the blood and body fat to guide us, we are now in a position to examine a group of known atherosclerotics and a similar-age group of true normals and to plot their dietary past. If there is a marked difference between these two groups in the amount of saturated and unsaturated fats, either in the blood or the body, it must be due to difference in previous diet. This research can provide a *new type of proof* of the value of the Prudent Diet.

Here are the conditions that a valid test of this type must fulfill:

1. The test group should consist of persons eating different types of diets.
2. All should be examined for the presence of coronary disease and atherosclerosis.
3. Body and blood fat should be analyzed for saturated and unsaturated fat.

The required findings for a valid test are as follows:

A. The "normals" must have blood and body fats of a predominantly unsaturated type.
B. The atherosclerotics must have blood and body fat which is mostly saturated.

If the first three requirements are met and if the results are as predicted, this would be *incontrovertible proof* of the value of the Prudent Diet.

For a complete study, including an examination of the body fats, we must go to the work of Dr. K. J. Kingsbury and his group at the St. Mary's Hospital in London. Dr. Kingsbury's tests were outstanding for the extraordinary measures taken to avoid all chance of error. The greatest possibility of error lay in the selection of normals and atherosclerotics. This type of error is the basis for much controversy in medical research.

"A major difficulty in human studies," writes Dr. J. A. Little of Sunnybrook Hospital, Toronto, "arises from the fact that subclinical atherosclerosis is universal in our adult population." Dr. Moses Wurm of St. Joseph's Hospital, Burbank, speaks of ". . . our inability to separate adequately the symptomless atherosclerotic individual from the true normal."

Dr. Herman E. Hilleboe, head of the New York State Department of Health, reminded a Conference on Coronary Prevention in 1959 that "The preclinical [hidden coronary] stages of atherosclerosis . . . appear to be occurring almost universally among our adult population in the United States." And he sums up: "The comparison of cases [of atherosclerosis] and non-cases, becomes almost impossible except in postmortem studies."

Which was exactly what Dr. K. J. Kingsbury intended to do. With this exception, his "autopsies" were to be on the living. The surgical team led by Dr. Kingsbury was in a strategic position for this study, because they were able to make careful examination of the visible conditions of blockage in the arteries of patients on the operating table. The normals were selected after the most rigid and careful tests, including vascular examinations, and the atherosclerotics were finally verified by microscopic study of sections of their arteries removed at operation.

With the selection of the two groups. Dr. Kingsbury moved swiftly into the core study: What was the percentage of unsaturated fats in normal blood and in atherosclerotic blood?

Kingsbury found that the percentage of polyunsaturated fats, especially the two-hinged and four-hinged fats, *were 50% greater in normal blood than in atherosclerotic* blood. In addition, blood-fat in the normals was mostly unsaturated, and in atherosclerotics it was mostly saturated.

In body fats the percentage of polyunsaturated fats was also 50% greater in normals than in atherosclerotics.

Dr. Kingsbury's test fulfills every requirement for the *final proof* of the value of the Prudent Diet.

The "normals" in this test were true normals, and age-matched to true atherosclerotics. So when the fat in the normal's body and blood was found to be 50% more unsaturated, there was only one possible source of this type of fat, a diet similar to the Prudent Diet.

The atherosclerotics, on the other hand, with their saturated blood and body fat, could only have obtained this from one source, a Western-type saturated-fat diet.

Dr. Kingsbury's indisputable blood fat research has been supported—although without his double check on body fat—by five other research surveys made in other countries.

The method used by Dr. W. Schrade and his associates at the University of Frankfort was to arrange the blood-test data on charts. Those with the highest blood fats were found, in general, to have the most coronary disease. As the severity of the atherosclerosis increased, and the blood fats rose higher and higher on Dr. Schrade's charts, *the increased blood fats were almost all saturated*.

From his researches in South Africa, Dr. A. Antonis' data shows a marked difference in the percentage of poly-unsaturated fats in the blood of atherosclerotic and normal Europeans. The atherosclerotics had only thirty per cent of the multi-hinged fats in their blood, but the "normal" men had forty-four per cent. Perhaps a better estimate of a true norm would be the results of Dr. Antonis' test on blood fats in his normal Bantu patients, which showed 55% polyunsaturated.

Dr. Barry Lewis of the University of Cape Town found similar differences in the percentages of the polyunsaturated fats "married" to the cholesterol (esters) in the blood of atherosclerotics compared to normals. The atherosclerotics had a significant excess of the saturated, and a relative deficiency of the multi-hinged fats.

From Holland and Poland comes further corroboration. Dr. G. Pol and Dr. Z. Wiktor have found distinct increases in the saturated content of the high blood fats of athero-sclerotics and angina patients and a decline in the poly-unsaturated percentage.

From the Prudent Diet . . . to the blood fats . . . and finally to the body fats . . . at all these stages the proper high ratio of multi-hinged unsaturated to saturated fats is necessary.

It is important to remember that Dr. Kingsbury's tests were made in England and the other tests in Europe and Africa, where a variety of diets were eaten, including the more frugal types, similar to that of the Prudent Diet.

In the United States, where virtually everyone partakes of the American Diet, high in calories and saturated fats, practically all now have the highly saturated type of blood and body fat.

That is, all except the members of the Anti-Coronary Clubs—and those changing over to the Prudent Diet.

THE PRUDENT DIET AND GOUT, DIABETES, GALLSTONES AND OTHER METABOLIC DISEASES

With the discovery and development of antibiotics, death from infectious diseases is now one of the minor medical problems. Today death and disability occur mostly from cancer and metabolic diseases such as (1) artery blockage of all types (2) diabetes (3) gout (4) obesity (5) gallstones (6) cataract and many others.

In general, these diseases are separate and distinct entities and affect different parts of the body. Yet curiously enough there is a statistical relationship between them, so that the occurrence of one often implies the presence of the other.

Take the supposedly very unusual illness of gout, which often shows itself by the painful and swollen big toe. Dr. L. M. Lockie of the University of Buffalo School of Medicine states that this once rare disease now afflicts one percent of our population. Since women are rarely afflicted, its occurrence is two per cent in men, with a higher prevalence in middle-aged men. The basic cause of gout is excess uric acid in the blood which deposits in the joints in the form of pointed crystals that cause excruciating pain.

The statistical relation of gout to coronary artery disease is now well known. Dr. P. M. Kahn has found that in heart attack patients, the occurrence of high uric acid was as frequent as high cholesterol in over two out of three cases. Drs. L. Salvini and G. Verdi of the University of Florence examined a group of men, and they found, "remarkable statistical significance relating cholesterol and uric acid serum levels in all normal subjects under observation."

As Medical Director of the heart-disease study unit at Framingham, Dr. T. R. Dawber also studied this subject. In the large group of people under his scrutiny, as the blood uric acid rose from less than four to a level of more than six milligrams, the death rate from coronary disease doubled.

Dr. D. W. Kramer of Philadelphia's Jefferson Medical College found that in a group of severe coronary patients, more than one out of four had high blood-uric acid. And of a large group with artery blockage in the legs, almost every one had high uric acid.

There also exists a relationship between gout and obesity. Drs. T. E. Weiss and C. Moore of the New Orleans Ochsner Clinic studied over a hundred gout cases and found 28% had high blood-sugar levels. None were yet diabetic. According to these doctors "certain features are common to gout and diabetes. Obesity is one of them."

Further evidence of this comes from Dr. F. Dudley Hart of London's Westminster Hospital who says, "Most of the gouty patients are, if anything, overweight."

The relation between obesity and high blood lipids is clear both statistically and as a cause and effect relationship, especially during the "gaining" period. The fact that insurance companies often increase premiums for overweights, shows that they regard the statistical relation between overweight, high blood lipids and coronary disease to be important.

Another metabolic disease is pre-diabetes. Usually persons with this problem drift into a diabetic state. The test for this condition is to give the suspect a large sugar or glucose "load," either by mouth or by injection directly into the blood. Dr. F. Wahlberg of the Karolinska Institute in Stockholm made a series of tests showing that most of the atherosclerotic patients had a poor ability to handle an injected glucose load, compared to matched controls who were patients in the same hospital. Dr. G. Reaven and his associates at Stanford found that three out of four coronary artery disease patients had poor glucose tolerance. Their tests showed that only one out of four with other diseases had the same pre-diabetic problem.

Dr. D. Aleksandrow of the Warsaw Medical Academy has reported tests in 1962 showing that four out of five of his atherosclerotic patients had a poor glucose tolerance and more than one third were in a pre-diabetic state. In the overweight atherosclerotics the situation was even worse; all were pre-diabetic.

With such a close statistical relationship between coronary disease, gout, diabetes, blood lipids, blood sugar and obesity, the suspicion of metabolic interrelationship increases. Of the group, obesity seems to be the common denominator, a fact which points to diet as a possible culprit.

The first clue to the answer had already been given by doctors who had noted a reduction in coronary disease after restrictions in fat, meat, sugar and other "luxury" type foods during World War II. Statistics had also shown that many other metabolic diseases were affected. For example, diabetes incidence was found to be reduced to half the prewar rate in Germany and other European countries. According to Dr. A. B. Gutman of the "Gout Clinic" of New York's Mount Sinai Hospital, the symptoms of gout "virtually disappeared during the austerities of World War II life, only to return promptly . . ." when the prewar diet was resumed.

Wartime diet restrictions have even affected the United States. The 1961 Diabetes Fact Book shows that both during World War I and World War II there was a significant and sharp drop in diabetes deaths, which in both cases immediately started to rise after the lifting of wartime restrictions.

Many medical scientists have studied this relationship and there is now a large body of evidence linking a rich diet to a high rate of metabolic disease of various types.

In England, according to Dr. A. J. Popert of Manchester's Royal Infirmary, "there is little doubt that richness of diet . . . is a characteristic attribute of the patient with gout." One of the basic steps in the treatment of gout used by Dr. Gutman is to place his patients on a low-saturated fat and low-meat diet.

As a matter of fact, in past years a fatty diet has been used as a provocative test for gout. Dr. L. M. Lockie of the University of Buffalo Medical School found that in nine out of ten cases suspected of gout, a high-fat diet precipitated the symptoms of a gouty attack. Dr. C. McEwen of the N.Y.U. College of Medicine used the high-fat diet as a provocative test for two weeks. If by this time no attack of gout resulted, it was regarded as a negative test. In Dr. V. J. Harding's survey very high fat meals caused the uric-acid level to double its previous amount in all cases. Other high-fat trials have resulted in increased blood uric acid depending on the amount of fat in the meals.

In all cases, a low-fat diet resulted in a drop in uric acid and the elimination of the gout symptoms.

Diabetes is regarded by Dr. F. S. P. van Buchen of The Netherlands as a result of an overabundant consumption of food, and his recommendation is a diet to reduce weight to less than normal. Dr. J. Lederer of France treats all his diabetics as cases of obesity, stressing the absolute necessity of weight reduction.

During World War II in Switzerland, Dr. A. Fleisch found that diabetes varied from 2 per 10,000 population to 10 per 10,000 depending on the location. He also found a close individual connection between income and diabetes. In the United States, with an incidence of over 150 per 10,000 and with everybody wealthy enough in food purchasing ability, surveys of diabetes show no relationship to income.

Dr. Timothy Leary of Boston, one of the pioneer pathologists who studied the causes of heart attack and artery blockage, wrote in 1936 that, "In connection with no other disease has there been such widespread experimentation in pathogenesis as was carried out in the feeding of diabetic diets high in fat, rich in cholesterol, in the decade 1920-1930. The results were as definite as those obtained in the experimental rabbit. The human lesions . . . [artery blockage] . . . were spectacular enough particularly in children. Moreover, the reverse procedure, a cutting down of the fats in the diet, including cholesterol resulted in a return to status quo . . ."

In the experience of the George F. Baker Clinic in Boston, the development of diabetes in pre-diabetics was four times as frequent in overweight individuals as in those of normal weight. It has also been shown by Dr. L. H. Newburgh that "Reducing obese middle-aged diabetics to normal weight resulted in a return to normal glucose tolerance in nearly 75%."

There have been many other reports of similar results. For instance, *Lancet* (Feb. 26, 1955) has a report from India, describing remarkable results which were achieved in normalizing diabetics, improving their sugar tolerance and decreasing their insulin requirements. More than two out of three patients could be taken off insulin within eight to eighteen weeks. The only diet change required was a reduction in fat to one ounce or less daily, and a reduction of calories in the diet.

There is no doubt that a whole revolution in the dietary treatment of diabetes is now taking place. In an editorial in *Diabetes* (July 1962) the Director of the Institute for Metabolic Research, Dr. L. W. Kinsell, declares that it is necessary to revise all previous diabetic diets. The new diets used by Dr. Kinsell and many other diabetic specialists are quite similar to the Prudent Diet. A bare minimum of dairy food, eggs and very lean meat are allowed. Recommended substitutions are fish, fowl, vegetable oil and nuts.

Dr. W. F. Van Eck reported in the August, 1959 *American Journal of Medicine* that he was able to cure the degenerative blood vessels in the eyes of his diabetic patients with a low-fat diet, and showed before-and-after photographs to prove it. Equally important was the fact that he was able to take many of these patients off insulin because of the great improvement in their glucose tolerance.

Blindness is not usually thought of as a metabolic disease. Yet this greatly feared affliction is more often the result of a metabolic disorder than any other cause. The 1961 United States Diabetes Fact Book gives the cause of perhaps half of all blindness as cataract, vascular diseases and diabetes. Since the best method for *both* the prevention and cure of all these three metabolic disorders is the Prudent Diet, it may be hoped that in the future blindness will be greatly reduced.

Another metabolic disease related to obesity is gallstones. This sometimes painful affliction exists in one out of six persons over fifty.

Dr. N. Watanabe has reported in *Archives of Surgery* that gallstones can be "dissolved" by the use of a diet high in polyunsaturated oils. The four-hinged oil found in walnuts was the best one because it caused the greatest increase in the capacity of the bile to dissolve these cholesterol-filled "stones." A diet containing saturated fat caused the stones to become "harder."

One method of research on metabolic disease is the study of groups known to be free of such afflictions. In Israel the newly arrived Yemenite Jews are such a group. We already know that their blood lipids and artery blockage increased when they adopted the Israeli diet, which is high in saturated-fat. Dr. A. M. Cohen of the Hadassah Hospital also studied diabetes in these people. On arrival they were practically free from diabetes, but after twenty years they too had the same high rate of diabetes as found in European settlers in Israel.

Not only Yemenites, but many other groups of people coming from countries in which diabetes is a non-existent disease acquire the high diabetic rates which prevail in the more highly industrialized countries to which they immigrate.

The world famous Dr. E. P. Joslin was eulogized in an editorial in the *New England Journal of Medicine* as having made his greatest contribution by teaching that "diabetic patients should themselves learn the basic principles and the application of their diabetic diet."

Based on Dr. Joslin's teachings, we should learn the unifying principle which lies behind the success of the Prudent Diet not only in heart attack and diabetes but in many other metabolic diseases. It is generally accepted that a major cause of diabetes is the exhaustion of the gland which manufactures the insulin enzyme, leading to a resultant excess of blood sugar. At one time it was the abundance of refined sugar in the diet that was thought to be the cause of diabetes, but today's medical research indicates that excess saturated fats must be given an equal, if not a larger, share of the blame.

It is important to reiterate at this point that the Prudent Diet is being accepted by the major diabetes clinics as the specific diet to control both the diabetic blood sugar condition and the high blood cholesterol which is recognized today as the most dangerous condition in diabetes which frequently leads to heart attack early in life. The bibliography lists a number of sources of this data.

In artery blockage there is, first, an exhaustion of enzymes in the heparin-clearing factor system in the blood and, second, an exhaustion in the fat digestive enzymes. Here it is definitely known that saturated fat is the major cause of enzyme exhaustion that results in an excess of fatty globules in the blood.

In the case of gout, saturated fat and excess purines (always found in a rich diet) are the main cause of the overload and exhaustion of the metabolic system with the resulting excess of uric acid in the blood.

Since all people are not equally affected by this exhaustion process, it has led to the theory that the metabolic diseases are hereditary, and that the basic weakness leading to the exhaustion is of genetic origin.

According to Dr. Roger J. Williams, no two people are born with identical biological systems. Great variations in the supply of enzymes have been found by him in different individuals. Some people are born with a very high capacity to manufacture enzymes that permits overeating well into old age. Others have such poor glands that they become victims of the metabolic diseases through over-eating at a very early age.

Today doctors are finding that babies already have diabetes at birth. The principle involved here seems to be that an overloaded and weakened enzyme system in the parents, caused by a rich diet, can result in a tendency to similar glandular weakness in the child.

One fallacy in any attempt at a hereditary explanation is that two generations ago such situations were unheard of.

But in general it is not possible to find out which specific individuals were born with a deficiency in any of the enzymes. This type of weakness can only be detected after the enzyme exhaustion has already started, as in the case of pre-diabetics and pre-atherosclerotics. Even here the telltale symptoms are not always found, and the final disaster of diabetes or coronary artery blockage occurs without warning.

The only prudent course in metabolic disease prevention is to assume that an average or even sub-average enzyme system exists, and to attempt to prevent dietary overloads that might lead to enzyme exhaustion.

The October 25, 1963 issue of *Medical World* carries the startling statistics that in Britain 14% of the population over fifty years of age have a diabetic abnormality. A leading scientific journal, *The New Scientist,* after the publication of the British data, editorially advocated that all those over forty should cut down on both calories and sugar.

One method of preventing dietary overloads is to cut down on our present large sumptuous meals.

Based on the research of Dr. Clarence Cohn of the Michael Reese Hospital, there may be some benefits in eating five small meals a day rather than our present one large and two medium meals.

The benefits of the new "nibbling" system may be important because it strengthens the "weak point" in our metabolic system. Nibbling causes an improvement in "glucose tolerance." The current "one large meal" system, according to Dr. Cohn's research, results in a poorer glucose tolerance.

Degenerative Deposits

In addition to excess weight, excess blood lipids and excess blood sugar, there is another major symptom of degenerative disease: the unnatural deposits which are the most evident effects of metabolic disorders.

Here are a few of the "deposit" problems:

• In gall bladder disease—the deposits are marble-sized "stones" in the gall bladder; their principal component is cholesterol.

• In gout—the deposits are the sharp pain-causing urate crystals.

• In obesity—the excess deposits are unwanted fat.

• In cataract—the clouding of the lens of the eye is caused by deposits mainly of lipids.

• In arcus seniles—the "white arc" in the outer rim of the iris of the eye consists mostly of cholesterol.

• In many of the "exotic" lipid diseases whose symptoms are "bumps" in the skin, elbow, tendons and other parts of the body—the deposits are fats and cholesterol.

• In yellow atrophy of the liver—the deposits are fats.

• In coronary artery disease—the deposits are fatty-fibrous-cholesterol debris that are later complicated by calcium deposits.

• In atherosclerosis—these deposits occur in all the large arteries of the body.

• In diabetes—the fatty cholesterol deposits occur not only in the large arteries of the body but also in the small arteries and even the minute arterioles.

As can be seen there are several types of substances which deposit in the body in metabolic disease. But there is a far greater number of diseases in which the *lipids* become unstable and form deposits, compared to those in which *non-lipid* substances are the cause of deposits.

Although there are other insoluble substances in the body, the lipids are the only totally insoluble substances which must travel, passing first through the intestines and other cell walls, then circulating through the blood and finally passing through the blood vessel walls and other tissues.

To do this nature has devised many ingenious vehicles for transportation, such as the fatty globules, but their excessive amounts and instability can cause deposition of insoluble contents in almost every part of the body, which all too frequently occurs.

But there are never any unnatural deposits of cholesterol, fats, fibrin, calcium, uric acid or any other substances when the body is in proper metabolic balance. In every one of these metabolic deposit diseases, medical research has shown that for prevention and cure the proper diet is the Prudent Diet.

It is a well known fact that the incidence of heart attack among doctors is more than double that of the general population. Logically, the results of a blood analysis in a representative group of doctors should show a large percentage of the types of abnormalities discussed in this chapter.

An opportunity to observe this relationship occurred at the 1963 American Medical Association Convention in Atlantic City. Over 1500 doctors volunteered to have their blood tested as part of a campaign in preventive medicine. According to a statement by Dr. T. M. Perry who conducted the survey, 80 percent of the tests revealed an abnormally high level in one or more of the following: blood cholesterol, blood sugar or blood uric acid.

According to Dr. Perry, such tests hold new promise for prolonging man's years of health, and his conclusion was that, ". . . modification of diet or habits may be all that is needed."

The past several decades have seen triumphs of research in the field of deficiency diseases: the discoveries of the basic requirements for vitamins, minerals, trace elements, food enzymes and other vital natural factors found in foods for maintaining adequate (maximum) health.

The past few years have introduced the new era of research in the field of metabolic and biochemical diseases.

Just as the *simple addition* of a few specific nutrients has resulted in tremendous benefits in the prevention and treatment of *deficiency diseases*, so may the *simple reduction* in the rich and refined foods result in tremendous benefits in the prevention and treatment of *metabolic disease*.

Dr. C. G. King, the former president of the Nutrition Foundation, has summed up the metabolic problem when he placed the blame squarely on ". . . the ease with which tempting food rich in sugars, fats or alcohol may be obtained by everyone big enough to reach or cry for something to eat."

HEART ATTACKS, SMOKING AND VITAMIN C

If you are in your fifties, and if throughout your coronary arteries the atheroma is thickening and spreading, then it is almost certain that you are now faced with the added danger of microscopic hemorrhages in the fragile new capillaries which are branching out and growing into the new artery blockage. These new capillaries are relatively weak, and if they burst, the hemorrhage can cause further growth of artery blockage, speeding the onset of occlusion or thrombosis.

In 1941, Dr. J. C. Patterson of the Department of Pathology, Ottawa Civic Hospital, made microscopic studies of artery blockage tissue in a group who had suffered a heart attack. He discovered positive evidence of capillary hemorrhages, and in four out of five of these coronary cases, Dr. Paterson found *a lack of Vitamin C*.

Among a control group of "normals" vitamin deficiency was noted in one out of two patients. Dr. Paterson concluded: To prevent capillaries from hemorrhaging, add Vitamin C to the diet.

However, since Paterson's experiments a new vitamin, Vitamin P, has been discovered. It's effect on hemorrhaging is much like that of Vitamin C.

"In dogs in which malignant hypertension [high blood pressure] is induced," explains *Nutrition Reviews* (May 1952), "hemorrhage in various parts of the body, especially the heart, is one of the serious complications and causes of death." The journal went on to add that the protection afforded to the animals by large amounts of Vitamin P (bioflavinoids) was sufficient to result in practically no hemorrhaging. On the other hand, when the Vitamin P dosage was reduced, hemorrhages continued.

But why not combine the two vitamins? In February 1953, *Geriatrics* published a report by Drs. E. T. Gale and M. W. Thewlis of a four-year experiment, the results of which show the value of this combination.

Thirty-two middle-aged and elderly people, with marked symptoms of diseased arteries, were given varying amounts of both Vitamin C and Vitamin P for periods of one to four years. The four patients who died—from coronary thrombosis and hemorrhage in the brain—were all from the group who had received the lowest supplements of Vitamins C and P.

Actually, Vitamins C and P are a *synergistic* team: a combination of two vitamins that makes the team more effective. That this combination does reduce the likelihood of capillary hemorrhaging is attested to by many medical reports.

One place in the body in which the effects of these vitamins can be most easily and directly observed is in the small blood vessels in the back of the eye. Dr. Walter R. Loewe of the New York City Hospital had many patients in his care with capillary hemorrhages in the eye. Here was a chance to watch the results of the combined vitamins with his own eyes.

Fifty of the patients were given medium to large doses of vitamins C and P. Later examinations showed that all hemorrhaging had stopped and that the effects of the old ruptures were gradually clearing up.

In the treatment of atherosclerosis, the beneficial function of Vitamin C does more than strengthen the capillaries —it also reduces high blood cholesterol.

Supporting evidence of this may be found in a summary published in the January, 1958 issue of the American Heart Association's journal, *Circulation*. The author is Dr. A. L. Myasnikov of the Russian Academy of Medical Science, and his article is an authoritative review of the research in the USSR using Vitamin C to prevent and treat atherosclerosis.

So impressed are the Russians with the many-sided benefits of Vitamin C that they have made this vitamin a major factor in their prevention work. The American medical publication *M.D.* comments that, "High in the Soviet armamentarium for the prophylaxis [prevention] and treatment of atherosclerosis is Vitamin C . . . in food or in doses of 500 mg. or 1000 mg. per day."

In 1952 a Canadian physician, Dr. G. C. Willis, became interested in the use of Vitamin C in the prevention of atherosclerosis. His five year research on this problem has provided answers to many questions concerning the value of this vitamin.

The question Dr. Willis first investigated was: Does Vitamin C prevent the increase of artery blockage caused by capillary hemorrhaging? After he studied fifty-two cases, his results, like Patterson's, demonstrated that Vitamin C does prevent this type of hemorrhaging.

A year later Dr. Willis tried to find out if Vitamin C added to the diet will affect the extent of the atheroma. X-ray photos taken before and after treatment with Vitamin C showed evidence of reduction of the atheroma.

If Vitamin C decreases atheroma, shouldn't there be an absence of Vitamin C in the actual artery blockage? In 1955, Willis examined atherosclerotic arteries and measured the Vitamin C content of the atheroma as well as the nearby clean sections. In the clean sections Vitamin C was present; in the atheroma it was absent.

Dr. Willis' new research on guinea pigs suffering from scurvy, a Vitamin C deficiency disease, showed atherosclerosis to be present. Couldn't atherosclerosis in those cases be cured by the addition of Vitamin C to the diet? Yes, additional vitamin C did cure it!

If Vitamin C *is* an anti-hemorrhaging factor, the American people, with their high Vitamin C diet, should show little or no capillary hemorrhaging. But the facts show that we have a vitamin C deficiency in many tissues and that hemorrhaging in the atheroma does occur. Why?

Vitamin C in our diet may be high, but, at the same time, there are many toxic substances which nullify its beneficial effects. Here's one report that may come as a shock. The Canadian Dr. W. J. McCormick, who is a Vitamin C specialist, has determined by laboratory and clinical tests that "the smoking of one cigarette neutralizes in the body approximately 25 milligrams of ascorbic acid [Vitamin C] or the amount in one medium sized orange. It will thus be seen how difficult it is to meet the bodily requirements of the pack a day smoker . . ." This report in the April 1952 issue of *Archives of Pediatrics* was verified a year later by a report in the *American Journal of Digestive Diseases*. Dr. A. Borquin showed the effects of adding nicotine to the blood. An equivalent amount of nicotine to that inhaled by a heavy smoker in one day caused a reduction of Vitamin C of almost 30%.

In July, 1957 in *Clinical Medicine* Dr. McCormick further reports that, "In hundreds of chemical tests for Vitamin C status in smokers, a normal level of this vitamin has yet to be found."

Only recently a report in *The Lancet* shows the harmful

effects of cigarette smoking in reducing Vitamin C in the blood. Dr. J. H. Calder in the March 9, 1963 issue reports that her tests show .91 milligrams of Vitamin C in the blood of non smokers. But in a mild cigarette smoking group, Vitamin C was down to .73 milligrams. And smokers of fifteen cigarettes a day or over had only .52 milligrams.

But tobacco isn't the only enemy of Vitamin C. The polluted city air we breathe and the foods which contain chemical preservatives also exhaust this essential vitamin. Other chemicals present in modern Western civilization also cause Vitamin C depletion to be widespread.

The use of anticoagulant drugs, is often part of the therapy after the occurrence of a heart attack. Among the doctors who advocate the use of these drugs in the prevention of further heart attacks is Dr. B. Manchester of the George Washington University School of Medicine. He has been able to report effective reductions in post-heart-attack mortality.

The greatest danger from the use of anticoagulant drugs is a possible hemorrhage. In order to prevent this disaster Dr. Manchester uses vitamin C in combination with his anticoagulant therapy.

In 1962 Dr. C. C. Saelhof reported his "Clinical Study of Little Strokes in 112 Cases," in the April issue of *Clinical Medicine*. He observed for a period of three years two groups of patients matched for age, blood pressure and their previous number of "little strokes." Dr. Saelhof placed one group on bioflavinoid therapy, the other group remained on their usual routine.

In the control group thirty six strokes occurred, seventeen "little," thirteen severe, and six mortalities.

But in the group protected by the bioflavinoids, only one severe and six "little strokes" occurred with no deaths.

It is likely that with added research Vitamin C will soon be assigned a far more important role in the prevention of coronary disease than it now holds. Unfortunately, the evidence is far from complete; all the results are not yet in. But we can summarize the known facts about Vitamin C in two ways: (1) Concerning its relation to coronary and general health, no harmful effects have ever been attributed to it. Whatever doubt remains concerning the precise functions Vitamin C performs, one thing is certain, its general effects can only be beneficial. (2) Concerning Vitamin C's relation to the capillaries, it is agreed by all authorities to be a powerful strengthening factor. The best protection against capillary hemorrhage inside the artery blockage is Vitamin C and its cousin, Vitamin P (Rutin and Bioflavinoids).

Dr. James Lind, the British naval officer who "rediscovered" the use of limes with their high Vitamin C content for scurvy prevention stated, in 1798, that almost 200,000 British sailors died needlessly of scurvy due to the 44-year delay in the general application of his discovery. The delay in the application of the knowledge of Vitamin C to counteract the "scurvy" of atheroma may well be the cause of much greater loss of life in adult American men.

"STICKY" BLOOD PLATELETS— TROUBLE IN YOUR BLOOD

The concept that an abundance of good fresh natural food—rich in vitamins, minerals and essential proteins—may be harmful is, for many people, difficult to understand.

However, this book has brought together enough scientific evidence to prove that a diet rich in dairy and other fatty animal foods is a major cause of our present high rate of coronary artery disease.

For further clarification the events that occur soon after eating a fatty meal must be fully described. This section will deal with the harmful effects of a fatty meal on the red blood cells, blood platelets and other elements which, together with the fatty globules, are the main constituents of a thrombotic blood clot.

We will start by showing how a fatty meal can turn the useful blood platelet into a cause of thrombotic blood and artery blockage. As seen through a microscope the platelets in normal blood are round, flat and smooth and about one third the diameter of a red blood cell. Earlier in the book it was described how, at the site of a cut or injury, these platelets become pointed and "sticky" and stop the bleeding by forming a clot. This stickiness is caused by a *chemical messenger* released from the injured tissues.

Now we are going to see how the chylomicron fatty

globules, which enter the blood stream after a fatty meal, may also contain a similar type of *chemical messenger,* which can cause some of the platelets to become "sticky."

In what ways do the sticky platelets cause trouble? Here is one discovered by the Canadian medical researcher, Dr. J. F. Mustard. He inserted a Y-shaped glass tube as a substitute for a joint in the artery system of swine. It is a known fact that artery blockage tends to form *particularly* at artery "joints."

Observations were begun on "supposedly" normal swine. At the junction of the Y-shaped tubes, surprisingly enough, there was some deposit of sticky platelets. The "civilized pig" is also often afflicted with atherosclerosis.

What happened when the pigs were fed a high-fat human diet?

The question was answered by Dr. Mustard at the Atherosclerosis Conference of the American Heart Association Annual Convention in 1961. On a high-fat diet "pigs . . . showed significantly more deposit formation than on a low-fat diet."

The advantage of the glass tubes was that Dr. Mustard could remove them and accurately measure any weight change. "The . . . weight of [sticky platelet] deposit formed in . . . egg and lard-fed pigs . . . was," he noted, "seven times that in the normal animals. The evidence indicates that diets high in fat increase the amount of encrustation." Obviously the rich human diet had caused the platelets to become much more sticky.

Here was a major breakthrough. Atherosclerosis was no longer a hidden and mysterious disease. Now it became possible to see and measure one of the early phases of artery blockage forming inside glass tubes.

It is also possible to see and measure this effect by motion pictures that have been taken of sticky platelets in the living arteries of animals. The work of the Japanese scientist and "cameraman," Dr. Takio Shimamoto, was independently conducted at approximately the same time as Dr. Mustard's. In the joints of living arteries, exactly as in the joints of Dr. Mustard's glass tubes, the camera recorded the formation of the sticky-platelet deposits.

The blood platelet was to become the atheroma detective. If, after a high butter-fat meal, the sticky platelets were attracted to and deposited on the walls of the arteries, our modern diet would be indicted, not only by circumstantial evidence, but by eye-witness testimony.

Micro-motion pictures (as reported in *Asian Medical Journal*, August, 1961) showed that within one hour after the special high-fat meal, many of the platelets became sticky and had adhered to the artery walls. The evidence was incontrovertible; the high-fat diet was the direct cause of this dual atherosclerotic-thrombotic effect.

Much other recent work has been reported which points to the same conclusion that, on a high-fat diet, platelets become sticky, deposit on artery walls and contribute to the build-up of artery blockage. This, then, is one way in which the platelet can cause trouble.

There is still another way. You have already seen that when the platelet undergoes its "sticky" metamorphosis, it releases a chemical messenger that helps to activate the formation of fibrin's treacherous web. What is that chemical messenger?

Back in 1936, a team of researchers headed by Dr. E. Chargaff separated the platelet out of the blood and tested all its "fractions" for clottability. One part of the platelet had an undeniable "activator effect on coagulation." That "fraction" was *cephalin*. Other research workers have since confirmed Chargaff's data.

Cephalin is not one substance but a group of fatty chemicals. They have rather unpronounceable names like phosphatidyl ethanolamine and phosphatidyl serine. Phosphorous-containing fatty substances, they are part of the family of phospholipids that cover the fatty globules in the blood stream.

Dr. Sylvan E. Moolten of the Cardiac Clinic of Middlesex General Hospital has for many years conducted research on the role of platelets in thrombosis. In his latest report he concludes that a high-fat meal increases platelet stickiness and that, "in addition the greater response of arteriosclerotic patients to a high-fat meal probably magnified the risk."

Nature's purpose in having the cephalins, which help initiate the blood clot, locked into the blood platelets, is to have a good supply of this material ready at the site of injury, yet not have it loose in the blood until it is needed in a natural clotting emergency.

The thin phospholipid protective cover of the "unstable" chylomicron fatty globule may be a second source of "loose" cephalin in the blood and so contribute to the trouble caused by chylomicrons in atherosclerosis.

In normal individuals there is little cephalin in the blood, but in atherosclerotics, according to Dr. Martin M. Nothmann of Tufts University Medical School, this is not true, because ". . . cephalins . . . in patients with coronary heart disease . . . are more than double that in normal subjects."

Others have confirmed this fact. For instance, Dr. T. Zemplini has reported in *Review of Czechoslovak Medicine* that in clinical atherosclerosis, ". . . an increase in the cephalin-serum fraction occurs."

Obviously excess free cephalin may be a source of chronic "clotty" trouble in the blood, and should be lowered to a safe level. Dr. Nothmann decided to try to reduce cephalins in the blood of his atherosclerotic patients.

In October, 1961, he announced his findings at the Annual Meeting of the American Heart Association: *At the end of only a few months on a low-saturated-fat diet, cephalin values were cut in half!*

But still the patients were not down to normal cephalin values. Additional treatment was necessary. Now Nothmann substituted a special type of concentrated unsaturated oil for the ordinary vegetable oils. Adding the new supplements to the diet resulted in a further drop in cephalins, down to *one fourth* of the original extremely high values! Within a period of five months, Dr. Nothmann had brought the cephalin values down to normal.

The name of the special unsaturated oil he added is arachidonic oil, the "four hinge" type obtained from the oil of walnuts.

It is interesting to note that in the special diets used in coronary-prevention programs, nuts are highly recommended because of their polyunsaturated content. In almost all cases, walnuts head the list of recommended nuts.

How about the foods which contain cephalin? Heading the list is eggs, with almost one per cent of the yolk consisting of this component. This may be one of the reasons for the thrombotic tendency caused by eggs.

Dr. S. E. Moolten, mentioned earlier, has reported a case which may illustrate this troublesome effect in a blood donor. He states that, "Difficulty was encountered in obtaining freely flowing blood from his vein because of unusually rapid clotting. On questioning, the donor said he had eaten 5 eggs for breakfast about four hours before."

It is not yet known whether the worst effects of some fatty foods are due to their excess content of cephalin, or to their excess of saturated fats or to the combined effects of both.

However, it is known that the sticky platelets in the blood become part of the atheroma blockage process when activated by a high-saturated-fat diet. The special clotting factor, cephalin, used by the platelet in its wound-repair process, is found to be excessively high in the blood of atherosclerotics.

The elimination of both these potentially harmful conditions is best achieved by the Prudent Diet.

PAIN AFTER HEAVY MEALS . . . INDIGESTION OR ANGINA?

Everybody knows what happens after we eat a heavy fatty meal. We become drowsy and dull, ready for a good nap. The popular belief is that the blood rushes from other parts of the body to the stomach and intestines, and that the loss of blood from the brain causes the dull and drowsy feeling.

But scientific studies made after a heavy fatty meal tell a different story. It is not so much the change in quantity of blood in different parts of the body that causes the drowsiness, but rather the change in the *quality* of the blood.

A leading scientist in this field of research is Dr. Roy L. Swank of the University of Oregon Medical School. In his work on neurology he made numerous studies of blood after a heavy fatty meal to trace its possible effects on the nervous system and the brain.

He found that about an hour or more after a fatty meal, when the chylomicrons entered the blood stream in quantity, the red blood cells began to stick to each other, and in some cases even to the white blood cells and blood-vessel walls. In most cases they formed stacks (the scientists call them *rouleaux*) that look like bank coin "rolls."

Watching the very small arteries and capillaries through his microscope Dr. Swank saw that "the blood flowed in great chunks." The flow in the small vessels slowed down and at times stopped completely for a short period of time.

After a heavy butter-fat meal the changes in shapes of the blood cells were extraordinary. Some of the normally dish-shaped red blood cells shrank in diameter and grew knobs on the surface. Then these knobby cells clumped together. Others swelled and rounded out but did not stick together. The cells changed slowly from one "sick" shape into another.

But as the chylomicrons began to be cleared out of the blood the adhesiveness of the red blood cells lessened. The abnormal sticky masses of red cells began to reform into normal individual cells. Within ten hours the circulation was back to normal.

These changes after a very high-fat meal seem pathological and dangerous. Though in some cases these acute changes can be felt, in most cases there is no awareness of them. We are protected, as Dr. Swank puts it, "because of the high factor of safety inherent in a normal vascular system." In other words, the normal person has more red blood cells than he needs, so that many of them must be put out of action before the effects are noticed.

The relation of these effects to clinical coronary disease was shown by Dr. E. H. Bloch, an established investigator for the American Heart Association. His microscope study showed that after a heart attack the red blood cells were found in clumps, plugging up the very small arteries, and that "such aggregates were not found in control groups." Dr. Bloch also found that during a mild cold or virus he could see this same effect but in a very mild form.

People under intense stress must be *specially* careful of what happens in the blood after rich meals. Dr. M. Friedman and Dr. R. H. Rosenman found that individuals under the greatest "time pressure" show the greatest amount of clumping and sticking of the red blood cells, causing many small arteries to be totally blocked after a high fat meal.

Many studies have been made on animals that showed enough red-blood-cell destruction after high fatty meals to cause anemia. After seeing this result in his laboratory dogs, Dr. A. L. Loewy actually came to the incorrect conclusion in 1943 that this was one of nature's methods of getting rid of unwanted red blood cells.

Another effect of a high-fat meal and the resulting myriad of "bumping chylomicrons" is the appearance of the so-called "buffy coat" on the red blood cells. This further reduces the oxygen-carrying capacity of the blood.

Now we can begin to understand the reason for our drowsiness and sluggishness after a heavy fat meal. It is because there is a deficiency of oxygen reaching the brain, due to the clumping of the red blood cells and the buffy coat, as well as the slowing down of the blood in the capillaries.

This reaction may be of great importance in the space program. Dr. G. Douglas Talbot made tests on himself and said, "As Cardiac Consultant to the Space Programs including Project Mercury, I have been responsible for the Human Safety Program. . . . I took heavy oral fat loads and flew in hypersonic aircraft. . . . It became obvious that one requires 34% more oxygen . . . with an elevated blood lipid."

Is this decrease in red-blood-cell efficiency immediately detrimental to the normal heart? No. The normal safety factor is large enough to protect the heart during the acute phase of fat digestion and the chylomicron clearing period.

But this is true only for the individual whose arteries are not seriously obstructed. In the atherosclerotic the safety factors may no longer provide adequate protection.

The pains after a heavy fat meal have often been diagnosed as acute indigestion, and in the past many deaths due to heart attack were also incorrectly blamed on a non-existent bout of acute indigestion. Later, with increased knowledge, doctors began to see that the pains were actually those of heart attack and angina.

But in discarding the incorrect diagnosis of acute indigestion, the possible relationship of the heavy meal to the heart attack was also lost sight of. Only during the last few years have clinicians re-established the connection between the heavy fatty meal, the heart attack and the anginal pains.

In a round table discussion on coronary disease (*Circulation*, June, 1960) Dr. Langendorf made this interesting aside: "Each of us who sees any number of coronary patients has encountered those who experience angina pectoris after a heavy meal."

Even Dr. James B. Herrick in his classic report which first introduced heart attack to the medical world in 1912 started his short list of cases with: "Case #1 . . . A man

. . . 55 supposedly in good health was seized an hour after a moderately full meal . . ."

During a recent survey on "Diet and Heart Disease of Rural Men," Dr. J. K. Boeck, of the New York State Department of Health, questioned a large group of farmers concerning chest pains after meals. Of those already known to have coronary heart disease, 23% said that they had chest pains similar to angina after meals.

There have been innumerable instances in medical literature of doctors having noticed the appearance of angina pains in their coronary patients after a fatty meal.

Dr. Oglesby Paul at a round table medical conference said, "I have had patients of my own in whom a high-fat meal has resulted in the appearance of angina. Therefore caution in the amount of fat taken is desirable."

Dr. H. J. Speedby of England has stated that "all doctors know from experience that year after year, many more heart attacks occur at Christmas and Easter time—when it is customary to eat a good deal of ham, sausage, egg, etc.

Dr. Ditlev Jensen of Sweden has shown by his detailed survey that heart attack is more common after a weekend and may be precipitated by a high-fat Sunday dinner.

These cyclical differences have been noticed less often by doctors in the United States. Due to our overabundance of food, there is now little difference between rich everyday eating and that which occurs on holidays.

Dr. Harry Sobel of the Aging Research Laboratory of the Veterans Administration says, concerning this problem that, "a high fat meal should only be ingested when increased physical activity will follow several hours later."

Added proof of this cause and effect relationship came with the publication of a report titled, "Angina Pectoris Induced by Fat Ingestion in Patients with Coronary Artery Disease" by Dr. P. T. Kuo. He fed fatty meals to volunteers at the hospital of the University of Pennsylvania and measured the amount of fatty cloudiness in their blood every hour. In most cases the maximum amount of fatty globules in the blood was reached within three hours. Dr. Kuo discovered that, ". . . attacks of anginal pain would invariably occur at or near the peak of the lipemic [blood fat] curve."

An even more definite proof would be provided if it

could be shown that clearing the fat out of the blood at its peak would simultaneously stop the anginal symptoms.

Two years later, in 1957, Dr. Kuo reported this critical experiment. At the time of the anginal pains after a fat meal, heparin was injected into the blood to reduce the amount of blood fats. Within a short time the cloudiness of the blood disappeared. And almost simultaneously the pains were gone too. "The tightness in the chest and difficulty in breathing began to ease off two to three minutes after heparin was injected."

Up to now, only the effects of a heavy meal, using saturated fat, has been shown. What might be the effect of a heavy *unsaturated* fat meal?

Dr. Swank investigated and reported his results to an International Conference on Blood Lipids and the Clearing Factor. His experiments showed that the most severe clumping of red cells occurred after a butter-rich meal. And after similar meals with unsaturated oils, the red blood cells showed only minor changes.

The practical value of this research was established a few years later. Dr. Swank observed that the blood of patients with atherosclerosis of the brain was thicker and slower moving than normal blood. In his opinion this thicker blood was due to a high-saturated-fat intake. Dr. Swank proved it by obtaining increased blood speed in his patients within two years, by means of a Prudent Diet.

"It is necessary to reduce fat intake," Dr. Swank said, "and at least half must contain a high percentage of highly unsaturated fats."

To sum up the effects of a high-fat meal:

1. A high-fat meal affects the red blood cells, leading to oxygen inefficiency and, in critical cases, to angina and even heart attack.
2. The platelets become "sticky."
3. The clot-dissolving activity of the blood is slowed down.
4. Saturated fat causes a much worse reaction than unsaturated fat.

The reason for the general scientific agreement on *these* results of a high-fat meal is that red blood cells and platelets are large enough for the microscope to clearly show changes in size and shape, and the dissolving of blood clots is slow and easy to observe.

But there is one effect which is somewhat more difficult to demonstrate. Are fatty meals a major cause of our clotty blood?

WHY YOUR BLOOD TODAY MAY BE MORE PRONE TO CORONARY THROMBOSIS

Medical experts are in general agreement that during the past half century our blood has become increasingly thrombotic. In the United States today, hundreds of thousands of men who have survived heart attacks are taking anticoagulant drugs in an attempt to prevent a recurrence.

In addition, there are hundreds of thousands who have not yet had a heart attack but whose blood is so hypercoagulable that they also require anticoagulants.

And scientific evidence indicates the existence of still another large group, of pre-hypercoagulables who, sooner or later, will need anticoagulants.

One reason for this increase in hypercoagulability was given by Dr. Ralph E. Knutti, Director of the United States National Heart Institute. In the Institute's publication, *Highlights of Heart Progress* (1961), Dr. Knutti states: "High-fat diets appear to increase the tendency of the blood to clot and also to impede the fibrinolytic mechanism by which the body dissolves clots." Dr. Knutti was in a position to have advance knowledge of research relating diet to hypercoagulable blood. The National Heart Institute is the largest single supporter of research in the fields of heart and circulatory diseases. Therefore, it has access to the reports of all current heart research.

Many other eminent medical authorities have expressed their opinions on hypercoagulability of the blood following a fatty meal. Among them is Dr. Frederick J. Stare, head of Harvard's Department of Nutrition. His statement on this problem at a Clinical Conference reported in *Circulation* in 1958 follows: "The avoidance of excessive fat particularly in the evening meal may be desirable from the viewpoint of decreasing the chances of intravascular clotting. It has been established that the blood is more likely to clot 2 to 7 hours following a high fat intake."

Dr. Richard Langendorf has stated at a clinical conference at the Michael Reese Hospital that, "It would therefore seem desirable to avoid heavy meals, particularly in the evening, to minimize the chances of intravascular clotting."

From another Clinical Conference in 1960 comes a similar report by Dr. Silver. He states that "The occurrence of coronary thrombosis after the ingestion of a heavy meal has been familiar to clinicians for years, but only recently has it been suggested that this may be due to hypercoagulability of the blood induced by alimentary lipemia."

Still another well-known authority, Dr. Herman E. Hilleboe, New York State Health Commissioner, has given his opinion in this answer to a question at a medical lecture: "Increased lipids in the blood after a fatty meal appear to make the blood more coagulable; this, in turn, may have a direct bearing on the development of thrombosis in the coronary arteries."

Back in 1935 the noted pediatric educator Dr. I. N. Kugelmass had reported the clinical use of a high fat and high protein diet to control excessive bleeding tendencies in children.

In 1949 Dr. S. E. Moolten noticed increased sticky platelets in the blood of those on a diet high in milk fat and egg yolk.

In 1953 Dr. Moolten went one step further. From the yolks of eggs he extracted the most active clotting factor, which he called "thrombocytosin," and used it with good results in correcting excessive bleeding tendencies.

In 1962, in preparing this chapter, the author asked Dr. Kugelmass if he had any further data "that might be of interest in this book." The answer was that his clinical results still showed the high fat diet to be useful in raising the clottability of the blood when it was found clinically necessary to do so.

Dr. George A. Mayer and his group at Queens University in Canada had been making blood coagulability tests on heart-attack patients. In 1958 Dr. Meyer announced that by means of the Prudent Diet, within a short period his patients' blood clottability had been sufficiently normalized so that the anticoagulant-drug dosage could be reduced to half the previous amount. This report has been verified by other controlled tests made on atherosclerotics, including such work as that of Dr. K. M. Lorie of the Moscow Therapeutic Nutrition Clinic, which showed a reduced hypercoagulability of the blood in patients on a low-fat, low-cholesterol, low-calorie diet.

A mass clinical trial on the effects of a Prudent Diet on blood coagulability was made in 1961 by Dr. M. J. Karvonen and his associates, who used two mental hospitals in Finland for their observations. In one the diet remained unchanged and in the other a change was made to the Prudent Diet. The doctors reported a "significant lengthening of the clotting time in the group whose diet had been changed."

The ideal test of the value of the Prudent Diet in reducing blood coagulability is the long-term mass test using control groups. Unfortunately, only a few such tests have been made.

Too little time, too few hospitals, too little money, and too few scientists are available for the "ideal" long-term type of tests which need to be performed on human beings. Therefore, many medical scientists who are interested in blood hypercoagulability have to use animals in order to study the effects of a fatty diet as it occurs inside living blood vessels.

Reports of such tests on dogs were made in 1960 by Dr. N. U. Bang and Dr. Cliffton of the Sloan-Kettering Institute for Cancer Research. They found that a fatty diet stimulated the formation of clots inside the dogs' blood vessels. Microscope slides showed platelets, chylomicrons and fibrin, all in close association in the blood clots.

In 1961, in Sweden, Dr. S. E. Bergentz made similar tests on rabbits at the University of Goteborg. Here, for five days, two groups of laboratory animals had been fed, one group on non-fatty and the other on fatty meals. An "isolated vein" in each animal was then examined. Almost three times as many clots were found in the veins from the rabbits on the fatty diet.

Dr. S. Naimi and a group at the Pratt Clinic in Boston investigated the clottability problem, and were satisfied with the correlations of the results of all their blood measurements. They stated, "In our studies, the three [factors], high blood fats, coagulation changes *in vitro* [in a test tube] and a tendency to thrombosis *in vivo* [in the living arteries] seemed to be associated."

Because laboratory animals are expensive, many medical scientists must cut costs by making simplified blood tests on human volunteers. In these cases, the coagulability of the blood is measured before and after varied types of fatty and non-fatty meals. To test a group of "human guinea pigs" very little equipment is needed: a typical American breakfast of eggs, bacon, buttered toast, and coffee with heavy cream; a hypodermic syringe; some test tubes; and a kitchen clock.

Although tests of this type were made as far back as 1940, there was much disagreement up to 1960 on the findings. The test was not as simple as it seemed, and the scientists found pitfalls at every step. Techniques for avoiding the many types of traps and pitfalls were slowly learned over a period of twenty years. Until recently the clotting test using whole blood was the most difficult and frustrating of all the blood tests.

Human blood is a complex mixture of chemical and biochemical substances—living bodies, semi-alive bodies, giant molecules with extraordinary shapes and properties, and finally the various sized and complicated fatty globules which are sent into the blood stream with each fatty meal.

The first defect found with the *in vitro* test was in the glass test tube. Some clotting factors in blood seem to "stick" to the smooth glass walls of test tubes. It was Dr. H. W. Fullerton's use of the super-smooth "artery-like" silicone coating on his test tubes that enabled him to affirm in 1953 that hypercoagulability occurred after a fatty meal. It took twenty-five minutes for blood to coagulate after a non-fatty meal, but, as Dr. Fullerton increased the amount of fat in the meals of the same subjects, the clotting time was shortened. With two ounces of fat in the meal it was six minutes shorter; and following a three-ounce fatty meal, the speed of blood clotting was almost double the normal rate.

Certain other pitfalls should have been obvious. One group, in 1957, instead of testing clottability of the blood in the same persons before and after fatty and non-fatty meals, used *different* groups chosen at random. Naturally, only inconclusive results could be obtained with such a method. Yet, in medical reviews of this problem, the above report has been cited as "disproving" the diet approach to reducing hypercoagulability in blood.

Of course excess fat in the diet is not the only cause of

clottability of the blood. Stressful emotions can be a pitfall which must be avoided in a valid test. Consequently, Dr. R.B. Goldrick of the Kanematsu Institute in Australia was careful to keep his "human guinea pigs" calm, confident, and comfortable. He even went to the trouble of administering "practice" blood punctures to instill confidence, so that the real tests conducted the next day would occur under minimal stress. Dr. Goldrick's results showed an average speedup in clotting time of about 20% after a fatty meal.

Some blood scientists will only consider large changes toward hypercoagulability as dangerous, and three major reports by well-established medical groups based their conclusions on this relatively arbitrary standard. Their findings have been frequently quoted to "disprove" the harmful effects of a fatty meal. Dr. J. F. Mustard, who is the head of the Canadian group of scientists with perhaps the widest experience in thrombotic-blood research in the world, has re-evaluated these reports. He concludes that, "Three of the studies frequently quoted in the literature as negative actually show that the ingestion of fat influences the clotting time of blood."

New methods are constantly being devised to measure the blood-clotting tendency. Dr. J. W. Hahn, of the Southwest Foundation for Research and Education, combined two clotting factors into a single index. After a fatty meal, Dr. Hahn found that this thrombotic index rose to double the pre-test level.

Actually every one of the very many clotting factors in blood should be considered. In 1962, Dr. E. Davidson of the University of Cambridge tested ten major clotting factors. Tests made on rats given a fatty diet showed a significant rise in seven out of ten clotting factors measured.

Most of the reported tests were made with dairy fats because these saturated animal fats have the greatest effect on blood coagulability. In Japan Dr. M. Matsuoka at Shinshu University showed that meals with vegetable oil caused blood to coagulate much more slowly than meals with animal fat.

In order to differentiate the effects of saturated fat from that of unsaturated oil in the diet, Dr. W. B. Rawls at St. Clares Hospital in New York introduced a more sensitive "retarded" test. He found that an intake of foods rich in saturated fats caused a marked acceleration in this sensitive clotting test, while vegetable oils had at most a slight effect.

Only the highlights in the story of the blood test pitfalls have been mentioned. Slowly the practice of testing the hypercoagulability of whole blood was becoming a science. By 1961 the last two pitfalls, the drying time for the silicone coat and the delicate skill needed in the hypodermic needle puncture, were overcome by the research studies of Dr. J. P. Dailey. Having now conquered the "last" of the pitfalls, Dr. Dailey had a blood-coagulation test of great accuracy, and he was able to show an increase in clottability after a fatty meal.

Every medical report in recent years shows that a fatty meal *does* cause hypercoagulability in the blood. But this knowledge is still new and has not been adequately communicated in the medical world. Unfortunately, the doubts of the 1950-to-1960 "pitfall" period still linger to some extent.

There are two ways in which blood hypercoagulability finally makes its presence known: (1) by the quiet, insidious deposits of platelets and fibrin, which slowly lead to increased artery blockage and (2) by the thrombotic blood clot.

The problem is not that of the blood being in immediate danger of a thrombosis following a fatty meal. (This has happened, but such cases are unusual.) It is the cumulative effect of small changes, caused by a lifetime of fatty meals, on the *many clotting factors* in the blood that first leads to atherosclerosis then perhaps to thrombosis. In the average case there is a combination of many factors: *First:* A reduction of the heparin circulating in the blood, thus weakening the blood's most important anti-clotting factor, thought by many research scientists to be caused by a lifelong fatty diet. *Second:* the effect of this diet in promoting stickiness of the blood platelets. *Third:* the harmful effects of this diet on the other thrombotic factors in the blood. *Fourth:* the accelerated growth of atherosclerosis as a result of these and other factors. These influences set the stage. Now a final "last straw" is needed. This may be a fatty meal, a stress situation, or a slowing down of the blood circulation. Depending on the combination of these and other factors, a small or large thrombosis may result.

Many other medical-research scientists are becoming concerned about the thrombotic effects of a fatty meal. One of them, Dr. J. Schmidt of Wayne State University College of Medicine, has added new data demonstrating an increase in blood coagulability after a fatty meal. His conclusion was that: "It seems reasonable to suppose that in patients with pre-existing vascular disease, such as atherosclerosis, moderate changes in coagulability induced by amounts of fat comparable to those ingested during a heavy meal, might produce thrombosis in a vessel with restricted caliber and reduced blood flow."

The only conclusive test of hypercoagulability on a high-fat diet, and of the prevention of this hypercoagulable state by the Prudent Diet, is a clinically oberved long-term mass test. The first of these mass tests was the five-year test of the New York Anti-Coronary Club which proved that the Prudent Diet not only reduced the number of heart attacks in the group, but also reduced the number of thrombotic events.

An even more dramatic trial on a mass scale was conducted on older patients in Denmark in 1962. It clearly proved the rapid effect of the Prudent Diet in reducing hypercoagulability of the blood. Here are the conditions for this test as it was set up by Drs. P. F. Hansen, T. Geill and E. Lund in the Geriatric section of the De Gamles By Hospital in Copenhagen. Since the 280 patients had been eating a high saturated-fat diet, the plan was to see if a prudent-type diet would reduce their known tendency to thrombosis. Two matched groups were set up, one to continue on the old fatty diet, the other to change to a diet free of butter, milk, cream and margarine.

Within five months, the value of the Prudent Diet was evident. Of the patients who continued with their old fatty diet, fourteen suffered thrombotic attacks in either veins or arteries. But the Prudent Diet group had only two such cases.

According to this research, it should be possible to observe the relation between diet and blood clots in autopsy investigations.

Dr. J. B. Enticknap of London spent four years making a series of examinations of the conditions of artery blockage found in the 750 autopsies at the Eastham Memorial Hospital. In addition, he examined the blood lipids of each cadaver for comparative analysis.

The cases of severe artery blockage always showed a much higher cholesterol count than matched normals and an even greater increase in beta fatty globules. And in addition "The more abnormal they [the lipids] are the more likely is a large thrombus to be present."

Diet is not the only cause for increased clottability of the blood. Most stress situations result in temporary hypercoagulability. This evolutionary method, which increased the possibility of quick wound repairs, was of value to the animal for jungle survival.

But even this reaction is related to the type of fats in the diet as will be shown in the next section.

TWELVE WAYS THAT HIGH-FAT MEALS INFLUENCE BLOOD-CLOTTING TENDENCY

There is a fourth very small fatty particle in the blood which is the major cause of stress hypercoagulability. In the last few years medical scientists have given it five different difficult-to-understand names. In this book, for simplicity's sake, these particles shall be named for their major function, *Energy Fatty Particles* or E.F.P.*

The E.F.P. are the actual small bits which are "burned up" when fats are used for fuel in the body. Although less in total quantity than the large fatty globules, they are far more active.

In a 1962 study of women during and after childbirth, Dr. H. L. Davis of the University of Nebraska Medical School found that the concentration of *Energy Fatty Particles* increased, and that clottability of the blood correlated with the increase in a step-by-step sequence. In this stress situation the E.F.P., more so than the other fatty globules, seemed to be the direct cause of clottability.

In any stress situation the E.F.P. are quickly released from the body's fat stores directly to the blood, and serve a twofold purpose by providing energy for the imminent

---

*Initials used by scientists are IFA, UFA, FFA, NEFA and ABFA.

"fight" and by introducing a temporary hypercoagulability to repair possible wounds.

The E.F.P. also enter the blood when chylomicrons are removed and so become a by-product of the "clearing process." Nature's method of protecting the blood from the hypercoagulable effect of these Energy Fatty Particles is to endow them with a short life, averaging less than seven minutes from birth until they are "burned up." A high-fat diet has the effect of keeping too many E.F.P. in the blood for too long a period.

Man's modern innovation is *immobilized stress*. Nature's method of *active stress* calls for a release of Energy Fatty Particles to supply concentrated fuel for fight or flight. Our modern immobilized stress usually takes place in a chair. This absence of physical effort increases the duration of hypercoagulability.

There are as many types of *Energy Fatty Particles* as there are different kinds of fat. For each of the primary types of saturated, monounsaturated and polyunsaturated fats, there is a special type of E.F.P. Dr. H. L. Davis, mentioned earlier in this chapter, has studied various types of *Energy Fatty Particles* to determine their specific effects on blood clottability. He has found that the *saturated* E.F.P. caused maximum coagulability and that the polyunsaturated E.F.P. has relatively little effect.

One source of the E.F.P. is body fat, whose content we can control by the type of fat that we admit in our diet. Hard saturated body fat can, during stress, be a source of hypercoagulable blood. But, if we eat and store more of the many-hinged (polyunsaturated) soft fats, the stress E.F.P. will be less saturated and cause less trouble.

It is now possible to bring up to date the neglected data on thrombosis reported during World War II. The first evidence noticed was a sudden and dramatic drop during this period in post-operative thrombosis and thromboembolisms, soon followed by the even more important decrease in coronary thrombosis.

Many medical specialists reported at that time that the lower blood coagulability was due to the marked decrease of saturated animal fats in the sparse wartime diets.

However, the short time interval between fat rationing and the dramatic reduction in thrombosis was the cause of much controversy. Many skeptics have questioned the data and doubted the possibility of such a quick change in rate of thrombosis. But now the latest research shows that this skepticism had no scientific basis.

Take the case of the De Gambles By Hospital experiment in Copenhagen. Within one month the protective effects of the Prudent Diet were already evident to Dr. Geill and his associates. The Canadian Queens University trial also showed the rapid effects of the Prudent Diet. It took only five weeks before Dr. Mayer saw that it was necessary to reduce the patient's dosage of anticoagulant drugs.

To sum up the knowledge concerning the effects of the various lipid (fatty) contents of the blood on blood coagulability:

1. The chylomicrons that enter the blood stream after a saturated fatty meal are larger in size and less stable than after a meal rich in vegetable oil.

2. The chylomicrons following a high saturated fat meal are the cause of many changes in the red blood cells.

3. Saturated fatty meals cause "sticky" platelets . . . the most important of the thrombotic factors.

4. Almost all of the many known clotting factors in the blood are increased by high fatty meals.

5. The cephalins in the platelets and blood are involved in thrombotic blood.

6. Egg yolk is one of the best food sources of cephalin.

7. Clot dissolving enzymes in blood are retarded by saturated fatty meals.

8. A retarded clot dissolving system eventually results in increased fibrinogen, which is a cause of hypercoagulable blood.

9. An increase in saturated E.F.P. will increase blood coagulability.

10. Stress exerts its effects on blood coagulability by mobilization of the fatty globules and the E.F.P. from the fat depots of the body.

11. Exercise exerts its beneficial effects on the clot-dissolving system by using up the excess lipids in the blood.

12. As will be shown later, all the above are inter-
    related to the exhaustion of heparin, the impor-
    tant regulator of almost every stage of the
    blood-clotting system.

UNNOTICED BLOOD CLOTS IN THE LEGS
A MAJOR CAUSE OF DISABILITY AND DEATH

Perhaps the clearest proof of our present hypercoagulable blood is the widespread occurrence of blood clots
in the deep veins of the legs. Dr. Roy J. Popkins of the
Cedars of Lebanon Hospital in Los Angeles made a special study of this problem and considers this type of
thrombosis to be "one of the commonest afflictions of
civilized people." According to Dr. Popkins' calculations
the aftereffects of these venous blood clots have caused a
reduction in work ability in over five per cent of our
adult population.

But this estimate shows only the known clinical facts.
Hidden in the deep veins of the legs may be clots which
have not made their damaging effects known. Pathologists
studying this problem have reported that at least half
of our adults will eventually have autopsy evidence of
thrombosis in the legs.

One of the events feared by surgeons is a thromboembolism in the lung which is caused by a "runaway" clot
first formed in the deep veins of the leg. This danger has
been reduced today by the anticoagulant drugs.

If Americans do have clotty blood as a result of a rich
diet, this should show up in hospital thrombosis data. Conversely, if the non-Western diet has a beneficial effect on
preventing blood clots and embolism, this should also show
up in hospital records in countries on a low-fat diet.

In the United States 30,000 sudden deaths occur annually from thrombo-embolism in the lung. Dr. Naide who
reported this statement to the American Academy of General Practice at their 1963 meeting, emphasized that this
is a "grave problem compared with the 40,000 people who
die in automobile accidents annually."

For a comparison figure there is the data by Dr. H.
Ueda of the University of Tokyo which he reported in the
American Journal of Cardiology (Sept. 1962). He states,
'Only two cases of fatal pulmonary embolisms can be

found in the statistics of autopsies from 20 pathology departments during the past 10 years."

Further comparison data comes from Africa. Dr. R. C. Franz of the King Edward VIII Hospital in Durban has presented data from a six year period showing that each year, from an average of 40,000 operations, there were only two fatal post-operative thromboembolisms.

In the United States the post-operative fatal thromboembolism rate is thirty times greater than the average of the Japanese, African and Indian figures.

And in addition to the 30,000 deaths from "runaway clots" in the United States, there are many more cases of embolism that are not fatal.

In the September 1963 issue of *Angiology* there appeared an estimate of the number of thromboembolisms which occur in the United States. Dr. J. C. Breneman in this report estimates that, "upwards of 400,000 unfortunate victims are afflicted each year."

This enormous figure for thromboembolisms may seem unbelievable but autopsy studies show that this may be an understatement.

Dr. S. Wessler at the Boston Beth Israel Hospital made a sample determination in 1961 on an unselected group of sixty autopsies. Of these, over 70% had some evidence of pulmonary thromboemboli.

Startling statistics from the Oxford Regional Hospital Board in England show that the embolism rate has increased five-fold compared to what it was ten years ago. In a *British Medical Journal* report of October 5, 1963, Dr. M. T. Morrell warns that deaths from "lung clots" are increasing to an "epidemic affecting Western society."

Thrombosis in the deep veins of the legs and thromboembolism in the lungs are caused by two conditions. First, a hypercoagulable state in the blood. Second, a slowing down of blood circulation in the veins caused usually by relative immobility following illness or operation.

WHY THE CORONARY ARTERIES ARE THE MOST VULNERABLE TO ARTERY BLOCKAGE

This explanation for thrombotic blood clots in veins may also help us to understand why the coronary artery is especially vulnerable to blockage. Strangely enough, the blood in these arteries is subjected to periodic "stoppage." The flow in the other arteries never stops, and the blood is constantly moving forward, impelled by the high pressure created by each beat of the heart. The coronary artery is the only exception, and in *certain portions* of this artery the blood stops its forward motion during the brief moment when the pumping action of the heart is at its *highest pressure*.

Unlike the other arteries in the body, the coronaries are subject to two opposing forces:

1. The pulsing pressure from the blood within the heart, flowing into the coronary artery via the aorta.

2. An *opposing* pressure from the other end, generated by the smaller branches of the coronary arteries which are embedded *inside* the heart muscle walls. This momentary pressure, which occurs only when the heart muscle contracts, tends to move the blood in the coronary artery *backward*.

For a fraction of a second, when these two opposing forces are approximately equal, the blood flow has a *standstill period* in the sections of the coronary arteries which are *outside* the heart muscle. The *standstill period* lasts about one fourth of the entire time required for the normal heart beat.

Just as the ocean deposits its flotsam and jetsam on its shores at the peak moment when the surge of the wave is at a standstill, so does the blood of the coronary arteries also deposit some of its excess thrombotic debris during a similar period in its ebb and flow.

Many medical researchers believe that this unusual set of circumstances is the major cause for the build up of serious blockage in the coronary arteries years before it occurs in other arteries.

The duration of the *normal standstill period* is approximately one quarter of a second per heart beat or about 15 seconds per minute. Each *standstill period* is about the same regardless of how fast the heart beats. If the heart rate doubles, the total of the standstill periods becomes 30 seconds per minute. The faster the heart beat, the longer the *overall standstill period*.

There are many causes for an increased heart beat rate. The principal ones are: stress, infection, allergy and exercise.

Increased heart beat rate during exercise is not harmful, since in this case the *increase in standstill period* is counterbalanced by a *natural increase in the blood clot dissolving factors*. But this protection is not present during stress and infection when, in fact, the blood is actually more coagulable than normally.

The only effective solution to the ever-present threat of the *normal standstill period* and the *added* threat, during an abnormal increase in heart rate, is to keep the blood "clean." This means to keep the amounts of the microscopic flotsam and jetsam of the blood—the unnatural excess of "sticky" platelets, fibrinogen, chylomicrons, unstable fatty globules and other lipid and thrombotic factors —as close to normal as possible.

And the only natural method of preventing this *excess debris*—and clearing it away if it is already present—has been shown to be the complete prevention program and especially the Prudent Diet.

CHAPTER FIFTEEN

Who Can Benefit Most From the Prudent Diet?

THE GAP BETWEEN SCIENTIFIC INFORMATION AND ITS APPLICATION

Coronary disease is so prevalent that almost everyone is becoming concerned about it. And sooner or later probably everyone will discuss the possibility of preventing heart attack with their family physician.

It would be useful therefore to know the present attitude of the average doctor toward the Prudent Diet. A recent survey based on answers to questionnaires sent to 500 doctors was published in the *Medical World News* of April 27, 1962. It contained the following summaries:

● ". . . most doctors agreed that cholesterol is a major

factor in coronary heart diseases, but fewer of them urge their patients to cut down on fats."

● Four out of five doctors considered elevated blood cholesterol a major contributing factor in heart disease.

● Three out of four doctors believed that high cholesterol was "a symptom predicting eventual atherosclerosis," yet only one out of four gave routine cholesterol tests even for patients over fifty-five years of age.

● Even in cases where the cholesterol was known to be high, only half the patients were placed on a low-fat diet.

● Finally, only one out of three doctors who prescribed a low-fat diet, asked their patients to adhere to a proper proportion of unsaturated to saturated fat.

What a gap between the scientific information known by doctors and their day-to-day application of it! One reason for this may be gleaned from a statement by Dr. William Dock, an outspoken Professor of Medicine at the State University of New York: "A challenging problem for the nutritionist is the fact that physicians who so often ascribe acute illness to a recent dietary mishap, have always hated to accept any theory of ascribing chronic disease to a bad food."

Another explanation for the lag was offered in 1962, by Dr. Jeremiah Stamler, head of the Heart Disease Control Program of the Chicago Board of Health. Referring to the attitude of general practitioners and internists in their work with adult patients, Dr. Stamler wrote: ". . . these key members of the medical profession are still overwhelmingly concerned with the care of the sick."

But the doctors are not the only ones indifferent to preventive medical care, Dr. Stamler continues, for, "Just as general practitioners and internists are, by and large, still unaccustomed to practicing preventive medicine, in their offices, so too, most adults have not yet been convinced of the wisdom of periodic check-ups, assessment for disease susceptibility and prevention intervention."

It is easy to see that the *cure-minded* general practitioners and internists, as well as their patients, are mostly concerned with the present acute condition and are thinking along different lines from those whose primary interest is in the *prevention* of heart disease. One can begin to understand the diversity of opinion on the subject of prevention of coronary disease by a brief survey of its unusual history.

At first there was almost no concept that prevention was possible. Indeed, very little was known about the cause of heart attack during the thirty year period after it was first recognized as a potentially important problem. Dr. James Herrick was the first to present a comprehensive account of heart attack to the world medical profession, in what is now an historic document, "Clinical Features of Sudden Obstruction of the Coronary Arteries," published in the *Journal of the American Medical Association* in 1912. During the following decade so few cases were being seen, even by specialists, that little attention was paid to his work.

Dr. Paul Dudley White made his first diagnosis of coronary thrombosis in 1921, and year by year, the percentage of such cases rose in his practice. For the next twenty-five years almost all of the heart specialists focused their attention on the pressing problems of diagnosis and emergency treatment of their ever-increasing number of heart-attack cases, but gave little thought to prevention. As recently as 1950, medical text books listed atherosclerosis as a "natural aging process." Very little has been added on heart-attack prevention to medical texts even during the past decade.

Doctors still must search medical journals to find relevant facts and new information; but the long lines of their anxiously waiting patients leave them little time and energy to attend meetings or to study thousands of medical research papers. The burden of communication rests on the associations of specialists who are doing the research on heart-attack prevention.

The American Heart Association is the foremost of such medical groups. And the American Heart Association is definitely urging a change to the Prudent Diet as is clearly indicated in the January 1961 report, (titled: DIETARY FAT AND ITS RELATION TO HEART ATTACKS AND STROKES) which was quoted in the fourth chapter of this book.

Although in this brief excerpt the A.H.A. may seem to be urging that almost every adult male in this country be placed on the low-fat Prudent Diet, this needs clarification. The official attitude of the A.H.A. report was that the doctor is urged to prescribe the Prudent Diet when there is an indication that the patient may have *more* than the "normal" expectancy of heart attack.

THE EIGHT "HIGH RISK" GROUPS FOR WHOM THE PRUDENT DIET CAN MEAN LIFE OR DEATH

In addition to known heart-attack patients, four groups were listed as those who would benefit most from a change to the Prudent Diet:

- Those with high blood cholesterol
- Those with high blood pressure
- Overweight persons
- Those with a family tendency to heart attack

Other medical groups and individual heart specialists have added to this list:

- Diabetics and pre-diabetics
- Individuals with any abnormality in their blood lipids
- Anyone with a higher-than-normal tendency toward blood clotting
- Those with any significant degree of atherosclerosis

What proportion of middle-aged American men fit at least one of the "maximum benefit" categories listed?

From a statistical point of view, virtually every one of them seems to be a good candidate for the Prudent Diet. Take each factor in turn:

1. High Blood Cholesterol: From thirty to seventy percent of American men are reported to have this trouble.

2. High Blood Pressure: From forty to sixty percent develop this condition by middle age.

3. Overweight: Anywhere from thirty to fifty percent of the total population.

4. Diabetes: Five percent or more of middle-aged men suffer from known diabetes and a larger group are in the undiagnosed diabetic group. A still more extensive fraction of the population are pre-diabetic.

5. Blood-lipid defects: May affect over fifty percent of our middle-aged men.

6. Hypercoagulability: The specific percentage of the population with a higher-than-normal tendency toward blood clotting is difficult to estimate, but it is probably high.

7. Atherosclerosis: Statistics indicate that two out of three middle-aged men have an important degree of atherosclerotic artery blockage.

Actually, the average middle-aged American male may suffer from *several* of the conditions listed. Of course there are some men who have miraculously reached middle age without any damage, but in the opinion of many eminent heart specialists, they are rare specimens. We have, therefore, a large segment of the population eligible for the Prudent Diet. Yet only ten years or so ago, many physicians who were interested in this diet as a method of heart-attack prevention limited its use to patients who suffered from angina or had a history of heart attack and who, in addition, had a high cholesterol level.

WHY EVERY MALE IS "A RISK"

More recently the requirement was stated as "two or more signs or symptoms." During the past two years, the limitations have been reduced by the American Heart Association to only one indication or to a "family tendency." Based on the evidence of statistics, the frequently voiced medical judgment is that, currently, every middle-aged American male is—as the heart specialists say—"a risk."

Dr. Thomas R. Dawber, head of the Framingham Study, made this broad statement concerning those who should receive the whole prevention program, including the Prudent Diet: "Selection of subjects for such a regimen should not be too difficult. Clearly, males carry considerably more risk than females and warrant first attention."

Dr. I .H. Page discussed the broad scope of the A.H.A. Report in a medical editorial in the *Review of Modern Medicine.* Since Dr. Page was the chairman of the committee who drafted the document, his analysis is important.

In summing up the meaning of the report and its general intent, he states that "it was primarily aimed at the coronary prone male but was made *permissive* for those normal people who like to *anticipate* by an educated guess."

For those doctors who have accepted this basic approach, the next logical step is to prevent artery blockage from starting in the young. Today there is a growing number of doctors who are in favor of *diet control from the cradle on.* This call for a lifetime of the Prudent Diet comes from some of the most eminent cardiologists in the United States.

An interesting item appeared in the January 1963 issue of the *American Heart Journal* by the well-known cardiologist, Dr. Myron Prinzmetal. It was a "Proposal on the Possibility of Improving Cow's Milk for the Purpose of

Lowering the Incidence of Atherosclerosis." But even if it were possible to breed cows whose milk contained less saturated and more *unsaturated* fat, it certainly would take many decades.

Other specialists envision quicker methods of introducing the Prudent Diet at an early age. In the *Journal of Clinical Nutrition*, Dr. Leon Swell of the Medical School of George Washington University says, in regard to his application of the Prudent Diet: "An important aspect of this diet was that it was readily accepted by the children of the family. This is of particular significance since such diets, if they are beneficial in reducing the incidence of atherosclerosis, should probably be started at an early age in the general population."

In the opinion of Dr. A. C. Corcoran of the United States National Heart Institute, "Possibly the procedure best directed toward delaying onset of coronary arteriosclerosis would be a wholesale fairly drastic change in exercise and dietary patterns *from youth on.*"

Another cardiologist who shares these opinions is Dr. M. S. Mazel, who is Medical Director at the Chicago Edgewater Hospital. Dr. Mazel has been specializing on the surgical rejuvenation of arteries of the atherosclerotic heart and, according to his educational exhibit at a recent annual meeting, of the American Medical Association, the proper diet *from infancy* should contain less than twenty per cent of fat if the need for his type of heart surgery in later life is to be avoided. Dr. G. de Takats, who is president of the Chicago Heart Association, spoke to the doctors about starting the Prudent Diet early in life and said that, "If we as physicians are convinced that too much tobacco, *too much bacon, too much fat is bad for our children—where the damage really starts—we must come out and say it, although it might alienate our financial supporters . . .* Why should we, and how can we prevent and treat cardiovascular disease when our population is unknowingly poisoning itself?"

Dr. Paul Dudley White in his address to the 1961 New Jersey Governors Conference suggested that "Milk should not be fed to children beyond the infant stage."

And a method of insuring the start of the Prudent Diet *at birth* was suggested in 1962 by two noted heart specialists, Drs. Lawrence W. Kinsell and Herbert Pollack. At a symposium on coronary disease, held at the Hahnemann Medical College, they stated—in a new interview—that the nursing mother can supply the right kind of milk to the new-born infant by eating foods high in polyunsaturated fats. If the baby must be on a bottle formula, they continued, it should be a form of skim milk with unsaturated oils added.

In 1962, Dr. Lars Soderhjelm of the East Bay Childrens Hospital in Oakland, California, completed a study on "The Role of Fats in the Child's Diet." His conclusion may come as a shock to those who think that milk fat is the most nutritious of all. He states: "Optimal results in infant feeding, however, seemed to be attained at linoleic acid [the polyunsaturated "two hinge" oil found in all vegetable oil] levels of four to five percent of dietary calories, such as in human milk or cow's milk mixtures in which the butter fat has been modified and a vegetable oil added."

Dr. Isadore Snapper, whose pioneering research among the Chinese before 1940 had uncovered the relationship between their low-saturated-fat diet and their complete freedom from coronary disease, has recently stated that the Prudent Diet, ". . . begun in early childhood as a life-long regimen will *prevent* the development of atherosclerosis, thrombosis and gall stones."

In his opinion the "myth" of the necessity of milk "can probably never be destroyed. This despite the fact that most clinicians today recognize that it is dangerous to encourage children to stuff themselves with milkshakes, ice cream and other foods with unsatisfactory [excess saturated fat] ratios."

HOW YOU CAN BENEFIT FROM THE PRUDENT DIET

A heart specialist who is fully aware of the entire situation is the present head of the New York City Coronary Club, Dr. George Christakis. In a recent radio-panel discussion the following question was put to him: "Is it necessary to get a doctor's permission before changing to the Prudent Diet?"

The essence of Dr. Christakis' answer was that *we are changing our diets every day, every time we go to the refrigerator, without our doctor's permission.*

It was Dr. Christakis' opinion that "when it comes to the Prudent Diet, we may do it ourselves, and it will be safe, effective in lowering cholesterol, and *more nutritive than our present diet."*

In other countries directives such as these are being issued by governmental medical authorities. For instance, according to an editorial in the *American Heart Journal,* "The National Board of Health of Sweden recently recommended to the people of that country a general restriction in fat intake."

In the *South African Medical Journal* there appeared an editorial by the National Nutritional Council which advised that "The desirable upper limit for fat intake is probably about 30% of the total calories."

In his book *Coronary Heart Disease,* Dr. J. W. Gofman sums up the situation as follows. "There will undoubtedly be those who say the idea of considering every adult as a patient or a potential patient with respect to a disease like coronary heart disease would mean a fabulous task for the medical profession. It will be a fabulous task for the medical profession, but one abundantly justified by the fabulous importance of the problem that lies before it in this field."

At the 1963 symposium on Atherosclerosis which was held in Minneapolis by the Minnesota Heart Association, a dinner was held in honor of the many medical research scientists who participated.

In front of each guest was a card which is reproduced below.

This evening's menu provides 1250 calories,
32% of them from fat. Polyunsaturated fats account for
16.2%, monounsaturated 7.1%, and saturated 8.7%.
The P:S ratio is 1.9.
If you start eating this way all of the time,
AND
you have previously been eating an average American diet,
AND
your blood cholesterol is now 225 mg.%,
AND
you respond in the average manner,
THEN
three weeks from now your blood cholesterol will be
197 mg.%,
AND
maybe you will live longer.

CHAPTER SIXTEEN

Myths and Misunderstandings About Heart Attack and Diet

EXCEPTIONAL CASES THAT DO NOT DISPROVE THE RULE

The voluminous body of facts supporting the Prudent Diet is so impressive that its value in the anti-coronary program seems irrefutable. Why then do some medical men still oppose it?

The opposition stems from confusion caused by the fact that coronary disease is the final result of a wide variety of disorders and conditions—some of which are beyond our control. The contributing factors which can be controlled and prevented include (1) diets high in saturated fats and excessive in calories (2) unstable fatty globules in the blood (3) high blood pressure (4) modern stress (5) pushbutton "exercise" (6) infections (7) metabolic illness (8) poor tissue tone (9) toxins in the environment and (10) the excess of blood-clotting factors. And most important is the length of time during which each specific condition was able to exert its influence. It is the total of all the years of damage from each specific cause that will finally determine each individual's accumulation of artery blockage.

It can easily be seen that in many cases it is impossible to trace the past history and the specific "active" period of each damaging cause. As a result, the real reason for the artery blockage may be obscured. This can create the illusion that some of the facts are "contradictory."

It was only a decade ago that the concept of the cause of heart attack was as shown in the chart below.

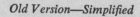

Old Version—Simplified

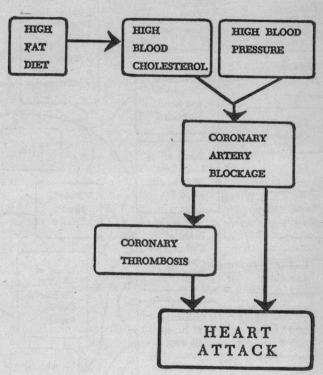

It is the very simplicity of this chart which led to the misconceptions that cause the many so called "exceptions."

During the past ten years, new research has added much more knowledge and a fully detailed understanding as seen in the Complete Chart of Coronary Disease.

COMPLETE CHART

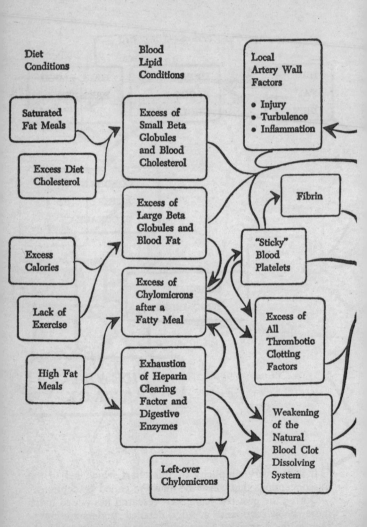

OF CORONARY DISEASE

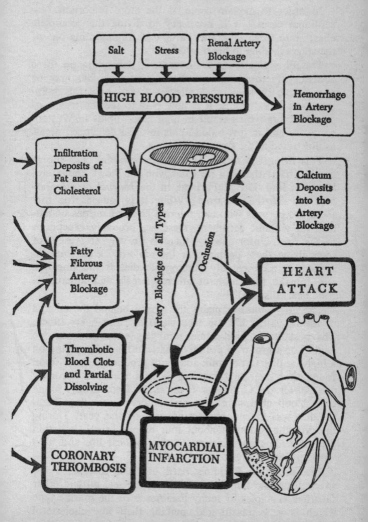

But even the "complete chart" with all its details can only give a *hint* of the extent to which the "exceptional cases" can occur and cause confusion in evaluating the Prudent Diet.

In order to explain some of the more important "exceptional cases," it is necessary to divide the "complete chart" into three separate charts, each representing one of the stages leading to heart attack.

The First Stage chart shows how, depending on three accessory factors, the bad effects of a rich diet may be aggravated, or sometimes alleviated, and how this influences the blood lipids. It is now easy to see the effects of many factors which result in high blood lipids in Western countries and in low blood lipids in underdeveloped areas, as illustrated in the first two columns.

This brings us to the Western exceptional case shown on the chart: the high fat eater with the "low" cholesterol level. Of him, Dr. McFarland, in the *Journal of the Germantown Hospital* warns: "While it is indeed true that there are persons who can tolerate large quantities of natural fat without detriment, these are probably exceptions to the rule. Unfortunately, there is no way at present of recognizing these people. For the majority, a habitual ingestion of a potentially atherogenic diet is the sine qua non for the formation of atherosclerosis and atherosclerotic heart disease."

The last column explains the reason behind the enigma of the fat-eating Eskimo who was free from heart attack. The best explanation came, strangely enough, from two studies of a group of primitive African herdsmen living on a high-fat diet (from milk and dairy products). Dr. Gibson found that their high-fat diet did not result in coronary disease. Dr. A. G. Shaper (*Lancet*, 16 Dec. 1962), found their blood cholesterol low and observed that their high-fat diet was eaten only during part of the year. During the drought period of about four months, semi-starvation prevailed. The combination of this cyclical life and hard work prevented excess blood lipids.

The primitive Eskimo's hard life also alternated between feast and famine. In addition, the seal oil and other fat used as staples by many Eskimos is of the marine type which is very unsaturated, making their low cholesterol easy to understand.

FIRST STAGE IN HEART ATTACK

From Diet to Blood Lipids

FACTORS THAT CONTROL BLOOD LIPIDS	GENERAL CASES		EXCEPTIONAL CASES	
	Low Fat Countries	Western Countries	Western Exception	Primitive Eskimos
TOTAL FOOD CALORIES	Low	High	High	Medium
TOTAL FAT IN THE DIET	Low	High	High	High
SATURATED FAT IN DIET	High	Low	High	Low
CHOLESTEROL IN THE DIET	Low	High	High	Medium
SUGAR IN THE DIET	Low	High	Low	None
CYCLICAL STARVATION	No	No	No	Important
THYROID METABOLISM	Normal	Lower in Middle Age	Very Good	Good
FAT ENZYME EXHAUSTION	No	Yes	No	No
EXERCISE	Good	Poor	Usually Good	Very Good
BLOOD LIPIDS	Low	High	Low or Medium	Low

Now, even without the aid of the chart it is possible to reconstruct the case of the low-calorie, medium fat-eating person who sometimes has high blood cholesterol. In this case, the factors of insufficient exercise and low metabolism may be decisive.

Still, there is one rule to which no scientist has yet found an exception: It is that the Prudent Diet, combined with other factors in the prevention program, will *always* tend to lower the blood cholesterol and all the other excess blood lipids.

In the Second Stage chart we see that the blood lipids are the *dominant* factors influencing the accumulation of artery blockage. However, many of the other factors listed may become a cause of "exceptions." Take that of time: In order to add up the total result of all contributing factors in artery blockage, one must not omit consideration of the years of damage for each specific cause. With this in mind we can examine the two general cases and the two types of "exceptions."

The main question skeptics ask is: How can you explain the case of an individual with excess artery blockage, yet a low blood cholesterol, and vice versa?

The answer to this question is shown on the "Second Stage" chart. There is much data available, showing, for example, that when young people suffer from coronary, they invariably have very high blood cholesterol. In middle-aged coronary cases the excess blood lipids have been causing trouble during a longer period, and such persons may have equivalent artery blockage even with a lower blood cholesterol.

And finally, some older coronary cases may have acquired most of their artery blockage years earlier and then, due to a change in diet, may show exceptionally low blood cholesterol.

This type of exceptional case has been summed up very well by Dr. W. Dock: "Atherosclerosis or coronary occlusion may be found in people who have low blood cholesterol at the time of death, but only in regions where high blood levels are often seen and may have existed for decades prior to the last years of life."

The stability of the fatty globule which carries the cholesterol is also important. Dr. B. M. Bloomberg of Johannesburg found that in the Bantu almost two-fifths of

SECOND STAGE IN HEART ATTACK

From Blood Lipids to Artery Blockage

CONDITIONS WHICH INFLUENCE ARTERY BLOCKAGE	GENERAL CASES		EXCEPTIONAL CASES	
	Frugal Diet Countries	Western Diet Countries	With High Blood Lipids	With Low Blood Lipids
• BETA GLOBULES • BLOOD FATS • CHOLESTEROL	Low	High	Probably Previously Low	Probably Previously High
• ALPHA GLOBULES • PHOSPHOLIPIDS	High	Low	May be High	May be Low
THROMBOTIC FACTORS IN BLOOD	Low	High		
CLOT DISSOLVING ACTIVITY	Good	Poor		
BLOOD PRESSURE	Usually Low	Rises with Age	Usually Low	Usually High
HEMORRHAGE INTO ARTERY BLOCKAGE	Rare	Frequent	May be Low	May be High
CALCIFICATION OF ARTERY BLOCKAGE	Not Present	Excessive		
THE TIME FACTOR	Less Important	Important	May be Short	May be Long
RESULTING ARTERY BLOCKAGE	Low	High	Less than Expected	More than Expected

their cholesterol is contained in the beneficial Alpha fatty globules, and the rest is in the Beta globules. But the average European is not that fortunate, and even when he has low blood cholesterol, he may still not be out of danger since his European diet usually results in a low proportion of cholesterol in the Alpha globules—only one-fifth. The balance of four-fifths is contained in the Beta fatty globules.

The harmful effect of high blood cholesterol is only

part of the story. The neutral fats which form part of the contents of the fatty globules are also of great importance in the formation of artery blockage. It is the excess blood fat that is the primary cause of the preponderance of the excessively large and physically unstable type of Beta fatty globules in the atherosclerotic. It is possible to have abnormally large quantities of neutral fats in the blood, yet have a normal blood cholesterol.

This does not minimize the importance of blood cholesterol, it only shows that *all* of the blood lipids in the fatty globules are important in the formation of artery blockage.

The Second Stage chart shows the accessory and the complicating factors in the growth of artery blockage. There are many damaging factors involved and they may have caused their damage over different lengths of time during a person's life. A large variety of combinations can occur which either accelerate or retard the atherosclerotic condition and this situation, when not completely understood, creates new "exceptional" cases.

The Third Stage chart shows that the growth of artery blockage eventually results in heart attack. But between the seemingly simple concept of blockade cause and heart attack effect are other factors that may hasten the heart attack or avert it for a long time. The factor of collateral circulation can often result in some of the most puzzling exceptions.

The quality and efficiency of the heart muscle also exerts an important influence in determining how much artery blockage can pile up before the heart attack results.

The collateral circulation is a natural safety factor that can lessen the effects of artery blockage or even prevent the heart attack. It is an interconnecting system of tiny arteries which are, so to speak, unused side roads interconnecting the coronary arteries in the heart. They are sometimes capable, under stimulation, of sufficient expansion in size to partially substitute for a seriously blocked artery. But there is no method of knowing until autopsy if this has happened.

Dr. T. D. Labecki, of the Heart-Disease Control Unit of the Mississippi State Board of Health, estimates that about ten percent of our population already have a collateral circulation sufficient to avert a heart attack. This

THIRD STAGE: From Artery Blockage to Heart Attack

CONDITIONS LEADING TO HEART ATTACK	Average middle-age male	Severe artery blockage exception	Moderate artery blockage exception
AMOUNT OF ARTERY BLOCKAGE	Severe	Severe	Moderate
LOCATION OF ARTERY BLOCKAGE	Average	May be harmless	May be strategic
OXYGEN EFFICENCY OF HEART MUSCLE	Poor	May be excellent	May be poor
COLLATERAL CIRCULATION	Average	May be good	May be poor
THROMBOTIC CONDITIONS IN THE BLOOD	Above normal	May be low	May be high
AGE AT WHICH HEART ATTACK OCCURS	"Average"	Later than expected	Earlier than expected

fortunate minority have what might be considered a complete set of spare parts and so can seemingly defy the rules of nature and still survive.

In addition there are other factors of chance which may decide when severe artery blockage will bring on a heart attack. Dr. Labecki's analysis is that "A man may have a strategically located plaque [artery blockage] and may die from coronary artery disease at age 35 years—while a person in whom atherosis gradually develops may live to the age of 75 or 80 years . . ."

Another factor in artery blockage where chance or luck plays a part is the area of location of the coronary occlusion on the surface of the heart. If the final result is a small scar on the outer working part of the heart muscle, there may be no signs or symptoms. This may not result in a "patient." But if the same scar is located in the area where the electrical conducting nerves pass, the victim may become seriously ill.

Until the explanation came at autopsy, cases of this type caused much confusion and frustration among those who sought an understanding of circulation and artery blockage in heart attack.

Some "exceptions" are best understood by considering all three charts together. Dr. Ancel Keys and his associates closely watched 281 Minnesota men for evidence of heart attack over a period of 15 years. They found that the cholesterol level was significantly prognostic in *most* cases.

Of the "exceptional" cases Dr. Keys states that, "The few men who developed coronary heart disease with low cholesterol values tended to be in the top 20 per cent of the distribution of blood pressure or relative weight or both."

In other words, those with lower levels of blood cholesterol are not safe from heart attack if their blood pressure is high. The effect of changes in blood pressure over the years is often a cause of confusion when these changes are not carefully observed.

The expectation of a consistent one-to-one relationship between blood cholesterol and heart attack, without taking the other factors into consideration, is the misconception that is the cause of most of the "exceptions."

Overemphasis of the "exceptional" cases, without full

knowledge of all the facts, which clearly explain them, leads to the defeatist "I'm from Missouri" attitude expressed as the desire to sit back and wait for more evidence.

But in the view of Dr. Albert E. Hirst, Jr., editor of *Medical Arts and Sciences,* waiting is dangerous. In his opinion, "Final proof of the protective action of unsaturated oils in atherosclerosis may not be available for a generation. In the meanwhile, those who wait until the evidence is convincing beyond any shadow of a doubt may not be around to reap the benefits of this knowledge."

THEORIES, FALLACIES AND CONFUSIONS

Some medical scientists have been seeking the main source of coronary disease in the artery wall itself. Among this group is Dr. N. T. Werthessen of the South West Foundation for Research and Education. His conclusion is that: "The primary factor leading to the atherosclerotic process is unknown but resident in the wall of the artery. It is further concluded that hypercholesterolemia and factors inducing it are of significance in determining the rate and degree of atherosclerotic change but could not alone precipitate the onset of the process."

So, in spite of his opposition to the idea that blood lipids are the *basic* origin of the trouble, Dr. Werthessen must logically conclude that a lower blood-lipid level is an intelligent method of prevention.

Other scientists have concentrated their attention upon the "ground substance" which holds together the cells within the artery wall. One of them is Dr. G. Schallock, Director of the Pathological Institute of the City Hospital of Mannheim, Germany. In a report issued in 1962, Dr. Schallock concluded: "With regard to the significance of dietary fat, it may be that when changes in the ground substance have occurred, the amount of fat ingested should be lowered if fats are not to be deposited excessively in the vessel wall."

Many others who have been searching for the answer inside the artery wall admit to the great importance of the excess blood lipids. This group, of course, cannot and does not take exception to the Prudent Diet. There are a few scientists who are so convinced that the yet-to-be-found "wall factor" will be an exclusive cause of coronary that they deny any value in the Prudent Diet. But they have not yet proposed any alternative prevention program.

Relevant to this controversy are the findings of Dr. H. F. Watts of the Temple University Medical Center in Philadelphia, who has spent the past five years taking electron-microscope photographs to find how lipids get into the artery wall.

Dr. Watts took innumerable sequential photographs which were almost equivalent to motion pictures—with enough enlargement to see the individual beta lipoprotein fatty globules traveling from the blood stream directly into the cell wall. Here an interesting and unexpected event took place. The blood lipids were actually used for energy in the vessel wall. When the additional amount of fatty globules was balanced by their use as energy, the wall remained normal. But when too many beta globules came into a section, or if too few were used up, there was an accumulation of lipids which gradually turned into the well known foam cells of atherosclerosis.

Other scientists have emphasized the role of stress in artery blockage and heart attack, and consider its role decisive. For this group it may be interesting to hear the opinion of Dr. M. Friedman, head of the Harold Brunn Institute where most of the atherosclerosis research connected with stress has been conducted.

Dr. Friedman says that, "It is our belief that whenever the plasma cholesterol is much beyond that observed at birth (i.e. above 100-125 milligrams) a situation has been created in the plasma that will enhance the rate of development of any atherosclerotic process regardless of its actual initial cause."

In the past, a few of those opposed to the Prudent Diet have tried to downgrade the value of some of the data used by certain proponents of the dietary origin of coronary disease.

One target was the cause-and-effect relationship in the data used by Dr. Ancel Keys for his many world surveys of diet and coronary disease.

Dr. Keys had published charts showing that in countries such as China, Japan, South Africa and Yugoslavia, the coronary disease rate, the blood cholesterol and the fats in the diet were correspondingly low.

By contrast, the figures for these three factors were all very high in the more industrialized countries such as U.S.A., England, Canada and New Zealand.

The Scandinavian and other European countries occupied a middle position in coronary rate. Their blood cholesterol and animal-fat consumption was moderate.

In an attempt to disprove the relationship of diet fat to coronary, Dr. Yerushalmy of California published a chart in 1957 showing a world-wide correlation between animal protein in the diet and coronary heart attack. Almost simultaneously, Dr. Yudkin of England published a chart showing a clear relationship between sugar in the diet and heart attack in the same countries.

These two charts were held to be a "scientific" knockout blow to the theory that the statistical parallel between a high-fat diet and coronary disease was due to a cause-and-effect relationship. For those who were seeking scientific data to downgrade the diet-prevention method, the charts seemed made to order. During the late 1950's dozens of medical review articles antagonistic to any diet change have used these two charts as a "refutation" of Dr. Keys' world surveys.

The fallacy in Yerushalmy's chart is so evident that it now seems strange that it could have been used as scientific refutation of the Prudent Diet. Consider the question: Where does animal protein come from? The answer is meat—eggs—milk—cheese, etc. And where do animal fats come from? Exactly the same foods. Consequently, Dr. Yerushalmy's chart was a proof rather than a disproof of the relationship of a high animal fat diet to coronary disease.

In the case of Dr. Yudkin's chart relating sugar to coronary disease, the explanation is more complicated. The fact is that sugar is the worst "hollow food" in our current diet. It is also conducive to poor tissue health, and for that reason, is a contributing factor in artery blockage. The deciding factor, however, is that the use of sugar usually increases directly in proportion to the prosperity of a country, which increase also results in more expenditures on the rich fatty foods.

In addition there has been research showing that sugar

increases cholesterol in the blood. Lifetime tests on rats have shown that when half the calories in the diet came in the form of sugar, their blood cholesterol was double that of the amount found in rats fed entirely on natural vegetable carbohydrates. The sugar diet also resulted in a 50% greater increase in body fat, compared to the vegetable eaters.

This was proven by research made by both Dr. Oscar W. Portman of Harvard in 1956 and by Drs. M. Womack and C. M. Coons of the U.S. Department of Agriculture at Beltsville in 1959.

One theory for these facts is that since sugar is digested with such unnatural rapidity, the overload causes its conversion into saturated fat for storage.

With unrefined vegetable carbohydrates such as whole grains forming most of the diet, the digestion is normal and gradual, and the body is able to handle the load.

In order to see if these results also applied to men, Dr. Ancel Keys and his associates used two basic diets. One, the "American type," was high in refined sugar and low in fruits and vegetables. The second, the "Italian type," was high in vegetables and fruits but lower in sugar and also low in milk intake.

The conclusion of Dr. Keys, after three months of tests, was "that sucrose [refined sugar] and milk sugar tend to produce higher [blood] cholesterol values than equal calories of . . . fruits, leafy vegetables and legumes." The average difference in cholesterol in the men using the two diets was twenty milligrams.

The use of sugar in the diet may also be the cause of the poor glucose tolerance (which was shown in Chapter 14 to frequently precede atherosclerosis). Dr. J. A. Uram of the Food and Drug Administration studied this problem using diets of either all cereal or part cereal part sugar.

Rats on the cereal diet had good glucose tolerance, but those which had been fed the "part sugar diet" had a very poor glucose tolerance.

This new data gives additional proof for the necessity to eliminate "hollow calories," especially sugar, but it is not evidence *against* the need to also eliminate hard saturated fat from the diet.

The facts which Drs. Yerushalmy and Yudkin relied

upon in constructing their charts were correct. However it was their incorrect interpretation of these charts that led them to the wrong conclusions.

During the past several years Dr. Keys and his group have greatly intensified and concentrated their international medical surveys of coronary disease. A summary of some of this work was given to a 1961 meeting of the New York Academy of Science by Dr. Grande, an associate of Dr. Keys.

About 8000 individuals in the same age range, from five different countries, had been carefully examined for blood cholesterol as well as heart abnormalities. Dr. Grande's report indicated an indisputable relationship between blood cholesterol levels and the percentage of abnormal electrocardiograms found in each national group. Starting from a low blood cholesterol of 180 in Yugoslavia with a low rate of only two per cent of heart abnormalities, the amount of heart defects rose with the blood-cholesterol values, step by step, until its maximum was reached in the United States where, in a similar age group, a cholesterol value of 240 and a six per cent rate of heart abnormality was found.

THE EGYPTIAN MUMMY MYTH

Each year new evidence has appeared in hundreds of medical journals, reporting and explaining the harmful effects of diets rich in saturated fats and "empty calories." Other reports have shown the value of the Prudent Diet in lowering blood lipids, preventing thrombotic blood conditions, and in inhibiting the growth of artery blockage.

One by one, the baffling exceptions have been explained and each of the puzzling questions answered.

But even after the exceptions are disposed of, there are four arguments still used in the attempt to refute or downgrade the value of the Prudent Diet. These arguments are:

1. There has been no increase in coronary disease because: "Atherosclerosis has been with us since the days of the Biblical Egyptians. It is inevitable, not preventable."

2. Even if the value of the Prudent Diet is unquestionable, it is difficult to indoctrinate a well person, and an immediate national educational cam-

    paign might result in a major economic disaster in the food industry.

3. Full and unconditional medical directives to change to the Prudent Diet might lead to overenthusiastic changes on the part of an impressionable public, with possible harmful effects.

4. Our present diet is so "nutritious" that it might be dangerous to tinker with it.

The "no increase" group has one favorite "proof," which is that atherosclerosis has been with us since Biblical days. This great Egyptian mummy myth is periodically introduced as a logical argument by scientists who are "too busy" to find out the actual facts.

The data on Egyptian mummy atherosclerosis came from a study made in 1911 by Sir Marc Armand Ruffer, who did find evidence of atherosclerosis in the half dozen Egyptian mummies available to him. He said, however, "The mummies examined were mostly those of priests and priestesses of Deir El-Bahri, who owing to their high position undoubtedly lived well." The historian W. Keller supports this view by describing the diet of ancient upper class Egyptians as a rich one. Also the Egyptian rulers were not "primarily vegetarians" as has been claimed by a few high-ranking medical-diet skeptics. According to the distinguished Egyptologist, Dr. J. H. Breasted, the illustrations in Egyptian tombs depict slaughter of cattle and geese for the royal table.

Artery blockage, then, is not an "inevitable destiny." It existed only in the wealthy Egyptian rulers whose diet was rich, although probably not as high in saturated fat as ours. And in addition, the atherosclerosis in these mummies was only equivalent to the 1911 "moderns" and not as severe as in our present-day "civilized" arteries.

The second argument is based on the fact that the rich American diet has become an ingrained habit which cannot be changed without a nationwide educational campaign.

In the opinion of many medical men, "A healthy person who has a sense of well being, vitality and self satisfaction is a poor subject for indoctrination with nutrition information." A healthy person requires specific proof of the hidden harm which he is inflicting upon himself. The argument continues with the statement that, "from a practical point of view the best patient for prevention indoctrination is one who is already chronically or severely ill and fearful for his recovery." But in the case of coronary disease, by the time symptoms are felt, most of the damage has been done and the "best patient" in the above report is in actuality a very sick patient.

But the argument takes still a new twist. The skeptical fatalist is now apt to say: "You are a middle-aged male and your arteries are already full of atherosclerosis and calcifications and scars. Is it worth losing so much eating pleasure just for the questionable possibility of a short increase in a dull life."

The inherent error of the fatalistic diet skeptic lies in overlooking the fact that, even if the atherosclerotic arteries cannot be improved by the Prudent Diet, at least the status quo can be maintained. The atherosclerotic is also a very good candidate for a thrombotic blood clot in one of his narrow, blocked, ulcerated arteries. He needs special care to keep his blood thin, clear and low in thrombotic factors. Aside from the anti-coagulant drugs, one proven method is the Prudent Diet which—according to recent clinical research—can prevent coronary thrombosis.

THE "ECONOMIC DISASTER" AND "DIET TAMPERING" ALARMISTS

So, for a successful prevention program, it is the healthy person who must be indoctrinated. But at this point a new delaying argument is introduced by the "economic disaster" skeptics, who advocate a "go-slow policy" in order to prevent a crisis in some parts of our food industry. These critics bring up the possibility that since indoctrination for change at an early age will have to be on a nationwide scale, this in turn may upset many important food industries.

However, for the individual, there is nothing more important than preventing further blockage in his coronary arteries. And those who have already changed their diets have already caused the sales of butter, cream and eggs to decline.

Dr. Luther L. Terry, the Surgeon General of the United States, has predicted that, "By 1973 several of the major causes of atherosclerosis will be understood and concern with the prophylaxis [prevention] will have affected the American agricultural economy. . ."

The problem of *possible* food industry distress must be considered as *secondary* to the *critical* heart attack situation, and should be solved by direct action, not by delaying tactics.

Next we come to those detractors of the Prudent Diet who began by claiming that the general public will not know how to follow the safe Prudent Diet, and that many individuals may try other "less safe" variations. They then assert that if variations are used, these individuals may be just as badly off as they were on their old rich diet.

Since a bit of a scientific stir is being made by these critics, we might examine their claims and find out if there is truth in their assertions.

One diet singled out for criticism is the *very low fat diet* which is high in calories. This diet should be called a "high carbohydrate diet."

The second diet is very rich in polyunsaturated fat, with vegetable oils supplying about forty percent or more of the calories. This diet should be called a "vegetable oil diet."

However it must be emphasized that neither of these two diets should be confused with the Prudent Diet. The Prudent Diet is low in calories, and low in saturated fat. The maximum fat intake of the Prudent Diet, including both the saturated and unsaturated fat, is twenty-five percent of the total calories.

To go back to the first variation . . . is there any danger in reducing the fats in the diet very much lower than in the Prudent Diet?

Medical data shows that in some individuals a high-carbohydrate, *very low-fat diet* can cause a rise in blood fats (triglycerides). But this happens only for a short time in a small percentage of those addicted to the high-saturated-fat diet whose blood lipids are already disturbed. It could be considered as a type of withdrawal symptom.

Dr. E. H. Ahrens of the Rockefeller Institute made tests in 1961 for relatively short periods on fifteen patients who were quite ill with hyperlipemia (excess blood fats). In this group all except two showed an increase in their already abnormally high blood lipids when they were put on a special diet, which replaced almost all fats with carbohydrates. From this and other similar short-term research came the incorrect conclusion that the *low-fat diet* is dangerous.

However, Dr. Ahrens mentions in his reports that a year before, Dr. A. Antonis had conducted *long-term very-low-fat tests* on prisoners in South Africa. These tests demonstrated that a temporary increase in blood fats sometimes occurs *for a short period, but only in those accustomed to living on a high-saturated-fat diet.* And he further added that within a few months the lipids decreased to a true normal level. Also, Dr. E. L. Bierman of the Rockefeller Institute Hospital tested a group of patients on a *very low-fat and high-carbohydrate diet.* He, too, found that the blood fats in his patients did increase, but that this was only temporary, and that within two months on the *very low-fat diet* the blood fats were down to a low normal.

Other researchers who investigated the effects of a very low-fat yet high-calorie diet have reported the same results.

Dr. W. E. Connor who "rediscovered" the low-cholesterol diet has made an extensive study of subjects on an extra low (20%) fat diet of the "Prudent type." At the Minnesota Heart Symposium in 1963 he reported that in *every person* on this diet the blood fats (triglycerides) quickly declined to a lower and safer level.

There is a well known fact which should have served to restrain the critics of the very low-fat diet. In all countries where the diet is *very low in fats* it has been found that the blood-fat levels are also in the low normal range. For instance, Dr. Kyu Taik Lee of the Kyungpook University in Korea measured the blood fats in a group of Buddhist monks living on a low-calorie diet extremely low in fats (7%). His measurements showed their blood fats to be less than half that found in a group of U.S. army officers of the same age.

Since it was Dr. Ahrens' research which initiated the unjustified fears of the very *low-fat diet*, it will be of interest to learn his views on an anti-coronary diet. As he stated in the 1961 *Review of Modern Medicine,* his recommendation is a change "to diets rich in fish, vegetables and fruits and poor in meats and dairy products." To this diet, Dr. Ahrens recommends the addition of supplementary vegetable oil, but warns, "It must be emphasized that liquid oils are exchanged for and not added to the saturated fats contained in egg yolks, meats, and butter."

The second "whipping boy" is the high-vegetable-oil diet. The supposed danger in this diet is the possible spoilage of the polyunsaturated fats to be consumed.

Although the high-vegetable-oil diet is not recommended for general use, but only prescribed occasionally by some physicians, it is still a better diet than our present high saturated fat diet. But since the criticisms concerning "spoilage" leveled against this diet can possibly be extended by inference to the Prudent Diet, it is important to explain the fallacy in the supposed spoilage problem.

In nature, spoilage of vegetable oil is prevented by the Vitamin E found in large quantities in the nuts and seeds which constitute the source of our dietary vegetable oils. So when one eats these natural vegetable oils, the Vitamin E protection is present.

The hypothetical case proposed by the skeptics is this. Modern man eats a diet already low in Vitamin E (refining causes its removal from whole wheat and other whole grain foods). Next, imagine adding to it a large quantity of *improperly refined* vegetable oil from which the Vitamin E has been *deliberately removed* by incorrect "purification" methods. Result: Vitamin E deficiency, plus oxidation of the oils due to the absence of the Vitamin E.

In order to "create" this problem, it is necessary to string together an improbable chain of events. First, an unwarranted switch from the moderate vegetable oil Prudent Diet to one excessively high in oils. Second, the excessive use of either rancid vegetable oil, or one from which the Vitamin E has been deliberately stripped.

The first mistake is possible although not probable; the second is almost impossible. Oil without Vitamin E becomes rancid and is inedible.

All the usual polyunsaturated vegetable oils on the market today are naturally rich in Vitamin E.

And the final point was cleared up by Dr. Snapper who speaks about "the remarkable resistance of unsaturated [fat] against metabolic oxidation in the human organism." In other words although vegetable oil can in time turn rancid on the grocery shelf it is a very stable fat inside the body.

The high vegetable-oil diet is rejected for general use by medical scientists, not because of the spoilage problem, but because a high-fat diet even from vegetable sources is an unnatural diet.

And finally we come to those who are against any tampering with our present diet because it is thought to be so nutritious. Their main argument is that eggs and dairy products are a good source of Vitamin A and calcium and that any curtailment might result in a national nutritional deficiency.

If we examine our national diet we find that more than half of the calories in our diet carry practically no vitamins or minerals. These foods are known as the "hollow" foods and include the sugars, highly refined carbohydrates, the hydrogenated oils and the meat fats.

Dr. Jolliffe was the author of the medical text book *Clinical Nutrition* which is the most detailed and most authoritative on this subject. In the formulation of the Prudent Diet, the replacement of the "hollow-foods" with the proper nutrient foods no longer make it necessary to use the previous large amounts of milk, butter and eggs for calcium and Vitamin A, etc. Dr. Jolliffe has published numerous medical papers emphasizing and reiterating the fact that the Prudent Diet contains far more of every vitamin and mineral (except calcium) than the previous "American diet."

The idea that milk, cheese, butter and cream may be a contributing factor in artery blockage and heart attack has been a source of emotional conflict to many who have been extolling the virtues of a quart of milk a day as a dietary necessity.

Dr. A. R. P. Walker, who has an international reputation for his heart research work, has stated that the dangerous calcification that often complicates artery blockage is a serious situation only in Western nations with a large intake of calcium in their diet. The World Health Organization's nutritional standard for calcium intake is about half the present average American consumption. Dr. Walker points out that in countries where calcium consumption is low, the calcification problem in artery blockage is seldom seen.

Another problem which milk creates is that it is often fortified with Vitamin D and is therefore partially responsible for the excessive amount of Vitamin D in our Western diet. Dr. C. D. DeLangen has reported in *Acta Medica Scandinavica* that feeding extra Vitamin D to adults is contributing to the development of calcification deposits in the artery blockage. Based on his extensive research he states that Vitamin D as a *supplement* is dangerous and "restriction of the use of Vitamin D is imperative."

Since the function of Vitamin D is to aid in the deposition of calcium in bone formation, the combination of *excessive amounts* of both nutrients, which is known to exist in our diet, is an unnecessary risk, to be viewed with concern.

Supplements of *all* the B complex vitamins, as well as vitamins A, C and E, are recommended because research has shown that they are all of value in the prevention of artery blockage.

However, the use of any vitamin supplement which contains Vitamin D should be avoided.

Even children can suffer from an excess of Vitamin D. The recommendation of the British Pediatric Society is that no food be fortified with Vitamin D. Any necessary doses of cod liver oil supplements are carefully prescribed to keep this potentially dangerous vitamin to a known low maximum.

Dr. Jolliffe, in his book *Clinical Nutrition*, shows that in those countries where the intake of calcium and Vitamin D is very low, there is no specific health problem due to lack of either.

The carbohydrate portion of milk (known as lactose) has also been reported in *Nutrition Reviews* (March 1960) to be a possible contributor to artery blockage. Dr. W. W. Wells' three research reports in 1957, 1958 and 1959 have shown that increased blood cholesterol and artery blockage occurs in animals fed diets high in milk carbohydrates. The increase in cholesterol and in artery blockage was worse in animals fed lactose than in those fed an equivalent amount of sugar.

It would seem that even though milk is regarded by some as the ideal food for human consumption, it is regarded by others as a food which contains an unusual combination of nutritional components which have all been suspected as possible contributory causes of artery blockage.

The answer to those who question the advisability of

"tampering" with our present "highly nutritious" diet is that:

1. Our present diet is so padded with "empty calories" that it is *not* as nutritious in essential vitamins and minerals as the Prudent Diet.

2. Our present diet is *not* as natural nor as safe as the Prudent Diet, which more closely resembles the time tested diets of some of the most healthy groups in the world.

3. Our present diet *does contain* many foods definitely proven to promote artery blockage that are eliminated in the Prudent Diet.

4. To sum up: The present diet is unsafe and imprudent, and Dr. Jolliffe's diet is truly prudent.

The place to look for danger is in the modern type of high saturated fat. Very few people have actually seen pure saturated fat such as either the natural 100% saturated fat or the chemically 100% hydrogenated fat.

In referring to hard animal fat, most people have in mind butter or the white fat of meat which is a combination of pure saturated fat and liquid unsaturated oils. But the hardness of a pure 100% saturated fat is almost beyond belief. Without identification, pure hard saturated fat would be rejected as a possible food and classified as a chemical or an extremely hard wax.

Pure saturated fat seems to be an artificial product, having the appearance and feeling of a brittle plastic rather than food. All attempts to induce individuals to "chew" and swallow a pea-sized particle of this white hard waxy "food" have met with indignant refusals.

Yet there are many Americans who eat enough of this 100% pure saturated fat in their diet to provide them with a large handful every day.

Simple or Complex

After the major objections to the Prudent Diet have been disposed of, there still remain sotto voce objections.

The first of these objections is suspicion of a single simple solution. In confronting the problem of heart attack, which is so complex and has so many interrelated causes, there are those who are dissatisfied with a seemingly simple solution. They have confidence only in a solution which is multifaceted and complex.

But merely because a solution to a complex problem is seemingly simple does not make it incorrect. One example is the very complex chain reaction which is often released by a deficiency of even one vitamin.

Also the Prudent Diet as the major factor in the coronary prevention program is not as simple as it appears. Consider the original change in diet which preceded the "coronary epidemic," the change from the frugal diet of our forefathers to the present rich Western diet. It involved not one simple change, but a number of them as shown in the "Historic Change" chart with the resulting complex changes in the blood.

Historic Changes in the American Diet

It is now the highest in the world in:

- Calories
- Cholesterol
- Saturated Fat
- Hydrogenated Fat
- Dairy Fat
- Sugar
- Refined Carbohydrates
- "Hollow" Foods
- Baked Goods
- Boxed Foods
- Canned Foods
- Pre-cooked Foods
- Preserved Foods
- Frozen Foods
- Chemical Preservatives
- Chemical Additives

These changes in diet have led to the many changes shown in the following list.

Historic Changes in the Blood and Arteries

Increases in:

- Cholesterol
- Beta Lipoprotein
- Blood Fats
- Saturation of Blood Fat
- Body Fat
- Saturation of Body Fat
- Thrombotic Factors
- Artery Blockage

Decreases in:

- Stability of Globules
- Alpha Lipoprotein
- Phospholipids
- Clearing Factor
- Heparin
- Fat Tolerance
- Glucose Tolerance
- Fat Digestive Enzymes

Therefore a return to the Prudent Diet will involve changes that are numerous and far reaching enough to satisfy those who seek a complex solution to the coronary problem.

But even though these changes are complex, they can be reduced to one essential key factor. All the reactions leading to artery blockage are related to the state of the lipids and the fatty globules in the blood.

Without excess lipids and unstable fatty globules we would not have modern hypercoagulable blood. And without these two blood conditions there would be no coronary epidemic. Consider all the factors known to affect the development of artery blockage and heart attack. Every one of these factors is known to exert its major effect—for better or worse—through the blood lipids.

All medical scientists agree that the most important of the "non-diet" conditions affecting heart attack include: high blood pressure—stress—exercise—age—sex—heredity —body build—obesity—hypothyroidism—other endocrine disorders—diabetes—other metabolic disorders—smoking and other toxic factors.

They have been mentioned before, under the headings of the "key" factor relationships and the "controllables."

THE UNIFICATION PRINCIPLE

Wherever these factors have been discussed in this book, research has proven that they influence artery blockage through changes in blood lipids and resultant thrombotic effects. In addition a survey of all the data from hundreds of research studies on the subject of prevention of coronary disease (which were not mentioned in this book) will show that practically all of them have measured the effect of each of the above 13 conditions by their influence on the lipids and the thrombotic factors in the blood.

At this point it can be clearly seen that those who still doubt the blood-cholesterol, blood-lipid explanation of artery blockage and heart attack are in a logical dilemma.

How can they accept the importance of the "non-diet" conditions and yet doubt and even deny the critical importance of excess cholesterol and lipids in the blood, since it is only through changes in the blood lipids that the effects of these conditions are usually measured?

Obviously one phase of the prevention program must be to lessen the harmful effects of the "non-diet" factors which increase cholesterol and blood lipids.

These factors, however, could not have exerted the full power of their *secondary* adverse effects if the *Historic Changes in the American Diet* had not prepared the way by the *primary* basic disturbance of the lipids and the thrombotic factors in the blood.

In completing the complex circle it can be seen that the solution is truly simple. The essence of the prevention method is to keep the blood free of the undesirable excess of lipids, cholesterol and fatty globules and all the attendant troubles they bring on.

INHERENT DANGERS IN THE DESIRE FOR ABSOLUTE CERTAINTY

The second problem is the desire for absolute certainty. This leads to an intolerance of the slightest inconsistency in the great volume of evidence supporting the Prudent Diet. Perhaps this is due to a misunderstanding, natural enough in lay persons, as to how the validity of a scientific theory is established.

Those demanding an absolute assurance imagine that the many proofs supporting the Prudent Diet form a *chain* of evidence *encircling* the problem, and holding it "captive"— so the final validity depends upon the integrity of each link in the *chain*. Should any link snap, should any single experiment be discredited, they imagine that the entire chain will burst and the problem will elude the solution.

But this is a mistaken notion, for the proof supporting the Prudent Diet is not a single chain but rather a group of independent chains or better still an interwoven set of chains.

Consider the proofs as a group of spotlights, differing in strength but all focused on a single center. Although one or two lights may dim or even go out, the test of validity is the *total* amount of light still cast and the accuracy with which they all converge and focus on the common center or solution to the problem. The many methods of proof are actually independent entities, each supported solely by its own merits.

Indeed, the many researches have shed their light from so many different angles and by so many different methods that it is surprising to find the consistent uniformity of the convergence of their light on the diet factor.

Should any part of the research be shown to be unimportant or even based on incorrect data, this will have *no* negative effect on the other proven theories, which constitute independent proof of the basic value of diet and exercise in the prevention program.

With the present interrelated research in support of the prevention program and the Prudent Diet, it seems incredible that only a short time ago the scientific picture was quite confused in many respects. Scores of critical medical reviews of only a few years ago were antagonistic to the very thought of the possibility of an overall unified prevention program because, at that time, there were so many contenders for the "honor" of being the "cause" of heart attack. How, asked the critics, could one single program possibly encompass the diverse effects of heredity, stress, exercise, metabolism, diet, environment, and a host of other factors?

In the light of the latest research, however, these reviews were found to be shortsighted, and so this type of "critical" analytical review has practically disappeared.

On a subject such as the prevention of heart attack, with its recently integrated theories, there are bound to be some remaining differences of opinion. I was surprised, therefore, to receive so few critical comments from the many eminent clinical, research and teaching cardiologists to whom I submitted this book for evaluation.

All, with the exception of one research scientist, were in general agreement with the choice of contents, intent and conclusions in the book. Since this "exception" is representative of the "desire for absolute certainty", a few comments on it are in order.

After first stating that, "I agree with much of this book. The author has done a great deal of careful work," he goes on to say that in his opinion, "we will not be justified to advocate any radical dietary changes for the general population until the relationship between diet and heart disease has been demonstrated *experimentally*." And since this is, of course, not immediately possible, he states, "Present evidence is suggestive, but does not justify the disruption of our economy that would be required to put the necessary changes into effect."

The evidence used in this book, however, was not originally researched from an economic point of view, but rather from a scientific and medical point of view. I cannot imagine any individual being concerned with the national economy if he were convinced that the evidence was sufficiently "suggestive" so that he considered his personal welfare involved.

When it is a question of a reasonable possibility of saving human lives, the question of economics should not be a factor at all.

Consider, from an inadmissibly cold business point of view, the economic benefits and financial gains resulting from preventing even a small percent of the millions of heart attacks which occur annually. The immense gain to the national economy from the availability of this manpower will more than offset the comparatively modest temporary subsidy needed to alleviate any financial disruption in the food industry which will probably occur anyway.

As to his final suggestion, "I would wait [ten years will be required] for the outcome of the National Diet-Heart Study," there are of course two schools of thought.

The inherent danger in the *desire for certainty* is, as has been shown earlier, the *wait and see policy*. Many eminent heart specialists have commented on this danger. Dr. George C. Griffith, President of the American Therapeutic Society, has said that as a practicing physician he is bound to ask himself:

"Can I afford to ignore the accumulated data and wait for the final proof—that is, the results of the mass field trials—or should I make my conviction known that measures for the prevention and control of coronary disease should at once be instituted?

"I believe the latter."

In a similar vein Drs. T. R. Dawber and W. B. Kannel, who are responsible for the historic Framingham Study, have said:

"In the absence of any conclusive proof of benefit, many physicians may choose to adopt a *wait-and-see policy*. If the measures described were those which entailed some hazard to the patient, such a policy would be justified. However, since the described procedures are consistent with good health practices and essentially void of any harm to the subject, it seems reasonable to recommend the necessary dietary changes, blood pressure reduction, discontinuance of cigarette smoking, weight loss, and increased physical activity in an effort to lessen the risk of CHD (Coronary Heart Disease) development. It also seems reasonable to recommend that these changes take place early in adult life rather than wait until a fibrotic, calcified, atherosclerotic plaque has been established."

There is no time to *wait-and-see*. Dr. Paul Dudley White says in his Convocation Address that while we continue ". . . vital cardiovascular research in progress and planned," the most important admonition is, "To begin *now* to apply simple and sensible positive rules of health before we can establish them statistically as 100 per cent valid."

CHAPTER SEVENTEEN

Breaking Through the Coronary Curtain

CENTRALIZED CLINICS TO TELL YOU YOUR CORONARY STATUS

Atherosclerosis is a hidden disease. But we have to draw aside the *Coronary Curtain* not only on an individual basis but also on a national scale and find out just how serious the hidden trouble is.

"A major difficulty in human studies arises from the fact that sub-clinical atherosclerosis is universal in our adult population."

"Indeed it is quite impossible at present to distinguish between the apparently normal adult and the very atheromatous individual who has not yet suffered recognizable complications of the atherosclerotic lesion."

These two statements, one by Dr. J. A. Little of Sunnybrook Hospital and the other by Dr. D. P. Barr of Cornell Medical Center, sum up the dilemma which confronts us:

We are *all* ill, but we don't all know it. We can't see it, and we are not yet psychologically prepared to face the problem until it is too late.

In all medical history there has never been a situation such as this: All previous plagues were easily recognized, by their terrible symptoms, but the coronary epidemic has no swollen glands, blackened skin, fever, or other tell-tale symptoms to disclose its presence.

If the ugly condition of the arteries of our middle-aged men were outwardly visible; if we could *see* the fibrous, fatty, knobby growths becoming encrusted with calcium deposits and ulcerating in the final stages; then there would be a tremendous public outcry for an immediate remedy.

But the arteries are well hidden, and until disaster strikes, there is usually a fatalistic attitude and even indifference. However, in the past few years there has been a greater awareness of this problem and a desire on the part of a fast growing section of the population to change this head-in-the-sand attitude.

Actually there are many holes in the "coronary curtain," some of which can be made wider with only a little know-how, through the Centralized Coronary Prevention Clinics.

This type of clinic does not yet exist, but its components do exist in separate laboratories in many countries, each specializing in tests for different specific indications of the hidden presence of atherosclerosis.

How about the popular tests, such as the electrocardio-graph and the X-ray?

These are of some value in cases where the patient has already had a heart attack, but even in the patients with *known* coronary atherosclerosis, these tests may fail to give a positive indication in fully half the cases, according to the report by Dr. R. E. Mason, in the *Journal of the American Geriatrics Society* (November 1953).

If in the more advanced stages of obvious coronary disease, these tests are only of partial value, then in the earlier stages of coronary they are of very little value. The specialized and definitive tests now available only in a handful of advanced research laboratories must all be standardized and perfected, so that they can all become economically available in centralized clinics throughout the country.

The coordination of knowledge now available, and its

wider application, should surely result in a big step forward in solving our nation's greatest medical problem.

We should have many centers in the United States where it will be possible to find out one's exact coronary status and be advised whether emergency measures are required or only routine prevention measures such as the Prudent Diet are necessary.

What should the program of such clinics be?

There are three major types of tests which the clinic could administer.

First: Blood tests such as beta globule stability, clearing-factor exhaustion, thrombotic and clot-dissolving factors, standard and unusual blood lipid content, and other blood tests. The blood tests will give a picture of the patient's current status and show the changes and improvements which should result from a proper preventive program.

Second: Electrical graphic recording of the vibration of the heart and body caused by the pumping movement of the heart and of the blood in the large arteries. When these are interpreted, they can give valuable information of the extent of damage which the heart and arteries have already suffered. These damages can also be mechanically and electrically measured by pulse-wave tests, ballistocardio-gram tests, and many other vibration tests.

Third: Direct observation tests by means of the opthal-moscope, the microscope, and camera, on the small capil-laries and arterioles close enough to the surface, such as those in the back of the eye and in the nail-bed.

To have all these tests made now would be enormously difficult, for it would involve thousands of miles of travel and the expenditure of many thousands of dollars. But if centralized blood clinics were set up, the costs could be brought within reason.

There are other good reasons, economic and political, for setting up such "Clinics" on a nationwide scale. The fact that the United States is the country with the highest rate of coronary disease in the world is a blemish on our national image.

And the great savings possible from years added to the life span of our scientific and political leaders will alone compensate many times over for the comparatively small cost of the centralized clinics. Each day's obituary columns

record the sudden and untimely deaths from heart attack
of many of our most prominent and valuable citizens.

ROAD BLOCKS IN THE PATH OF RESEARCH

One important and urgently needed service which the
central clinic could undertake is the coordination of the
knowledge available from extensive research now being
carried out in many foreign countries. At present almost
nothing is being done to make the tremendous fund of
knowledge available to the busy researchers, cardiologists,
and medical practitioners.

Much valuable work relating to coronary prevention is
being published in Chinese, French, German, Hungarian,
Japanese, Polish, Spanish, Rumanian, Russian, and many
other languages.

There is some publication of translations of these scientific works, but compared to what is needed, this is an
insignificant contribution.

Dr. W. Raab has commented that, "It is a disturbing
phenomenon even in our present world of irrational con-
tradictions, that, in the face of a great deal of verbal
emphasis on 'international cooperation,' 'exchange of ideas,'
etc., and despite much academic concern about our stag-
gering cardiac mortality, the momentous development of
preventive medicine abroad against the 'diseases of civilization' have remained unnoticed by the American medical
and lay public alike."

A hundred times as much manpower as that now available should be used to make the international data of
actual scientific use, by translation and publication in at
least a condensed form. The effort required will be great,
but the need is even greater.

The cost of bringing this important data, neglected at
present, to the elbow of many thousands of interested
scientists in this country is insignificant compared to the
great help it will certainly be in the final solution of the
coronary problem.

To a large extent the value of much of the material on
coronary-prevention research which is being published in
English is being dissipated by scattering it throughout
many dozens of medical journals.

Too much time and effort is required of the hardworking

individual research specialist without a large staff to gather a proper reference library, even for the narrow sector of his sub-specialty.

Valuable time in realizing the Prevention Program is now being lost because the complete picture of progress in the entire field of atherosclerosis is not easily available to the busy research specialists.

In a critical situation such as the one created by the coronary epidemic, each medical library throughout the country should immediately establish a section devoted exclusively to the national and international data on coronary heart disease. The Centralized Coronary Prevention Clinics should be in a position to organize this data.

In addition, special monthly summaries of all the latest research must be made available by the "Clinics" to any interested scientists and medical practitioners.

The importance of this problem was emphasized by Dr. C. E. Kossmann of the N.Y.U. School of Medicine when he stated: "I consider that the significant development in cardiovascular diseases in the next ten years will be in the area of communication between scientists."

BLOOD TESTS THAT IDENTIFY THE CORONARY PRONE INDIVIDUAL

The Blood Lipid Tests

There is no longer any doubt that it is the blood lipids which are the active factors in causing much of the artery blockage. There are many ways to observe and study these lipids—we can measure the amounts of the different sized globules, their many components and chemical contents, their stability, their dynamic actions after a meal, and their critical interrelations with other blood factors. All in all, the lipid variables are too numerous even to list.

Yet at the present time it is only the simple cholesterol test which is being used by the average physician to help him visualize this very complex and dynamically changing situation in the blood.

The cholesterol test, although it is a very valuable low cost test, can no longer be considered adequate to reveal all the abnormal conditions that are now known to exist in the various blood lipids and associated factors.

Take, for instance, the triglyceride test. This test is just as valuable, and in most instances even more prognostic, than the cholesterol test. But neither truly substitutes for the other. In order to get even a partial view of the blood-lipid conditions, both tests are necessary.

However, there are still too few commercial laboratories that are able to provide the doctor with this very valuable test. And the few that can make this test have not yet established a uniformly reproducible method. This situation should be remedied quickly.

In regard to the determination of the quantity of each of the different groups of fatty globules, the situation is even more difficult. Unfortunately there is only one institution in the entire country, a *non profit* laboratory, that is able to furnish the interested physician with data obtained by the Gofman Mechanical-Centrifugal method. This test gives the full quantity spectrum of chylomicrons, large and small beta globules and alpha globules.

Accurate determination of the amount of alpha as well as beta globules is the best method of evaluation of blood-lipid disorders. All tests on coronary-free groups such as young women, Yemenite Jews, Bantus, and other similar groups have shown a relatively high proportion of alpha globules and a low quantity of beta globules in their blood.

This type of test is much more valuable than the combined cholesterol-triglyceride test and would probably be the main quantitative blood lipid test in the centralized clinics. In addition to knowing the quantity of the various blood globules, it is important to know their *quality*, or their *stability*.

One definition of stability of the fatty globules is the ability of the "protective coat" of the globule to prevent "leakage" of its fatty-cholesterol contents. It has been found that by adding a fat solvent to blood, the "leaky" cholesterol inside the fatty globule is dissolved and the *readily extractable cholesterol* can be measured.

The tighter and more firmly the lipid core of the globule is protected, the less the amount of cholesterol that can be extracted. Conversely, a larger quantity of cholesterol extracted from the blood indicates a greater instability of the globules. This is an indication of a poor blood-lipid condition in an individual. These tests have been performed by Drs. D. H. Sherber and M. Marcus. The rat and dog, which are resistant to artery blockage, have very stable fatty globules. Tests indicate that they have only four units of "leaky" cholesterol in the blood. The baboon is intermediate, with fourteen units, while man has the least stable globules, with fifty units of "leaky" cholesterol.

An even more accurate method of testing the stability of the blood was devised by Dr. Louis Horlick (*Circulation*, July 1954). A special enzyme added to a blood sample slowly removes the protective coat around the fatty globules.

The resultant instability causes the fatty globules to "stick together" and form still larger globules. The change in size causes increased cloudiness of the blood serum. The time required for the instability to start—and the amount of cloudiness which occurs—is the index of the basic stability of the fatty globules. This index accurately differentiates the atherosclerotic pre-coronary individual with unstable globules from the true normal who has stable fatty globules.

Using a method similar to Dr. Sherber's "Freely Extractable Cholesterol," Dr. D. S. Amatuzio of the Minnesota Mount Sinai Hospital measured *all* the extracted lipids. The individual results also clearly indicated that those with an excess of lipids extracted from the globules were the atherosclerotics.

Medical scientists no longer doubt that the atherosclerotic, coronary-prone individual has unstable fatty globules. The next problem would be to see if a long-term improvement in stability could be achieved by the Prudent Diet. Only one small hint of what may be expected was given by the short-term tests used by Dr. George Michaels and his associates at the Institute for Metabolic Research. First, the amount of free extractable lipids of twenty-one-individuals was measured. Next they were fed a saturated fatty meal. Three hours later, when the stability tests were repeated, there was a 25% increase in the freely extractable lipids. But when the same group was again tested after a vegetable-oil, unsaturated-fatty meal, the "leaky lipids" actually decreased 18% from the original test level.

In other words, saturated-fatty meals seem to result in

unstable chylomicron globules. Yet, vegetable oil in the diet seems to make them more stable.

Another important blood-lipid test, which shows up the weakest spot in the fat metabolism of the atherosclerotic, is one used by Dr. Barrit, which was described in Chapter 6.

Today this test is known as the *Fat Tolerance Test* because atherosclerotics cannot "tolerate" a large amount of diet fat without a resulting excessively dangerous peak amount of chylomicron fatty globules in their blood. Much of this type of research has been done, during the past few years, by Dr. D. Berkowitz and his group at Philadelphia's Hahnemann Hospital. It has also been verified by other research studies, and today it is acknowledged to be a very accurate method of identifying the coronary-prone individual.

As an extension and further development of the *Fat Tolerance Test*, there is a second test which is also of great value in identifying the coronary-prone individual. In general, within three hours after a fatty meal the maximum amount of chylomicrons is present in the blood. At this stage heparin is injected, which results in an exaggerated increase in the speed of removal of chylomicrons from the blood.

Since the removal of chylomicrons in the atherosclerotic was not nearly as great as that in the normal person, the heparin reaction is another excellent test for the separation of the two groups.

This brings up an important question. What causes this difference in chylomicron removal? One group of scientists claims that there is an exhaustion of the clearing system in the blood of the atherosclerotic. The other group points to research which indicates the importance of the exhaustion of the pancreatic fat-digestive enzymes as well.

However, the fact that atherosclerotics need larger quantities of injected heparin to produce an equivalent amount of clearance of chylomicron globules seems to prove that the exhaustion is mainly in the heparin-clearing-system. Dr. D. Aleksandrow of Poland has reported in *Circulation* (Nov. 1959) that the clearing effect after a heparin injection definitely separates the normal from the atherosclerotic with relatively little overlapping.

The research of Dr. E. Klein and his group at the Harvard Medical School in 1959 has added to the validity of the previous research. His report concludes that "Equivalent amounts of heparin induce less clearing activity in patients with hyperlipemia than in normal individuals."

In 1962 came further data from Brazil's Dr. Italo Martirani and his group working at the University of Sao Paulo Medical School. At least three out of four in a group of known atherosclerotics could be quickly detected by the simple fact that their chylomicrons did not clear out fast enough after an injection of heparin.

Finally, in 1963 came the U.S.S.R. report by Dr. M. P. Stepanova of the Novokuznetsk Medical Institute that after a small injection of heparin, a group of atherosclerotics could be accurately differentiated from a control group of normals by the difference in clearing reaction time.

There is no doubt that the fat tolerance test and the heparin clearing test will be among the most important tests used by the centralized clinics to detect the pre-coronary individual.

An important problem for those living on a Western-type diet is the longer time span needed for the clearance of chylomicrons after a saturated-fatty meal than after a vegetable-oil meal.

Research which proves this fact came in 1958 from Drs. M. Eggstein and G. Schettler in Germany and Dr. L. W. Kinsell in the United States. Their tests showed fewer chylomicrons in the blood (and lingering for a shorter time) after a vegetable-oil meal, compared to an equivalent saturated-fat meal.

Further research along this line showing similar results was reported in 1959 by Dr. P. F. Kuo in the United States, by Dr. M. B. Bronte-Stewart in England, and in 1961 by Dr. E. Bohle in Germany.

In 1963 Dr. R. L. Jones reported that the replacement of dairy fat with corn oil for two weeks causes a two hour delay in the chylomicron inrush after a fat meal.

Very many factors are involved in this process. Although many of them have already been discussed in this and previous chapters, for clarification and simplicity the complete process is shown in the accompanying chart.

HOW THE BODY HANDLES FAT

The Critical Chylomicron Balance

INTAKE   INTERFERENCE   REMOVAL

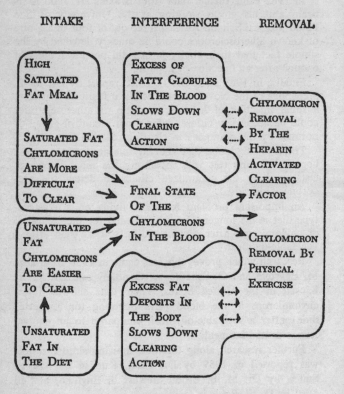

- *Intake Problem:* Exhaustion of the fat digestive enzymes results in a type of chylomicrons which are difficult to clear.
- *Removal Problem:* Exhaustion of the heparin and clearing factor causes inefficient removal of the chylomicrons from the blood.
- *Cause of Both Problems:* A lifetime of rich fatty meals.

Thrombotic Blood Tests

One of the most important advances in medical science has been the use of heparin and other anti-clotting drugs in controlling excessive thrombotic factors in the blood.

But overdosage of these drugs can result in a dangerous deficiency in the many vital clotting factors. Therefore proper and frequent tests are necessary.

The medical practitioner should have available a test for blood clottability which is (1) accurate and consistent; (2) quick; (3) inexpensive; (4) requires little apparatus; (5) doesn't require an expert technician; and (6) really shows the proper sum of *all* the many clotting factors.

Several clottability tests are in use today. But as yet none of them adequately fulfills the necessary requirements. The clotting test problem is complicated by the fact that there are over a dozen different factors in the blood, each of which contributes—separately and in combination—to the complex clotting process.

These tests are highly useful, but since the present need is so great no effort should be spared to improve this critical situation.

The result today is that although the anti-coagulant drugs are undoubtedly saving lives, there is a difference in opinion as to how much of each of the potentially dangerous drugs to use in an individual case.

For this reason many doctors hesitate to use them until the test situation is solved.

Dr. M. J. Seide in his report "The Laboratory Control of [anti-coagulant] Therapy: The Clinicians Dilemma" brings out in detail some of the problems just mentioned. In his conclusion he suggests the establishment of a "Central Anti-Coagulation Laboratory" to establish and test standards. Dr. Seide's proposed Laboratory should, of course, be part of the Centralized Coronary Prevention Clinics.

HOW TO PREDICT
THE INDIVIDUAL HEART ATTACK

In addition to its other activities, the Prevention Clinic would have another major function, to evaluate the *coronary status* of the individual. This evaluation, which would be based on a synthesis of the many known prognostic tests, could indicate a person's heart-attack expectancy.

The problem is to perfect a simple formula that could summarize and interpret the meaning of all the combined test results in the form of a simple numerical ratio. This ratio would indicate whether the individual is in serious, average, or mild danger of increased atherosclerosis or in the safe zone.

Blood lipid and metabolic abnormalities can be evaluated by testing for: (1) Cholesterol, (2) Blood fat, (3) Beta globules, (4) Alpha globules, (5) Phospholipids and (6) Stability of globules. In addition there are the dynamic tests which show the condition of the fat metabolism, such as the tests for fat tolerance and heparin induced clearing. The problem for the "Clinic" will be to find the smallest number and least expensive combination of these tests.

In addition, various thrombotic blood tests should be used such as those that determine fibrinogen, sticky platelets and the many other known blood-coagulation factors. Again the problem will be to determine the most practical and inexpensive tests that will accurately evaluate a possible pre-thrombotic condition.

The other known pre-coronary conditions such as high blood uric acid, high blood sugar and low sugar tolerance should be routinely investigated.

Other important tests in the evaluation of heart attack status are: (1) Blood pressure, (2) Vital capacity, (3) Percent overweight, (4) Percent body fat and (5) Thyroid metabolism.

Next are the graphically recorded tests which indicate the actual damage which may have already occurred to the artery wall and heart muscle. These are: (1) Ballisto-cardiogram, (2) Heart vibration, (3) Arterial pulse, (4) Venous pulse, and (4) Electrocardiogram.

Finally, there is the problem of fitting the results obtained into a single or multiple index for evaluation:

1. From the Framingham study it is known that groups with the highest cholesterol levels had six times the heart attack expectancy of those with the lowest levels.

2. The highest readings in blood pressure tests can predict a ratio of five to one in heart-attack expectancy.

3. An obese group has twice the heart-attack rate of a normal weight group.

4. Groups high in uric acid show double the heart-attack probability of those low in uric acid.

5. Other relationships have also been noted. Those with the lowest ballistocardiogram movement have three times the heart-attack probability of those with the normal higher movements shown on the graph.

6. Those with the lowest vital capacity have double the heart-attack expectancy rate of those with normal high vital capacity.

The six tests mentioned are the only ones for which long term records have been kept with any degree of accuracy. If there were no interrelationships, the six tests could show ratios of up to 500 to 1 based on individuals with the worst or best test results. Since many of the tests, however, are interrelated, this will lower the ratio, but the use of these six simple tests should provide the ability to predict ratios of 60 to 1.

By the use of tests in addition to the six previously mentioned, the total ratio swing could be extended to far over 100 to 1.

At the end of a Coronary Prevention Clinic test each person could be provided with an evaluation based on his age and test results that would indicate his heart-attack expectancy.

If the result is in the low-index range of less than 2 to 1, the fortunate individual will probably be a young woman. The most coronary free of the men will have an index ratio of perhaps 4 to 1. Such persons are statistically relatively safe, but a change to the Prudent Diet would be urged for still greater safety. Those in the range of 8 to 1 are already in the modern, civilized dangerous range.

Those found to have a ratio index of over 16 to 1 will be in urgent need of prevention treatment in addition to the Prudent Diet, and those in the very high ranges may require more drastic medical treatment, depending upon each individual case.

But for those in the less dangerous but definite pre-coronary ranges the proper treatment on a mass base has already been worked out in thousands of rehabilitation centers in Europe. In the United States, with its great economic wealth, it should be a matter o fa moment's decision to set up similar reconditioning centers. We already have an expert consultant in Dr. W. Raab, who has devoted years to the study of these centers and whose book *Organized Prevention of Degenerative Heart Disease* should be read by all.

CHAPTER EIGHTEEN

If You Have Already Had a Heart Attack

PROS AND CONS OF ANTICOAGULANTS AND HEPARIN

I have been asked on many occasions, what I would do if I suffered a heart attack.

To begin with, having followed the prevention program for the past fifteen years, my chances of having a heart attack have been reduced, in all probability, to a low figure.

The question, however, does introduce some thoughts concerning anticoagulant therapy. The problems related to this therapy are usually discussed only among doctors but I think that it is now important for everyone, whether he has had a heart attack or not, to become acquainted with a new approach to this subject.

This chapter is not a do-it-yourself story on how to treat a heart attack. I will only discuss a few of the methods for its treatment which are under special study at this time, and my own personal reactions to them.

First, there is the need for special bed rest following an attack. The purpose of this treatment is to permit nature time for repairing the damaged heart tissues. In this repair process, nature uses fibrin strands as a natural thread to sew up the injury. Ironically, these fibrin strands consist of the same dumbbell-shaped molecules which, due to imbalances in the blood, are partly responsible for the clogging of the artery and the reduction of the flow of blood, which brought on the heart attack.

The old school of treatment relied almost entirely on immobilizing the patient. For myself, I would choose the new "Boston school" of treatment which allows the patient to sit up earlier and to have more freedom of movement. With new methods of treatment based on the latest research on prevention, strict immobility has been found to be unnecessary and is now considered by some doctors to introduce factors which may be more harmful than beneficial.

At this point the important question is: Does the complete prevention program apply just as well to those who have had a heart attack as to those who have not yet been afflicted?

The answer is "Yes."

Indeed, for heart-attack patients, it is most important that they closely adhere to the prevention program described in this book. It is now the most widely prescribed regimen by doctors for their heart-attack patients.

It might help here to recapitulate, briefly, the four most important causes of heart attack with an emphasis on their interrelationship.

First: Consider one of the causes emphasized at the October 1963 Scientific Sessions in Los Angeles held by the American Society for the Study of Arteriosclerosis. There, a group of researchers heard a discussion by Dr. Meyer Friedman, who emphasized that his group's latest research, which had just been presented by his associate, Dr. R. Rosenman, showed the necessity of paying greater attention to the special problems of individuals with an intense stress pattern.

"True," Dr. Friedman said, "the American diet of today is a *Witches Brew*. But it is with the addition of our self-imposed stresses that the *brew* is transformed into a truly deadly concoction."

Second: Consider the causes pointed up by Dr. Paul Dudley White who is constantly trying to bring them to the attention of the American public. His latest warning is that, "We now have so many pushbuttons that we have stopped using our muscles. Also our diet has become richer and richer. We are becoming a soft race. The 'Life of Riley' favors the earlier occurrence of heart disease, hypertension and diabetes."

Dr. J. N. Morris, who occupies an important position in

the British school of heart-attack prevention, has often seconded Dr. White on these points. During a recent visit he warned this country that, "Inactivity and overeating are imbedded in our behavior patterns, and there is little sign that the medical profession can successfully introduce environmental controls. Physical inactivity is integral in our social progress, and overeating is integral in its affluency. Social progress will increase the amount of cardiovascular disease."

Third: Practically all medical-research scientists in the field of heart-attack prevention now are in agreement that high blood pressure is detrimental to the artery wall. Many of these same researchers attribute to excess salt in our diet an important or at least a permissive role in elevating blood pressure.

It is well to note that the major artery-clogging effects which result from high blood pressure can only be clearly seen when superimposed on those resulting from over-rich diets found in highly industrialized countries like our own.

With this brief presentation of three important culprits, we find that the fourth and principal offender, invariably mentioned as the necessary co-factor, is our high-calorie and high-saturated-fat diet. The important point, frequently overlooked by many who seek the decisive answer to this four-way problem, can be found in the recent report by Dr. W. M. Kannel of the National Heart Institute and the Framingham Study:

"In a population that has been saturated with fat . . . some threshold (of safety) has been passed."

Although stress, sloth and excess systolic and diastolic blood pressure are individually harmful to the coronary arteries, they become lethal when stirred into the "witches brew" of our present-day luxury diet.

Here then is the deadly quartet—truly the four horsemen of the present-day apocalyptic coronary crisis.

There is no doubt, to put it in the simplest possible language, that our diet has too long been too rich for our blood. The understanding of the harmful effects of over-rich blood on the arteries, especially when compounded by the three other factors, enables us to see the best possible starting point for the prevention of the second heart attack as well as the first.

My principal concern, after a heart attack, would be to

prevent this blood with clotting tendencies from congealing into a lethal clot in one of the clogged and narrowed coronary arteries. I have pointed out in previous chapters the numerous research studies which show the possibility of accomplishing this before the heart attack through normal and natural physiologic methods.

But, after a heart attack, doctors must resort to more drastic means of solving this problem. They no longer rely on our body to handle it in a simple physiological manner.

The problem now is whether to prescribe drugs which can quickly restore the blood to a more normal state of clottability. To put it briefly, to anticoagulate or not to anticoagulate is the question which must be answered by both doctor and patient.

Anticoagulants are being used after most heart attacks, but there is still a difference of opinion as to the long term use of these life-saving drugs.

One misconception which has grown up around the use of anticoagulants is the exaggerated fear of hemorrhage. This is due to a misleading association of a minor and controllable hemorrhage with the eventually fatal hemorrhage of the hereditary disease, hemophilia.

The simple truth is that reducing the coagulability of the blood results in a much less dangerous state than the status quo in which the blood is allowed to remain in the hypercoagulable condition which usually exists after a heart attack.

Ironically, when a second coronary thrombosis strikes, it usually is attributed to an act of God, yet on the very rare occasion when a hemorrhage occurs during anticoagulant treatment it may become attributed to incorrect therapy.

Even if the blood coagulability should become excessively low, the condition is easily recognized and remedied. Only in unusual cases does it become serious, but almost never fatal. High coagulability, on the other hand, is insidious and not usually recognized until the all too frequently fatal coronary thrombosis shows that the dangerous state had been present for some time.

An important event that strengthened my personal decision in favor of anticoagulants occurred at the 1963 American Heart Association convention where, along with over a thousand intent cardiologists, I listened to a historic "debate" on this problem. Dr. Tage Hilden of Copenhagen had been invited to give the negative view: Dr. I. S. Wright of New York City was chosen to present the affirmative.

Dr. Wright cited many research reports which proved that mortality rates from heart attack were being lowered in this country by the use of anticlotting drugs. There are probably technical reasons for the lack of success of the Copenhagen group. But from the data of Dr. G. C. Griffith of the University of Southern California, and Dr. H. Engleberg of the Cedars of Lebanon Hospital, as well as from reports by Dr. B. Manchester of George Washington University, Dr. Nichol of Miami, and approximately 100 others mentioned by Dr. Wright, there seemed to be no doubt that the great majority have found that many lives are being saved by the use of these drugs.

The discussion continued at a less formal evening session. At its conclusion the question was put by one of the doctors present: Who among them would want anticoagulants if heart attack were to strike him? In answer, almost 95 percent raised their hands.

There are two main types of anticoagulants. One is the "natural" *blood policeman,* heparin, which in addition performs other physiological tasks in the body. The others are synthetic drugs which reduce excess blood clotting factors, but without the extra benefits obtainable from the physiologic heparin.

From one point of view it is unfortunate the heparin was discovered long before the present widespread use of anticlotting drugs. At that time fear of hemorrhage was greater than it is today, and so the stigma of danger was incorrectly attached to heparin—the most natural and safest anticoagulant of them all. Even today, unfortunately, the misleading stigma clings, despite the many research reports attesting the safety of heparin.

The benefits of heparin in preventing a second heart attack are so many and so varied, it will be simpler to understand them when listed in four groups:

FIRST: Anticoagulant Actions.

1. Heparin lowers coagulability of the blood.
2. It reduces "stickiness" of the blood platelets and so prevents the start of a thrombus.
3. It prevents the red blood cells from sticking togther after a fatty meal.

4. The total of the above factors, as well as others too complex to include here, makes heparin a potent preventive of coronary thrombosis.

SECOND: Blood Lipid Normalizing Actions.

5. Heparin cooperates with the "clearing-factor" and quickly removes most of the dangerous excess of leftover chylomicrons.

6. It also reduces high levels of beta fatty globules as well as cholesterol and blood fats (triglycerides).

7. It lowers the excessively high viscosity of the blood which may be caused by excess blood lipids.

8. It improves the efficiency of oxygen usage in the blood.

9. It improves "fat tolerance."

THIRD: Other Actions.

10. Heparin acts against the allergic effects of histamine and reduces inflammation, both of which cause trouble to the coronary-prone individual.

11. Reports from doctors indicate that patients claim to feel better after a heparin injection.

FOURTH: Safety of Heparin.

12. After a suitable dosage is established, heparin does not necessitate laboratory determinations of blood coagulability which other drugs require.

13. The short "life" of heparin in the blood acts as a safety valve. An accidental overdose is easily controlled by discontinuance for a period. This usually prevents further symptoms.

The above list should not come as a surprise since heparin is normally an essential factor in many reactions involving blood-fat metabolism, blood clotting, blood-clot dissolving and atherosclerosis. In all of these conditions it acts as a normalizing factor, a true *"Policeman Of The Blood."*

Based on all these facts it is not difficult to understand why I would favor the use of heparin for myself in the event of heart attack, despite its higher cost and even though each dose of heparin has to be injected, which is certainly more trouble than taking a pill.

The question may be asked: Since the data so far presented earlier in the book has been against drugs in the prevention of heart attack, why then am I personally for the use of heparin?

The answer is that the use of heparin *after* a heart attack is quite a different question. It has been proven valuable saving lives in this *new* and *critical* situation. That by its use a maximum number of lives can be saved is attested by reports after many years of clinical use by such outstanding specialists as Dr. G. C. Griffith, Dr. H. Engelberg, Dr. R. T. Wagner, and many others.

Another reason is that, from one point of view, heparin can be regarded as a natural factor rather than an artificial drug. It is a natural organic compound extracted from animal tissues, and it's utilized by the body in the same physiologic fashion as the natural heparin. This is probably why no harmful "side effects" have ever been reported even after ten years of continuous use of heparin therapy.

Despite the important values of heparin, of all the tremendous number of men in this country who are on anticoagulant therapy, only a small percentage are given heparin. A complex set of reasons seems to be involved. The higher cost of heparin is no doubt one very important reason for many but certainly could not be a decisive factor in a country of planned obsolescence and two cars in the garage of so many heart attack victims.

The need for self injection is a second important factor, but since the injections of B$_{12}$ or insulin are so prevalent, this difficulty cannot be valid in a possibly fatal illness.

The above reasons, understandably, influence the patient, but there is also a scientific reason which influences many doctors. The action of heparin in the blood as an anticoagulant is only ten hours, but that of the oral anticoagulant is a whole day. However, in the opinion of many, this is offset by the combined beneficial effects of heparin which, over many years of use, results in the maximum saving of lives, clearly statistically greater than by the single purpose oral anticoagulant.

The only conclusion one can come to is that, in the history of the development of anticoagulant therapy, the inexpensive and easy to take pill caught on and became popular. The difficulties and expense involved in heparin therapy, and the lack of communications as to its many values, has kept it in the background where it has unfortunately remained.

The interest in heparin therapy, however, is increasing rapidly on the West Coast. This can be seen from the large attendance at the recent "First International Conference on Heparin" at the University of Southern California which over 700 doctors attended. A major interest in heparin therapy was also evident at the 1964 Miami Anticoagulant Symposium.

In many respects the deficiency of heparin in severe atherosclerotics and heart attack victims has a parallel in the deficiency of insulin found in diabetics. Both heparin and insulin are natural compounds manufactured by glands in the body. Both become exhausted as a result of a long period of the same type of incorrect living. It is purely an accident of individual physiology as to which misfortune strikes first.

But what are the specific causes of heparin deficiency? The answer leads to another interrelationship between three of the four horsemen of the coronary apocalypse. Stress, sloth and saturated fat—each acts to exhaust our heparin reserves.

Our over-rich diet is the major cause of heparin exhaustion by introducing excessive amounts of fatty chylomicrons into the blood stream with each meal. Sloth robs us of the exercise and activity needed to use up the excess fatty contents of the blood and thereby causes increased use of heparin by the body. Similarly, civilized stress causes heparin exhaustion when physical activity does not immediately use up the excess fatty contents mobilized and released into the blood by the stress emergency.

Research has shown that the deficiency of insulin and heparin are both preventable, and that the long-term use of the Prudent Diet is the best insurance against both deficiencies. In previous chapters it has been documented that the Prudent Diet has reduced the daily requirements for both insulin and anticoagulants.

In the field of research relating a rich diet to heparin exhaustion, Italian researchers and clinical cardiologists have forged ahead of our medical scientists. Their early studies have enabled them to pioneer in natural enzyme-type drugs, some of which imitate the action of the heparin "clearing-factor" in the blood, and others the special fat-digestive enzymes which become exhausted in the gastric system.

I have recently had discussions with research cardiologists who have treated their patients first with anticoagulants alone and later also introduced the Prudent Diet. It was found that, in many cases, the requirement for the drug was reduced after use of the diet.

In my opinion more corroborative clinical and laboratory data will be accumulated in the next few years, and new research reports will support those described earlier in the book.

The human body is so infinitely complex that the attempt to compress the truth by the necessary simplifications used in this chapter is bound to cause some loss in perspective. It should be mentioned, for instance, that stress, sloth and "civilized" diet also act through other channels than the fatty-thrombotic contents of the blood and the exhaustion of the heparin reserves. But an attempt to cover these other, less critical, factors might confuse the issue, which calls for a clear understanding, on an unprecedented mass scale, of the basis for prevention both before and after the heart attack.

Heparin is not the sole key to the coronary crisis, but its understanding does make it easier to disentangle some of the knots into which we have tied ourselves by the complexities of modern civilization.

For instance, Dr. G. C. Griffiths' microscopic chylomicron counts show that smoking only two cigarettes by his coronary patients can tie up and inactivate much of the supply of heparin which has just been injected. Dr. H. J. White has recently reported similar research entitled "Heparin Inhibition by Nicotine." This is but one of the many ways that cigarette smoking exerts its harmful effects on the heart.

To sum up, this is my answer to the question posed at the start of this chapter. Although my choice of curative measures after my improbable heart attack would be heparin, the reasons for this choice emphasize the importance of prevention rather than cure.

How much better it would be for us if the body stores of heparin were regarded as one of our body's most precious assets. Instead of squandering it by rich meals, sloth and stress, as if it were inexhaustible, it should be conserved so that its true function will always be available to us.

For years the individual key factors of stress, lack of exercise and our rich diet have had individual scientific protagonists who usually chose one or the other as the preferred basis for a prevention program against coronary heart disease.

Today, however, it is clearly recognized that these, along with less important factors, are not independent culprits but are all interrelated and simultaneously affect the same elements in our blood to bring on clogged arteries and coronary thrombosis.

The scientific controversy which, in the past, was the greatest stumbling block to the formulation and popularization of an acceptable prevention program no longer exists.

We are now at the frontiers of scientific knowledge of heart attack prevention. This is providing each of us with enough understanding to see his individual problems clearly. It is now possible to use personal judgment in placing the correct emphasis on those factors of the prevention program which will be most effective in reducing our individual chances of heart attack.

* * * * *

The use of anticoagulants is perhaps the most potent heart-attack therapy which the physician has available today. But there are still many medical differences of opinion as to the possible dangers which may be involved in its long term use. A final official decision on this important problem may not be forthcoming in the near future.

I have given my personal opinions on this question because I thought it might help the reader to understand the ramifications of the pros and cons of the decision which the reader and his physician may some day be confronted with.

CHAPTER NINETEEN

What You Can Do, Right Now, To Reduce Heart-Attack Vulnerability

Since reports indicate that in the United States up to ten thousand heart attacks may occur daily, the obvious question from the intelligent reader would be: is there anything I can do *right now* to reduce my vulnerability?

The answer is yes.

Although the prevention of heart attack is basically a lifetime project of avoiding the slow deposits of artery blockage, some beneficial reactions in the blood can take place relatively rapidly. For instance, many of the reported reductions in thrombotic hypercoagulability, as a result of the Prudent Diet, occurred within a month.

The culmination of all the conditions leading to heart attack is the final critical reduction in oxygen which is supplied to the heart muscle by the red blood cells.

The principal cause of this oxygen reduction is the slow growth of atherosclerotic blockage which can eventually become severe enough to completely shut off the supply of blood in a coronary artery branch. A more sudden and dramatic reduction in oxygen occurs when a thrombotic clot forms in a clogged coronary artery. Methods for preventing both of these types of heart attack have already been discussed in previous chapters.

But heart attack can also occur when the coronary arteries are only half blocked, and no thrombotic clot has formed. It is evident that simple mechanical blockage is not the only cause of critical oxygen reduction.

There must be secondary contributing conditions affecting the heart muscle and the blood. These, when combined with the primary obstructive slow down of the blood, are the cause of the three-way squeeze which results in the final oxygen bankruptcy and leads to the heart attack.

Your program *right now* should be to improve your "oxygen safety margin" by increasing the critical difference between oxygen supply by the blood and oxygen demand of the heart muscle.

On the one hand, it is vital to decrease the *critical minimum oxygen demand* of your inefficient and oxygen-wasting heart muscle. On the other, you must improve all the conditions relating to *oxygen supply* by the red cells of the blood.

For ways and means to prevent oxygen wasting by the inefficient heart muscle, we must go to the studies and recommendations of Dr. W. Raab. His research shows that heart-muscle inefficiency can be a result of reduced physical activity which normally provides the stimulation needed to balance the autonomic nervous system. A state of imbalance results in an excess release of oxygen-wasting hormones from nerve endings.

Dr. Raab has reported on the practical application of this principle by thousands of "cure centers" in West and East Europe. In these centers regular exercise conducted in outdoor surroundings, combined with supervised diets similar to the Prudent Diet, has helped to increase heart-muscle efficiency in millions of mildly afflicted patients.

Until such centers are made available in this country, you can set up a "do-it-yourself" cure center in your own home with your own outdoor exercise program and your own dietary control.

In addition to reducing your vulnerability by increasing your heart-muscle efficiency, the next step is to eliminate a possible condition of "thick blood."

It is a generally accepted fact that those with the greatest percentage of red cells have thicker and consequently slower-moving blood, and are usually more vulnerable to coronary thrombosis and heart attack.

Dr. George E. Burch of Tulane University has studied a large random group of heart-attack cases whose red-cell percentages had been measured and recorded before their heart attack occurred. Compared to a normal group of similar age, the heart-attack group included too many with high red-cell counts. Statistically, according to Dr. Burch, there was only one possibility in 10,000 that this large number was due to chance or accident.

There are many reasons for changes in your red-cell count. Stress frequently causes a rapid rise. Illness may cause changes in the red-cell quantity. Lack of oxygen in the air at high altitudes is compensated by a higher quantity of red cells in the blood.

Dr. Milton Eisen of New York City has presented evidence that smoking causes an increase of red blood cells. His clinical research reports indicate that when his patients stopped smoking their red-cell counts dropped, and it increased again when they resumed smoking. Other tests made at the same time showed that cigarette smoking caused an increase in "sticky" platelets and hypercoagulability of the blood.

One explanation presented is that the carbon monoxide reduces the red-blood-cell efficiency and as a consequence more red cells are produced. Dr. Eisen also finds that cigarettes cause a dehydration resulting in a relatively increased percentage of red cells in the blood. The rapid weight gain, after smoking is discontinued, is not always due to an increase in food consumption, but is often due to rehydration of the body with a resultant thinner blood.

More research is needed to clarify the specific reasons for these effects caused by smoking. The above evidence against smoking, however, when added to those previously described in this book as well as to a multitude of other evidence, makes it urgent not to wait for further confirmation before giving up smoking.

In clinical practice it is the patients with the very low blood counts who have to be treated to *increase* their amount of red cells and hemoglobin. Unfortunately there has not been enough research, as yet, to determine at what stage an increase of red cells ceases to be desirable and actually becomes a source of danger.

The lack of oxygen at high altitudes as well as lack of oxygen due to smoking and in fact lack of oxygen due to any cause is known to result in a crowded condition of red cells in the blood. This leads to a rational method by which you may be able to reduce the need for the excess number required in your blood. Our present day sedentary life leads to shallow breathing with a low oxygen intake. Logically, it would seem that deep breathing exercises with an increased oxygen intake should increase the efficiency of the red cells which may result in a reduction of the amount of red cells required.

Some medical scientists believe that another possible cause of "thickened blood" is to be found in their observation that those with the highest red-cell counts were usually "well nourished."

Women have much less red-cell crowding in their blood. This may be an important factor, along with their lower blood cholesterol and lower blood fats, in their relatively low rate of heart attack.

The well known Boston cardiologist, Dr. S. A. Levine, has stated that, "Plethora [excess red cells] and increased viscosity or turbidity of the blood must play important roles in the production of coronary thrombosis, and I wonder whether development of mild chronic anemia might not be of value for certain vulnerable persons."

The study of red-blood-cell excess is especially important because of the light it sheds on a critical but easily preventable red-blood-cell problem. This is the temporary clumping of red cells and the blocking of minute arteries which occurs frequently as an aftermath of a heavy fatty meal.

The large inrush of chylomicrons after a fatty meal and the subsequent transformation of the smooth and slippery surfaces of the red cells into buffy and sticky coats have already been described. It is easy to visualize how an excess of red cells combined with an excess of fatty chylomicrons in the blood can cause more bumping and greater aggregation of red cells.

It is of interest to note that red-cell-blocked arterioles, after a fatty meal, are found more frequently in individuals who have a high stress-coronary profile.

Dr. Melvin H. Knisley of the Medical College of South Carolina has pioneered in the study of red-blood-cell sludging and sticking. After thousands of observations on animals and humans, he proposes the idea that this process, in vulnerable individuals, may be an important "last straw" in causing a heart attack. After death, however, the red-cell masses break up and fall apart, leaving no trace of this cause of oxygen loss which, in combination with the effects of artery blockage and reduced heart-muscle efficiency, was the cause of the final critical deficit in oxygen.

This may sound like a scientific detective story to the lay person. But Dr. F. T. Zugibe of the University of Pittsburgh Medical School has made experiments which can be studied in the light of Dr. Knisley's theories, and the results lead to another concept in heart attack prevention.

At the 1963 A.H.A. Convention, Dr. Zugibe reported his research on dogs and human subjects. His experiments on dogs show that if the oxygen supply to a heart muscle is reduced below the critical minimum for only 12 minutes, tissue death occurs. His autopsy studies on human subjects show that many deaths, biochemically proven to have been caused by heart attack, occurred in patients whose coronary arteries had less than 50% blockage and no occlusion or thrombosis.

It is important to note that, by a new technique, Dr. Zugibe showed that one of the conditions of vulnerability for this type of heart attack was the absence of a secondary or collateral circulation to the affected heart muscle.

The logical explanation for this type of heart attack is based on a combination of all the conditions of vulnerability described in this chapter.

In addition to a "Standing Room Only" condition of red blood cells there may be an excess of large fatty globules and, to make matters worse, an over abundance of "sticky" platelets and other thrombotic factors may exist in the blood. Another important condition of vulnerability is partial exhaustion of the heparin-clearing-factor system discussed earlier in the book.

In the highly vulnerable individual, the red-cell clumping, triggered by a high fat meal, will be much greater than in normal individuals. The resulting oxygen loss, caused by the combination of all the conditions described, may now be decisive. The final result can be that of choking off the primary oxygen supply to some part of an inefficient heart muscle to below its critical level and for longer than the critical period.

Considering the number of factors which may be involved in creating a fully vulnerable condition for this "non-occlusive" type of heart attack, it is difficult to point out the most important one. The question still remains to be answered: How many factors are needed to load the "red cell revolver"?

You never know if the "red cell revolver" has 1000 empty chambers or only a dozen. But if you are a vulnerable candidate, you may be playing "coronary roulette" every time you take a chance with a high-fat meal.

It is obvious that as your artery blockage becomes more extensive fewer of the contributing conditions mentioned are necessary for a vulnerable state to exist. When your artery blockage is truly serious, then the red-cell clumping combined with almost any one of the many changes which may occur even during rest or sleep, can cause the decisive reduction in oxygen supply. For those who have already had a heart attack, this knowledge is of critical importance, and it is the modern corroborating evidence for the long accepted medical practice of forbidding high-fat meals after a heart attack.

The greatest value of the facts and ideas which have been discussed here is that they refute the pessimists who say that by the time the average American male is past middle age his arteries are clogged, blocked, calcified and possibly ulcerated, and so why should he give up the known pleasures of eating in a vain attempt to repair what they have termed an "irreparable situation."

The problem is not only in your hardened arteries but in the equally important condition of your fatty, thickened and thrombotic blood, the normalization of which is to a large extent under your own control.

Heart surgeons have coined an expression, "Hearts too young to die," for the undamaged hearts they consider worth saving by their delicate artery operations.

Based on the possibility of reducing the vulnerability to heart attack by the combined short and long term prevention methods, I believe that no matter how badly scarred the heart muscle, no matter how clogged and blocked their coronary arteries: ALL HEARTS ARE TOO YOUNG TO DIE.

Partial List of References

This list does not include the references which are adequately identified in the book. References are listed in the same sequence as they appear in the book. Asterisks indicate references of value which were not specifically mentioned.

For simplification, the names of associate authors were not listed.

Pages 15-28

WHY CORONARY THROMBOSIS IS INCREASING

Gorlin, R. *American Journal of Cardiology,* March 1962.

Gordon, H. "Dietetics of Coronary Heart Disease," *South African Medical Journal,* 6 July 1957.

Puffer, R. *"Bulletin of the World Health Organization,"* 9: 315, 1958.

Cassidy, Sir M. "The Harveian Oration," *The Lancet,* 26 October 1946.

White, P. D. "Heart Disease a Generation Ago . . . and Now," *Cardiologia,* 21: 218, 1952.

Flint, A. Cited by White, P. D., "Coronaries Through the Ages," Minnesota Medicine, 71-78, 1956.

Herrick, J. B. *J.A.M.A.,* 59: 2015, 1912.

Parrish, H. M. "Autopsy Incidence of Ischemic Heart Disease," *Journal of Chronic Disease,* September 1961.

Spain, D. M. "The Relationship of Coronary Thrombosis to Coronary Atherosclerosis and Ischemic Heart Disease (a Necropsy Study Covering a Period of 25 years)," *American Journal of the Medical Sciences,* December 1960.

Editorial. *The Lancet,* 26 November 1955.

Shanoff, H. *Canadian Medical Association Journal,* 11 March 1961.

Hucheson, J. M., Jr. "Changes in the Incidence and Types of Heart Disease," *American Heart Journal,* 46: 565, 1953.

Spiekerman, R. E. "The Spectrum of Coronary Heart Disease in a Community of 30,000," *Circulation,* January 1962.

Drake, R.M. "An Epidemiological Investigation of Coronary Heart Disease," *American Journal of Public Health,* April 1957, No. 2.

Wright, I. S. *American Journal of Public Health,* March 1960.

Jett, J. D. "Studies on Age and Sex Incidence of Various Diseases Resulting From Atherosclerosis," *Journal of the American Geriatrics Society,*" April 1960.

Pages 28-34

ARTERY BLOCKAGE—10 SYMPTOMS

Torok, F. "Vestibular Reactions in Atherosclerosis," *Archives of Otolaryngology,* March, 1962.

Fabrykant, M. *Journal of the American Geriatrics Society,* September, 1962.

Hallberg, O. E. "Sudden Deafness and its Relation to Atherosclerosis," *Journal of the American Medical Association,* 30 November, 1957.

Pope, C. H. *Diabetes,* January, 1960.

Wertheimer, P. *Journal of Cardiovascular Surgery,* August, 1962.

"Little Strokes," U. S. Public Health Service Publication No. 689.

Miasnikov, A. L. Atherosclerosis, National Institute of Health, Bethesda, 1962.

*Gal, P. "Mental Disorders of Advanced Years," *Geriatrics,* April 1959.

*Beckett, H. D. "Corn Oil in Atherosclerosis Dementia," *Journal of Mental Science,* March 1962.

Pages 34-38

WORLD'S MOST IMPORTANT HEALTH DOCUMENT

Special Communication: "Dietary Fat and its Relation to Heart Attacks and Strokes," *Journal of the American Medical Association,* 4 February, 1961.

Report by the Central Committee for Medical and Community Program of the American Heart Association: "Dietary Fat and Its Relation to Heart Attacks and Strokes," *Circulation,* January 1961.

Pages 39-44

AN UNEXPECTED LIFE-SAVING DISCOVERY

Raab, W. Via Rosenthal, S. R. *Archives of Pathology*, November, 1934.

Raab, W. "Diet Hormones and Arteriosclerosis," (Pamphlet) Burlington, Vt.

Raab, W. "Aliment äre Faktoren in der Enstehung von Arteriosklerose und Hypertonie," *Medizinische Klink*, 28: 487, 521, 1932.

Schornagel, H. E. "The Connection Between Nutrition and Mortality from Coronary Sclerosis During and After World War II," *Documenta Medicina Geographica Trophica*, 5: 173, 1953.

Sivertssen, E. *Acta Medica Scandinavica*, 461, 1957.

Vartianen, I. *Ann. Med. Int. Fenniae*, 36: 748, 1957

Schettler, G. Report at Symposium on Coronary Artery Disease, at the New York Academy of Sciences, October, 1961.

Okinaka, S. Report at Symposium on Coronary Artery Disease, at the New York Academy of Sciences, October, 1961.

USA, WW II, Diabetes Data from: *Diabetes Fact Book*, U.S. Public Health Service Publication, No. 890.

Pezold, F. A. Arteriosclerosis and Nutrition, Verlag D. Steinkopf, Darmstadt, 1959.

Sinclair, H. M. Address to the Newspaper Food Editors Conference, New York City, October 3, 1960.

Strom, A. "Mortality from Circulatory Diseases in Norway 1940—1945," *The Lancet*, 20 January, 1951.

Wertheman, A. Thrombosis and Embolism, B. Schwabe, Basel, 1955.

Dedichen, J. "Incidence of Atherosclerotic Disease During War Years," in Factors Regulating Blood Pressure, Josiah Macy, Jr. Foundation, New York, 1951.

Eisenreich, F. X. Thrombosis and Embolism, B. Schwabe, Basel, 1955.

Zeitlhoffer, J. *Wein. Klin. Wschr.*, 446, 1952.

Van Unnik, J. "Rarity of Thromboembolic Disease in the Dutch East Indies," *Documenta Medicina Geographica Tropica*, 5:261, 1953.

Henschen, F. "Geographic and Historic Pathology of Arteriosclerosis," *Journal of Gerontology*, January, 1953.

Pages 44-54

VITAL DIET FACTORS REVEALED IN ASIA AND AFRICA

Oppenheim, F. *Chinese Medical Journal,* 39: 1067, 1925.

Tung, C. L. "The Relative Incidence of Atherosclerotic Heart Disease in East China and its Relationship to Cholesterol," *Chinese Medical Journal,* December 1958.

Steiner, P. E. *Archives of Pathology,* October 1946.

*Snapper, I. Bedside Medicine, Grune and Stratton, New York, 1960.

Scott, R. F., Davies, J. N. P. "Comparison of the Amount of Coronary Arteriosclerosis in Autopsied East Africans and New Yorkers," *American Journal of Cardiology,* August 1961.

Hannah, J. B. "Civilization, Race and Coronary Atheroma." *Central African Journal of Medicine,* January 1958.

Higginson, J. *Journal of Clinical Investigation,* 33: 1366, 1954.

Sachs, M. I. *Circulation,* July 1960.

Gelfand, M. *West African Medical Journal,* 1: 91, 1952.

Edington, G. M. *Tr. Roy. Soc. Trop. Med. Hyq.,* 48: 419, 1954.

Trowell, H. D. "A Case of Coronary Heart Disease in an African," *East African Medical Journal,* October 1956.

Gore, I. "Coronary Atherosclerosis and Myocardial Infarction in Kyushu, Japan, and Boston, Massachusetts," *American Journal of Cardiology,* August 1962.

Mathur, K. S. *Circulation,* July 1961.

Miller, D. C., White, P. D. "Survey of Cardiovascular Disease Among Africans in the Vicinity of the Albert Schweitzer Hospital in 1960," *American Journal of Cardiology,* September 1962.

Tejada, C. *Circulation,* July 1958.

*Ferro-Luzzi, G. "Food Patterns and Nutrition in French Polynesia," *American Journal of Clinical Nutrition,* October 1962.

*Hunter, J. D. "Diet, Body Build, Blood Pressure, and Serum Cholesterol Levels in Coconut-Eating Polynesians," *Federation Proceedings,* July-August, Part 2, Supplement 2, 1962.

White, P. D. "Convocation Address," *American Journal of Cardiology,* March 1963.

*Chi, K. L. "Cardiovascular Diseases in China," *American Journal of Cardiology*, September 1962.

*Ueda, H. "Cardiovascular Diseases in Japan," *American Journal of Cardiology*, September 1962.

Lee, K. T. "Critical Level of Dietary Fat and Myocardial Infarction in Koreans," *Experimental Molecular Pathology*, February, 1963.

Pages 54-57

INSIDIOUS FIFTH COLUMN IN THE MESS HALL

Enos, W. F. "Coronary Disease Among United States Soldiers Killed in Action in Korea," *Journal of the American Medical Assn.*, 18 July 1953.

Glantz, W. M. "Coronary Artery Disease as a Factor in Aircraft Fatalities," *Journal of Aviation Medicine*, February 1959.

Sinclair, H. M. *British Medical Journal*, December 1957.

Andrews, J. S. "The Lipids of Arcus Senilis," *Archives of Opthalmology*, August 1962.

Stare, F. J. Symposium on Atherosclerosis, Washington: National Academy of Sciences, Pub. No. 338.

Graybiel, A. "Diet in Treatment of Asymptomatic Coronary Heart Disease in Military Pilots," *Journal of the American Medical Association*, 30 April 1960.

Walker, W. J. "Atherosclerosis in the Armed Forces: Should the Military Diet be Altered?" *Military Medicine*, March 1962.

Preston, W. D. "Atherosclerosis in the U. S. Air Force," *Military Medicine*, March 1962.

Enos, W. E. *"American Journal of Cardiology,"* March 1962.

Pages 58-61

THE MILK ULCER DIET

Sippy, B. W. *J.A.M.A.*, 15 May 1915.

Sandweiss, D. J. "The Sippy Diet for Peptic Ulcer—Fifty Years Later," *American Journal of Digestive Diseases*, October 1961.

Plotz, M. "Possible Hazards of High Fat Diets in Coronary Disease," *Journal of the American Medical Association*, 5 March 1949.

Briggs, R. D. "Myocardial Infarction in Patients Treated with Sippy and Other High Milk Diets," *Circulation*, April 1960.

Miller, W. R. "Iatrogenic Atherosclerosis," *Minnesota Medicine*, October 1957.

Hartroft, W. S. "Coronary Thrombosis," *Archives of Surgery*, January 1961.

Sandweiss, D. J. "Do Ulcer Diets Promote Coronary Heart Disease in Peptic Ulcer Patients?" *Harper Hospital Bulletin*, January 1959.

Sandweiss, D. J. "Peptic Ulcer, Ulcer Diets and Arteriosclerotic (Coronary) Heart Disease," *Hebrew Medical Journal*, Vol. 1 and 2, 1960.

*Morrison, L. "The Increased Incidence of Coronary Thrombosis in Chronic Peptic Ulcer," *Review of Gastroenterology*, May 1951.

Pages 62-69

STRESS

Berkson, D. M. *Annals of the New York Academy of Sciences*, 8 December 1960.

Carroll, V. P. "Serum Lipoprotein Responses to Repeated Mental Stress," *Circulation*, October 1961.

Becker, G. H. *Gastroenterology*, 14: 80, 1950.

Cannon, W. B. The Wisdom of the Body, W. W. Norton, New York, 1932.

Uhley, H. N. "Blood Lipids, Clotting and Coronary Atherosclerosis in Rats Exposed to a Particular Form of Stress," *American Journal of Physiology*, August 1959.

Groover, M. E. "Variations in Serum Lipid Concentration and Clinical Coronary Disease," *American Journal of the Medical Sciences*, February 1960.

Russek, H. I. "Role of Heredity, Diet and Emotional Stress in Coronary Heart Disease," *Journal of the American Medical Association*, 3 October 1959.

Russek, H. I. "Emotional Stress and Coronary Heart Disease in American Physicians," *American Journal of the Medical Sciences*, December 1960.

Pages 69-74

HOW EFFECTIVE IS EXERCISE

Rakestraw, N. W. *Journal of Biological Chemistry*, 47: 565, 1921.

Brunner, D. "Influence of Labor on Lipid Values and Their Relation to the Incidence of Coronary Artery Disease," *Circulation*, October (Part II) 1961.

Adelstein, A. M. *British Journal of Preventive and Social Medicine*, January 1963.

Chapman, J. M. *American Journal of Public Health*, 47: 33, 1957.

Keys, A. *Science*, 123: 29, 1956.

Golding, L. A. News Item, *Herald Tribune*, New York, 19 April 1962.

Spain, D. M. "Occupational Activity and the Degree of Coronary Atherosclerosis in Normal Men," *Circulation*, August 1960.

Mann, G. V. *New England Journal of Medicine*, 253: 349, 1955.

Raab, W. "Loafers Heart," *Archives of Internal Medicine*, February 1958.

Pages 74-82

CAN HEART ATTACK BE INHERITED

Vecchi, G. P. "Dietary Consumption in Patients with Myocardial Infarction," *Nutritio et Dieta*, January 1959.

Mustard, J. F. Blood Coagulation During Alimentary Lipaemia in Subjects With and Without Evidence of Atherosclerosis," *Canadian Medical Association Journal*, 1 November 1958.

Bassett, A. R. "Serum Lipids in Young Adults with Parental Atherosclerosis," *American Journal of the Medical Sciences*, June 1962.

Moses, C. Atherosclerosis, Lea and Febiger, Philadelphia, 1963.

Toor, M. "Serum Lipids and Atherosclerosis among Yemenite Immigrants in Israel," *The Lancet*, 22 June 1957.

Toor, M. "Atherosclerosis in Aged Yemenite and European Immigrants to Israel," *Geriatrics*, March 1962.

Larsen, N. P. "Atherosclerosis: a Comparative Study of Caucasian and Japanese Citizens in the Hawaiian Islands— 1959," *Journal American Geriatrics Society*, November 1960.

Puddu, V. *American Journal of Cardiology*, September 1962.

Keen, H. "Diet and Arterial Disease in a Population Sample," *British Medical Journal*, 28 June 1958.

Morris, J. N. *The Practitioner*, April 1962.

Wearn, J. T. *American Journal of the Medical Sciences,* 165: 250, 1923.

Boas, E. P. *Journal of Chronic Diseases,* 5: 300, 1957.

Murphy, E. A. "Genetics and Atherosclerosis," in Coronary Heart Disease, Grune and Stratton, New York 1963.

Pages 82-88

HEART-ATTACK PROTECTION IN WOMEN

Kurland, G. S. "Hormones, Cholesterol and Coronary Atherosclerosis," *Circulation,* September 1960.

Oliver, M. F. *Minnesota Medicine,* Nov.-Dec. 1955.

Stander, R. W. "Serum Lipid Patterns Before and After Castration of the Human Female," *Surgery Gynecology and Obstetrics,* April 1961.

Oliver, M. F. "Effect of Bilateral Ovariectomy on Coronary Artery Disease and Serum Lipid Levels, *The Lancet,* 31 October 1959.

Pages 89-93

THE FAMOUS FRAMINGHAM EXPERIMENT

White, P. D., Sprague, H. B., Stamler, J., Stare, F. J., Wright, I. S., Katz, L. N., Levine, S. L., Page, I. H., and 106 Members of the American Society for the Study of Arteriosclerosis. (Pamphlet) National Health Education Committee, Inc., New York, 1959.

Dock, W. *J.A.M.A.,* 170: 2199, 1959.

Groover, M. E. *Trans. Coll. Phys. Phila.,* February 1957.

Jolliffe, N. *J. Amer. Geriat. Soc.,* November 1958.

Nahum, L. H. *Connecticut Medicine,* October 1960.

Schroeder, H. A. Mechanisms of Hypertension, C. C. Thomas, Springfield, 1957.

Shaper, A. G. *The Lancet,* 10 October 1959.

Wright, W. D. *Nebraska S.M.J.,* January 1961.

Groen, J. *Ned. Tijdschrift Voor Geneeskunde,* 18 March 1950.

Moynihan, B. *British Medical Journal,* 1: 393, 1925.

Searcy, R. L. *Osteopathic Profession,* March 1961.

Stamler, J. "Symposium on the Prevention and Control of Heart Disease," *American Journal of Public Health,* March 1960.

Pages 94-98

WHAT MEDICAL RESEARCH FINALLY REVEALED ABOUT THE LOW-CHOLESTEROL DIET

Cook, R. P. "Cholesterol Absorption and Excretion in Man," *Biochemical J.*, 62: 225, 1956.

Taylor, C. B. "Diet as a Source of Serum Cholesterol in Man," *Proc. Soc. Exper. Biol. and Med.*, April 1960.

Taylor, C. B. "Meager Capacity to Compensate for Dietary Cholesterol," *Circulation, October* (Part 2) 1961.

Connor, W. E. *Circulation,* October (Part 2) 1960.

Connor, W. E. "Effect of Dietary Cholesterol upon Serum Lipids in Man," *Journal of Laboratory and Clinical Medicine,* March 1961.

Connor, W. E. "Dietary Cholesterol and the Pathogenesis of Atherosclerosis," *Geriatrics,* August 1961.

Nutrition Reviews: "Importance of Cholesterol in the Human Diet," November 1960.

Nutrition Reviews: "Dietary Cholesterol and Serum Lipids in Man," October 1961.

Steiner, A. "Importance of Dietary Cholesterol," *Circulation,* October (Part 2) 1961.

Steiner, A. "Importance of Dietary Cholesterol in Man," *Journal of the American Medical Association,* 21 July 1962.

Wells, V. M. "Egg Yolk and Serum-Cholesterol Levels: Importance of Dietary Cholesterol Intake," *The Lancet,* 2 March 1963.

Pages 98-106

UNSATURATED FAT . . . KEY TO THE CHOLESTEROL MYSTERY

Groen, J. "The Influence of Nutrition, Individuality and some other Factors, Including Various Forms of Stress, on the Serum Cholesterol; An Experiment of Nine Months Duration in 60 Normal Human Volunteers," *Voeding,* November 1952.

Kingsbury, K. J. Drugs Affecting Lipid Metabolism, Elsevier, Milan, 1961.

Lewis, B. *The Lancet,* 24 May 1958.

Camien, M. N. *Arch. Biochem. Biophys.,* 70: 327, 1957.

Goldsmith, G. A. *Arch. Int. Med.,* April 1960.
*Other Relationships:

*Wilkins, J. A. *South African Medical Journal*, 33: 1076, 1959.

*Schroeder, H. A. Mechanisms of Hypertension, C. C. Thomas, Springfield, 1957.

Pages 107-111

FAT BLOOD CELLS

Gofman, J. W. "The Role of Lipids and Lipoproteins in Atherosclerosis," *Science*, 111: 166, 1950.

Gofman, J. W. Coronary Heart Disease, C. C. Thomas, Springfield, 1959.

Davis, H. L. "Blood Particle Agglomeration and Fat Embolism," *Int. Rec. of Med. and Gen. Pract. Clin.*, August 1954.

Gordon, I. "Chylomicron: Clue to Atherosclerosis and Coronary Disease," *Journal of Atherosclerosis Research*, 3: 1, 1963.

Pages 111-115

"BLOOD POLICEMAN"

Engelberg, H. "Long-Term Observations of Intermittent Heparin Therapy for the Prevention of Coronary Atherosclerosis," *Circulation*, October (Part 2) 1960.

Oliver, M. F. *Clinical Science*, 12: 293, 1953.

Engelberg, H. "The Rate of Lipolysis of Saturated and Unsaturated Fats by Post-Heparin and Endogenous Plasma Lipoprotein Lipase," *Circulation*, September 1958.

Engelberg, H. Heparin, Springfield, C. C. Thomas, 1963.

Pages 116-120

TESTS FOR CHOLESTEROL-FAT PARTNERSHIP

Technical Group of the Committee on Lipoproteins and Atherosclerosis, *Circulation*, 14: 691, 1956.

Albrink, M. J. "Triglycerides, Lipoproteins and Coronary Artery Disease," *Arch. Int. Med.*, March 1962.

Albrink, M. J. "Serum Lipids, Hypertension and Coronary Artery Disease," *American Journal of Medicine*, July 1961.

Metz, J. *British Medical Journal,* October 1960.

Schwartz, M. J. "A Study of Lipid Metabolism and Arteriosclerotic Heart Disease in Israelis of European and Yemenite Origin," *Journal of Atherosclerosis Research,* 2: 68, 1962.

Pages 120-128

TODAY'S FAT

White, P. D. "Convocation Address," *American Journal of Cardiology,* May 1963. "Reflections of a Pioneer in Cardiology."

Drummond, J. C. The Englishman's Food, J. Cape, London, 1939.

Van Slyke. C. *J. Am. Dietetic Assn.,* 21: 508, 1945.

Epstein, F. H. "Fat Consumption in the United States," *Public Health Reports,* April 1960.

Reiser, R. *Journal of Nutrition,* 44: 159, 1951.

Nichols, C. W. *Journal of Atherosclerosis Research,* 1: 133, 1961.

Sinclair, H. *The Lancet,* 28 January 1961.

Williams, H. H. *J.A.M.A.,* 14 January 1961.

Holman, R. T. "Polyunsaturated Fatty Acids in Milk," Annual Meeting of the American Medical Association, June 1961.

Editorial, *The Lancet,* 2: 557, 1956.

Brown, J. B. "The Fats of Life and Soybean Oil," *Soybean Digest,* November 1957.

Medical Journal Low Fat Meat Advertisements: American Meat Institute, 59 E. Van Buren St., Chicago, Illinois.

New Meat Grading: News clipping, *New York Times,* 15 April 1962.

Pages 128-131

YOUR BODY'S EMERGENCY REPAIR SYSTEM

Friedman, M. *Circulation,* May 1958.

Hall, C. E. *Jour. Biophysics Biochemistry,* January 1959.

Pages 132-136

PEOPLE WITH THICK BLOOD

Alexander, E. *New England Journal of Medicine,* 252: 432, 1955.

Mustard, J. F. "Blood Coagulation in Subjects With and Without Clinical Evidence of Atherosclerotic Blood Vessel Disease," *Canad. M. A. J.*, 1 October 1958.

McDonald, L. "Studies on Blood Coagulation and Thrombosis and on the Action of Heparin in Ischemic Heart Disease," *American Journal of Cardiology*, March 1962.

Pavlov, I. P. Anticlotting Factor, in Excerpts from Biochemistry of Blood Coagulation, U.S.S.R. Reprinted O.T.S. Washington, February, 1959.

Pages 137-141
UNCLOTTING THE BLOOD CLOT

Sandberg, H. *American Journal of Cardiology*, May 1960.

Sarkas, N. "Reduced Fibrinolytic Activity of Atherosclerotic Sera Caused by an Increase in Low-Density Lipoproteins in Blood." *Nature*, 18 March 1961.

Greig, H. B. W. "Inhibition of Fibrinolysis by Alimentary Lipemia," *The Lancet*, 7 July 1956.

Greig, H. B. W. "Studies on the Inhibition of Fibrinolysis by Lipids," *The Lancet*, 7 September 1957.

Merigan, T. C. "The Effect of Chylomicrons on the Fibrinolytic Activity of Human Blood," *Clinical Research*, 6: 46, 1958.

Merigan, T. C. *Circulation Research*, March 1959.

Nestel, P. J. "The Relationship Between Blood Fibrinolytic Activity, Serum Lipoproteins and Serum Cholesterol in Atherosclerotic Arterial Disease," *Australasian Annals of Medicine*, August 1960.

Gajewski, J. "Effect of the Ingestion of Various Fats on the Fibrinolytic Activity in Normal Subjects and Patients with Coronary Heart Disease," *Journal of Atherosclerosis Research*, May 1961.

Cliffton, E. E. "Inhibition of Fibrinolysis by Hyperlipemia," *Thrombosis et Diath. Haem.*, 5: 463, 1961.

Kwann, H. C. *Nature*, 2 February 1957.

Thomas, W. A. "Dietary Lipids and the Clotting Mechanism with Particular Reference to Lysis," in Blood Platelets, Little, Brown, Boston 1961.

Bang, N., Cliffton, E. E. "The Effect of Alimentary Hyperlipemia on Thombolysis in Vivo," *Thrombosis et Diath. Haem.*, February 1960.

Cliffton, E. E. in Anticoagulants and Fibrinolysins, Page 173, Lea & Febiger, Philadelphia, 1961.

Pages 142-147

HOW ARTERY BLOCKAGE BEGINS

Rutstein, D. "Effects of Linolenic and Stearic Acids on Cholesterol-Induced Lipoid Deposition in Human Aortic Cells in Tissue Culture," *The Lancet,* 15 March 1958.

Blaustein, A. U. *Circulation,* October (Part 2) 1960.

Lazarini-Robertson, A. in Drugs Affecting Lipid Metabolism, Elsevier, Amsterdam, 1961.

Microvilli data: in Branwood, A. W. *Journal of Atherosclerosis Research,* 1: 358, 1961.

Tuna, N. "The Fatty Acids of Total Lipids and Cholesterol Esters from Normal Plasma and Atheromatous Plaques," *Journal of Clinical Investigation,* August 1958.

Still, W. J. S. "Role of the Macrophage in Experimental Atherosclerosis," *Circulation,* October (Part 2) 1961.

O'Neal, R. M., Still, W. J. S. *Federation Proceedings,* July, Part 2, No. 2, 1962.

Simon, R. C. "The Circulating Lipophage and Experimental Atherosclerosis," *Journal of Atherosclerosis Research,* 1: 395, 1961.

Adams, C. W. M. "A Hypothesis to Explain the Accumulation of Cholesterol in Atherosclerosis," *The Lancet,* 28 April 1962.

Butter Macrophage Data: in Hartroft, W. S. *American Journal of Cardiology,* March 1962.

Hirsch, E. F. *Physiological Reviews,* 23: 185, 1943.

Enos, W. E. "Pathology of Coronary Atherosclerosis," *American Journal of Cardiology,* March 1962.

Tarizzo, R. A. "Atherosclerosis in Synthetic Vascular Grafts," *Archives of Surgery,* June 1961.

Royal Victoria Infirmary Data: in *British Medical Journal,* 5 May 1962, Page 1244.

Shimamoto, T. "The Relationship of Edematous Reaction in Arteries to Atherosclerosis and Thrombosis," *Journal of Atherosclerosis Research,* 3: 87, 1963.

Sandler, M. "Some New Observations on Human Aortic Atheroma and the Possible Role of Essential Fatty Acids vention, June 1961.
in its Development," American Medical Association Con-

Pages 148-153

SIX COMPONENTS OF ATHEROSCLEROSIS

Duguid, J. B. in Morgan, A. D. Pathogenesis of Coronary Occlusion, C. C. Thomas, Springfield, 1956.

Woolf, N. "The Distribution of Fibrin within the Aortic Intima," *American Journal of Pathology*, November 1961.

O'Neal, R. M., Thomas, W. A., Hartroft, W. S. "Affinity between Fibrin and Fat," *Circulation*, October (Part 2) 1962.

Mustard, J. F. "Platelets, Thrombosis and Vascular Disease," *Canadian Medical Association Journal*, 9 September 1961.

Mustard, J. F. "Lipids, Platelets and Atherosclerosis," in: Blood Platelets, Little Brown, Boston 1961.

Beadenkopf, W. G. *Journal of Chronic Diseases*, November 1960.

Hyaline Reference: McKinney, B. "The Pathogenesis of Hyaline Arteriosclerosis," *Journal of Pathological Bacteriology*, April 1962.

Pages 153-159

TO SALT OR NOT TO SALT

Meneely, G. R. in "Panel Discussion," *American Journal of Cardiology*, October 1961.

Dawber, T. R. *Annals of Internal Medicine*, July 1961.

Brown, R. G. *The Lancet*, 1073, 1957.

Blood Pressure, "Insurance Experience and its Implications," Metropolitan Life Insurance Company, New York.

Dahl, L. K., Love, R. A. "Salt and Hypertension," *Archives of Internal Medicine*, 94: 525, 1954.

Fallis, N. *Nature*, 196: 74, 1962.

Meneely, G. R. "Experimental Epidemiology of Chronic Sodium Chloride Toxicity," *American Journal of Medicine*, November 1958.

Ross, E. J. *Clinical Science*, 15: 81, 1953.

Babadzhanov, S. H. "Sodium Chloride and Inorganic Phosphorus Levels in the Blood of Hypertensive Patients Living in Tashkent," Feration Proceedings, Translation Supplement, July 1963.

McDonough, J. "Effect of Excess Salt Intake on Human Blood Pressure," *American Journal of Digestive Diseases*, July 1954.

New England Journal of Medicine, 12 June 1958, "The Role of Salt in the Fall of Blood Pressure Accompanying Reduction in Obesity," Dahl, L. K.

Tobian, L., Jr. *Circulation,* 7: 754, 1952.

DeLangen, C. D. "Sodium Chloride and the Capillary System," *Koninkl. Nederl. Akademie Van Wetenschappen —Amsterdam,* Proceedings C 56 No. 5, 1953.

DeLangen, C. D. "Sodium Chloride in Geographical Pathology and its Influence on the Capillary System," *Acta Medica Scandinavica,* 149: 75, 1954.

Talbott, G. D. "Effects of Excess Sodium Chloride on Blood Lipids: A Possible Factor in Coronary Heart Disease," *Annals of Internal Medicine,* February 1961.

Meneely, G. R. *American Journal of Medicine,* November 1958.

DeLangen, C. D. "Changes in the Vascular Wall and Sodium Chloride," in Symposium on Arteriosclerosis, B. Schwabe Verlag, Basel, 1957.

Patton, A. R. "Letter to the Editor," *Nutrition Reviews,* May 1953.

"Salt Sick" Data: in Gilbert, F. A. Mineral Nutrition and the Balance of Life, University of Oklahoma Press, Norman, 1957.

Pages 160-164

ARE SALT TABLETS NECESSARY

Allen, F. M. "Hypertension and Nutrition," *"Nutrition Reviews,* September 1949.

Stefansson, V. Not by Bread Alone, Macmillan, New York, 1954.

Schweitzer, A. in: Preface to book "Cancer" by Berglas A. Institute Pasteur, Paris, 1957.

Data on Human Requirement for Salt: in Meneeley, G. R. "Electrolytes in Hypertension: The Effects of Sodium Chloride," *Medical Clinics of North America,* March, 1961.

Dahl, L. K. "Role of Dietary Sodium in Essential Hypertension," *Journal of the American Dietetic Association,* June 1958.

Abrahams, D. G. *West African Medical Journal,* 8: 45, 1960.

Lancet, "Editorial" 18 February 1961.

Lowenstein, F. W. *The Lancet,* 18 February 1961.

Grollman, A. "The Role of Salt in Health and Disease," *American Journal of Cardiology,* October 1961.

Dahl, L. K. "Salt, Fat and Hypertension: The Japanese Experience," *Nutrition Reviews,* April 1960.

Sasaki, N. "High Blood Pressure and the Salt Intake of the Japanese," *Japanese Heart Journal,* July 1962.

Dahl, L. K. "Possible Role of Chronic Excess Salt Consumption in the Pathogenesis of Essential Hypertension," *American Journal of Cardiology,* October 1961.

*Corroboration of Dahl's Five Point Curve: Isaacson, L. C. "Sodium Intake in Hypertension," *The Lancet,* 27 April 1963.

Weller, J. M. "Importance of Dietary Sodium in the Etiology of Essential Hypertension," *Illinois Medical Journal,* March 1959.

DE-SALTING DRUGS

Brest, Grollman, Freis, Hollander: in "Panel Discussion," Page 283, Hypertension, Lea & Febiger, Philadelphia, 1961.

Corcoran, A. C. "Changing Status of Sodium Restriction in the Therapy of High Blood Pressure," *American Journal of Cardiology,* December 1961.

Conway, J. in: Hypertension, Lea & Febiger, Philadelphia, 1961.

Fuchs, M. *American Journal of Cardiology,* June 1962.

Fishberg, A. M. *Journal of the American Geriatrics Society,* October 1958.

*Additional Reports on Salt and its Relation to High Blood Pressure:

*Kinsey, D. "Incidence of Hyperuricemia in 400 Hypertensive Patients," *Circulation,* October (Part 2) 1961.

*Healey, L. A. "Uric Acid Retention Due to Hydrochloro Thiazide," *New England Journal of Medicine* 261: 1358, 1959.

*Zatuchni, J. "The Diabetogenic Effects of Thiazide Diuretics," *American Journal of Cardiology* 7: 565, 1961.

*Koletsky, S. "Hypertensive Vascular Diseases Reduced by Salt," *Laboratory Investigation,* 7: 377, 1958.

*"High Blood Pressure Seen from Salt in Baby Foods," *Science News Letter,* July 6, 1963.

*"Sodium Chloride and Myocardial Infarcts in Rats," *Nutrition Reviews,* November 1961.

*Fregly, M. J. "Specificity of Sodium Chloride Aversion of Hypertensive Rats," *American Journal of Physiology,* 196: 1326, 1959.

*Dahl, L. K. "The Enhanced Hypertensogenic Effect of Sea Salt over Sodium Chloride," *American Journal of Cardiology,* November 1961.

*Kohlstaedt, K. G. Panel Discussion on Genetic and Environmental Factors in Human Hypertension, *Circulation,* April 1958.

*Sodium-Restricted Diets, National Research Council, Publication 325, Washington, D. C., July 1954.

*Yorke, E. T. Salt and the Heart, Drapkin Books, Linden, N. J., 1953.

Pages 166-172

ANTI-HEART-ATTACK DRUGS

Achor, W. P. *Circulation,* October (Part 2) 1961.

Engelberg, H. *Circulation,* October (Part 2) 1961.

Parsons, W. B. *Archives of Internal Medicine,* 107: 653, 1961.

Pollack, H. Editorial: "Nicotinic Acid and Diabetes," *Diabetes,* March 1962.

Birge, K. G. "Side Effects of Nicotinic Acid in Treatment of Hypercholesteremia," *Geriatrics,* August 1961.

Steinberg, D. in: Drugs Affecting Lipid Metabolism, Elsevier, Amsterdam, 1961.

Lown, B. Editorial in: *Clinical Pharmacology and Therapeutics,* July 1962.

Pages 173-176

TWENTY FACTORS IN CORONARY DISEASE

*Data on Relationship of Blood Lipids to Toxic Environment:

*Effects of D. D. T. on Blood Lipids: in Worne, H. E. *American Journal of the Medical Sciences,* July 1959.

*Bicknell, F. Chemicals in Your Food, Emerson, New York, 1961.

*Problems in the Evaluation of Carcinogenic Hazard from Use of Food Additives, Publication No. 749, National Academy of Sciences, Washington, D. C., 1960.

Cigarette Smoking and Cardiovascular Disease: Report by the American Heart Association, *Circulation*, July, 1960.

Doyle, J. F. "Cigarette Smoking and Coronary Disease," *New England Journal of Medicine*, 19 April 1962.

*Data on Constipation and Cholesterol:

*Walker, A. R. P. in Hormones and Atherosclerosis, Academic Press, New York, 1959.

*Portman, O. W. "Constipation," *American Journal Clinical Nutrition*, 8: 462, 1960.

*Antonis, A. "The Influence of Diet on Fecal Lipids in South African White and Bantu Prisoners," *American Journal Clinical Nutrition*, August 1962.

Pages 176-194

DR. JOLLIFFE'S ANTI-CORONARY CLUB

Jolliffe, N. "Fats, Cholesterol and Coronary Heart Disease," *N. Y. State Journal of Medicine*, 15 August 1957.

Jolliffe, N.   *J. Chronic Disease*, June 1959.

Jolliffe, N. "The Anti-Coronary Club," *American Journal of Clinical Nutrition*, July 1959.

Jolliffe, N. "Fats, Cholesterol and Coronary Heart Disease," *Circulation*, July 1959.

Jolliffe, N. "Dietary Control of Serum Cholesterol in Clinical Practice," *Circulation*, December 1961.

Jolliffe, N. Clinical Nutrition, Hoeber-Harper, New York, 1962.

Jolliffe, N. "Prudent Diet," *N. Y. State Journal of Medicine*, 1 January 1963.

James, G. Heart Newsletter, June 1963.

Dayton, S. *New England Journal of Medicine*, 17 May 1962.

Rinzler, S. H. "Lessons from the Anti-Coronary Club Study," *Federation Proceedings*, July, Part 2, No. 2, 1962.

Pages 194-202

MEDICAL FACTS ABOUT REDUCING WEIGHT

Pilkington, T. R. E. "Diet and Weight-Reduction in the Obese," *The Lancet*, 16 April 1960.

Zuntz, N. in: Pennington, A. W. *American Journal of Digestive Disease*, February 1955.

Bloom, W. L. "Inhibition of Salt Excretion by Carbohydrate," *Archives of Internal Medicine*, January 1962.

Benedict, F. G. U. S. Dept. Agr. Office Exp. Sta. Bull. 175, 1907, Page 225.

Lusk, G. The Science of Nutrition, Saunders, Philadelphia, 1921.

Fineberg, S. K. *Journal of the American Medical Association*, 18 September 1962.

Duncan, G. G. in *Science News Letter*, 29 June 1963.

Roracher, H. in "Body Vibrations Found, May be Key to Warmth," *Science News Letter*, 2 June 1962.

Gubner, R. S. "Fatness, Fat and Coronary Heart Disease," *Nutrition Reviews*, December 1957.

Sanders, K. "Coronary-Artery Disease and Obesity," *The Lancet*, 29 September 1959.

Russell, G. F. M. "Effect of Diets of Different Composition on Weight Loss, Water and Sodium Balance in Obese Patients," *Clinical Science*, April 1962.

Elsbach, P. "Salt and Water Metabolism During Weight Reduction," *Metabolism*, August 1961.

Pages 203-206

SATURATED BODY FAT IS DANGEROUS

Christakis, G. "Effect of a Cholesterol Lowering Diet on Fatty Acid Composition of Subcutaneous Fat in Man," *Circulation*, October (Part 2) 1962.

Dayton, S. *New England Journal of Medicine*, 17 May 1962.

Kingsbury, K. J. "A Comparison of the Plasma Cholesterol Esters and Subcutaneous Depot Fats of Atheromatous and Normal People," *Clinical Science*, April 1962.

Little, J. A. "Diet and Degeneration," *Canadian Medical Association Journal*, 3 December 1960.

Hilleboe, H. E. *American Journal of Public Health*, October (Suppl.) 1960.

Schrade, W. *Journal of Atherosclerosis Research*, 1: 47, 1961.

Schrade, W. "Humoral Changes in Arteriosclerosis, Investigations on Lipids . . . in the Blood," *The Lancet*, 31 December 1960.

Antonis, A. in: Essential Fatty Acids, Academic Press, New York, 1968.

Lewis, B. "Composition of Plasma Cholesterol Ester in Relation to Coronary-Artery Disease and Dietary Fat," *The Lancet*, 12 July 1958.

Wiktor, Z. "Diagnostic Value of the Determination of Fatty Acid Serum Level and of the Degree of their Unsaturation in Atherosclerosis," *Polski Tygodn.*, 13: 853, 1958.

Pol, G. "Polyunsaturated Acids in Relation to . . . Complaints of Angina Pectoris," *Journal of Nutrition*, July 1962.

Hammond, E. G. *Archives of Biochemistry and Biophysics*, 57: 517, 1955.

*Supplementary References to Kingsbury:

*Tanaka, K. cited by: Oshima, *Japanese Circulation Journal*, February 1963.

*Lee, K. T. "Long Term Effects of Seven Percent Fat Diets on General Health," *Circulation*, October (Part 2) 1952.

Pages 207-209

THE PRUDENT DIET AND METABOLIC DISEASE

Kahn, P. M. "Hyperuricemia—Relationship to Hypercholesteremia and Acute Myocardial Infarction," *Journal American Medical Association*, 15 August 1959.

Salvini, L. "Statistical Study on Correlation between Blood Level of Cholesterol, Beta/Alpha Lipoprotein Ratio and Uric Acid of Normal and Arteriosclerotic Subjects," *Gerentologia*, 3: 327, 1959.

*Schoenfeld, M. R. "Serum Cholesterol—Uric Acid Correlations," *Metabolism*, August 1963.

*Dreyfuss, F. "Role of Hyperuricemia in Coronary Heart Disease," *Diseases of the Chest*, September 1960.

Dawber, T. R. *Journal of the American Geriatrics Society*, October 1962.

*Moore, C. B. "Uric Acid Metabolism and Myocardial Infarction," in: Etiology of Myocardial Infarction, Little Brown, Boston, 1963.

Kramer, D. W. "Metabolic Influence in Vascular Disorders," *Angiology*, June 1958.

Weiss, T. E., Moore, C. "Gout and Diabetes," *Metabolism*, 6: 103, 1957.

Wahlberg, F. "The Intravenous Glucose Tolerance Test in Atherosclerotic Disease," *Acta Medica Scandinavica*, 171: 1, 1962.

Reaven, G. "Glucose Tolerance in Patients with Myocardial Infarction," *American Heart Association,* October (Part 2) 1962.

Aleksandrow, D. "Studies on Disturbances of Carbohydrate Metabolism in Atherosclerosis," *Journal of Atherosclerosis Research,* 2: 171, 1962.

Gutman, A. B. *American Journal of Medicine,* October 1960.

Diabetes Fact Book, Public Health Service Pub. No. 890, 1961.

Popert, A. J. "Gout and Hyperuricaemia in Rural and Urban Populations," *Annals of the Rheumatic Diseases,* June 1962.

Gutman, A. B. "Prevention and Treatment of Chronic Gouty Arthritis," *Journal of the American Medical Association,* 157: 1096: 1955.

Lockie, L. M. *Journal of the American Medical Association,* 104: 2072, 1935.

McEwen, C. "High Fat and High Purine Diets in the Diagnosis of Gout," *Journal of Mt. Sinai Hospital,* 8: 854, 1942.

Harding, V. J. "The Effect of High Fat Diets on the Content of Uric Acid in the Blood," *Journal of Biological Chemistry,* 63: 37, 1925.

van Buchen, F.S.P. "Frequency of Diabetes Mellitus in the Netherlands," *Med. et Hygiene,* 11 (250); 339, 1953.

Lederer, J. "Nutrition Education, Social Problem in the Prevention and Treatment of Diabetes," *Med. et Hygiene,* 11: 337, 1953.

Fleisch, A. "Diabetes Mellitus, a Disease of the Well-to-do," *Gaz. Med.* 60: 31, 1953.

*Armstrong, D. B. "Obesity and Its Relation to Health and Disease," *Journal of the American Medical Association,* 10 November 1951.

Pages 210-215

Leary, T. *Archives of Pathology,* April 1936.

Data From George F. Baker Clinic: in Marble, A. *Am. J. Med. Sci.,* April 1939.

Singh, L. "Low-fat Diet and Therapeutic Doses of Insulin in Diabetes Mellitus," *The Lancet,* 26 February 1955.

Kinsell, L. W. "The Case for the Routine Use of Diets High in Polyunsaturated Fat for Diabetics," Editorial. *Diabetes,* July 1962.

Van Eck, W. F. "Effect of a Low Fat Diet on the Serum Lipids and Lipoproteins in Diabetes and its Significance in Diabetic Retinopathy," *American Journal of Medicine,* August 1959.

Data on Gallstones: in *Gastroenterology*, 29: 377, 1955.

Watanabe, N. "Effect of Polyunsaturated and Saturated Fatty Acids on the Cholesterol Holding Capacity of Human Bile," *Archives of Surgery*, July 1962.

Cohen, A. M. "Prevalence of Diabetes among Different Ethnic Jewish Groups in Israel," *Metabolism*, January 1961.

New England Journal of Medicine, 28 January 1962.

*Data on Prudent Diet in Diabetes:

*Southwood, A. R. "Prediabetes," *The Lancet*, 6 April 1963.

*Hackedorn, H. M. "Polyunsaturated Fat in Diets for Diabetics," *Northwest Medicine*, December 1962.

*Stone, D. B. "Prolonged Effects of a Low Cholesterol, High Carbohydrate Diet upon Serum Lipids in Diabetic Patients," *Diabetes*, March 1963.

Williams, R. J. Free and Unequal, University of Texas Press, Austin 1953.

*Data on Enzyme Overload:

*Long, C. N. H. *The Lancet*, 2: 106, 1951.

*Solez, C. "Overeating and Vascular Degeneration," *Journal of the American Geriatrics Society*, December 1958.

Cohn, C. "Fats, Rats, Chickens and Men—Results of Feeding Frequency," *American Journal of Clinical Nutrition*, March 1963.

Cohn, C. "Nutritional Effect of Feeding Frequency," *American Journal of Clinical Nutrition*, November 1962.

Cohn, C. "Nutrition Effect of Feeding Frequency," *American Journal of Clinical Nutrition*, November 1962.

King, C. G. in: Symposium on Foods, Oregon State University, 11 September 1961.

King, C. G. Certified Milk, July 1953.

HEART ATTACKS, SMOKING AND VITAMIN C

Patterson, J. C. *Canadian Medical Association Journal*, February 1941.

Gale, E. T. "Vitamins C and P in Cardiovascular and Cerebrovascular Disease," *Geriatrics*, February 1953.

Loewe, W. R. *Eye, Ear, Nose and Throat Monthly*, February 1955.

Simonson, E. "Research in Russia on Vitamins and Atherosclerosis," *Circulation*, November 1961.

Data on Vitamin C in Atherosclerosis in *M.D.* January 1957.

Willis, G. C. *Canadian Medical Association Journal,* December 1952: January 1953: December 1954: 1 April 1955: 15 July 1957.

Borquin, A. *American Journal of Digestive Disease,* 20: 75, 1953.

Calder, J. H. "Comparison of Vitamin C in Plasma and Leucocytes of Smokers and Non-Smokers," *The Lancet,* 9 March 1963.

Manchester, B. "Anticoagulant Prophylaxis Following Coronary Occlusion," in: Anticoagulants and Fibrinolysis, Lea and Febiger, Philadelphia, 1961.

Pages 220-223

STICKY BLOOD PLATELETS

Mustard, J. F. "Blood Coagulation and the Formation of Deposits in Extracorporeal Shunts," *Circulation,* October 1961.

Mustard, J. F. "Effect of Different Dietary Fats on Blood Coagulation, Platelet Economy and Blood Lipids," *British Medical Journal,* 16 June 1962.

Shimamoto, T. "Acute Vascular Endothelial Reaction," *Asian Medical Journal,* August 1961.

Moolton, S. E. *Archives of Internal Medicine,* 84: 667, 1949.

Chargaff, E. *Journal of Biological Chemistry,* 116: 237, 1936.

Nothman, M. M. "Cephalins in the Blood of Patients with Coronary Heart Disease," Annual Meeting of the American Medical Association, June 1961.

Zemplini, T. "Some Recent Advances in Lipid Metabolism in Relation to Atherosclerosis," *Review of Czechoslovak Medicine,* January 1960.

Nothman, M. M. "Cephalins in the Blood," *The Journal of the Medical Association,* 6 January 1962.

Moolten, S. E. "Dietary Fat and Platelet Adhesiveness in Arteriosclerosis and Diabetes," *American Journal of Cardiology,* March 1963.

*Additional Reports on the Possible Relationship between Blood Platelets, Cephalin, Atherosclerosis and the Excessive Dietary use of Egg Yolks:

*Mustard, J. F. "Dietary Fat and Platelet Survival in Man," *Circulation,* October (Part 2), 1961.

*Mustard, J. F. "Lipids, Platelets and Atherosclerosis," in: Blood Platelets, Little Brown, Boston, 1961.

*Mustard, J. F. "Effects of Material Rich in Phosphatidyl Ethanolamine or Phosphatidyl Serine on Clotting and Cholesterol Levels," *Circulation*, November, 1959.

*Mills, C. A. "The Role of Platelets in Blood Clotting," *Chinese Journal of Physiology*, 1: 235, 1927.

*Howell, W. H. "Nature and Action of Thromboplastic (zymoplastic) Substances of Tissues," *American Journal of Physiology*, 31: 1, 1912.

Pages 224-228

PAIN AFTER HEAVY MEALS

Swank, R. L. "Changes in Blood of Dogs and Rabbits by High Fat Intake," *American Journal of Physiology*, March 1959.

Cullen, C. F., Swank, R. L. "Intravascular Aggregation and Adhesiveness of the Blood Elements Associated with Alimentary Lipemia," *Circulation*, March 1954.

Bloch, E. H. *American Journal of the Medical Sciences*, 229: 280, 1955.

Friedman, M. "Changes in Serum Lipids and Capillary Circulation after Fat Ingestion in Men Exhibiting a Behavior Pattern (A) Associated with Coronary Arterial Disease." *Circulation*, October 1963.

Loewy, A. L. "Increased Erythrocyte Destruction on a High Fat Diet," *American Journal of Physiology*, 138: 230, 1943.

Talbott, G. D. in *Conference* Serum Lipids and Other Factors in Coronary Atherosclerosis, June 1962.

Boeck, J. K. "A Restudy of the Diet and Heart Disease of Rural Men," Pamphlet, New York State Department of Health, Albany, 1961.

Speedby, H. J. The 20th Century and Your Heart, Centaur Press, London, 1960.

Jensen, D. *Nordisk Medicin*, 62: 1051, 1959.

Sobel, H. "Physical Activity and Lipemia Clearance," *American Journal of Clinical Nutrition*, May 1963.

Kuo, P. T. "Angina Pectoris Induced by Fat Ingestion in Patients with Coronary Artery Disease," *J.A.M.A.*, 23 July 1955.

Kuo, P. T. "Effect of Heparin on Lipemia Induced Angina Pectoris," *J.A.M.A.*, 2 March 1957.

Kuo, P. T. "Effect of Lipemia upon Coronary and Peripheral Arterial Circulation," *American Journal of Medicine,* January 1959.

Swank, R. L. "Effects of Large Fat Intake on the Physical State of the Blood," Third International Conference on Biochemical Problems of Lipids, Brussels, 1956.

Williams, A. V. "Increased Blood Cell Agglutination Following Ingestion of Fat, a Factor Contributing to Cardiac Ischemia, Coronary Insufficiency, and Anginal Pain," *Angiology,* February 1957.

Pages 229-238

WHY YOUR BLOOD TODAY MAY BE MORE PRONE TO CORONARY THROMBOSIS

Stare, F. *Circulation,* May 1958.

Silver, E. "Clinical Conference," *Circulation,* June 1960.

Kugelmass, I. N. "Clinical Control of Chronic Hemorrhagic States in Childhood," *J.A.M.A.,* 20 January 1934.

Kugelmass, I. N. "Bleeding and Clotting Diets," *Medical Clinics of North America,* 19: 989, 1935.

Moolten, S. E. "Dietary Fat and Platelet Adhesiveness in Arteriosclerosis and Diabetes," *The American Journal of Cardiology,* March 1963.

Hilleboe, H. E. "Some Epidemiologic Aspects of Coronary Artery Disease," *Journal of Chronic Diseases,* September 1957.

Mayer, G. A. "Environmental Factors Influencing Blood Clotting," *Circulation,* September 1958.

Lorie, K. M. "Changes in Blood Coagulation in Atherosclerotic Patients Under Varying Diets," *Institute for Contemporary Russian Studies,* April-June 1962.

Karvonen, M. J. *Proc. Royal Society Medicine,* April 1962.

Bang, N. U. *Thrombosis et Diatheisis Hemorrhagica,* 4: 149, 1960.

Bergentz, S. E. "Fats and Thrombus Formation," *Thrombosis et Diathesis Hemorrhagica,* 5: 474, 1961.

Naimi, S. "Cardiovascular Lesions and Changes in Blood Coagulation and Fibrinolysis Associated with Diet Induced Lipemia in the Rat," *Journal of Clinical Investigation,* September 1962.

Fullerton, H. W. "Relationship of Alimentary Lipaemia to Blood Coagulability," *British Medical Journal,* August 1953.

Goldrick, R. B. "The Effects of Diet on the Blood Coagulation Response to Alimentary Lipaemia in Healthy and Atherosclerotic Men," *Australasian Annals of Medicine*, May 1960.

Mustard, J. F. "Platelets, Thrombosis and Vascular Disease," *The Canadian Medical Association Journal*, 9 September 1961.

Hahn, J. W. "The Effect of Hyperlipemia on a Thromic Index," *Circulation*, October 1960.

Davidson, E. *British Journal of Experimental Pathology*, April 1962.

Matsuoka, M. *Japanese Circulation Journal*, June 1962.

Rawls, W. B. *Journal of the American Geriatric Society*, November 1959.

Dailey, J. P. "Lipid Induced Coagulation Changes in Normal Subjects and in Patients with Atherosclerosis," *American Journal of Clinical Nutrition*, January 1960.

Schmidt, J. "Influence of Fat on Blood Coagulation," *The Journal of Laboratory and Clinical Medicine*, February 1962.

Hansen, P. F., Geill, T., Lund, E. "Dietary Fats and Thrombosis," *The Lancet*, 8 December 1962.

Enticknap, J. B. "Lipids in Cadaver Sera After Fatal Heart Attacks," *Journal Clinical Pathology*, 14: 496, 1961.

Olney, R. C., Davis, H. L. "Serum Lipids in the Etiology of Thromboembolism," *Nebraska State Medical Journal*, March 1962.

Davis, H. L. "The Influence of Fatty Acids on Blood Coagulability," *Circulation*, September 1958.

Pages 239-242

UNNOTICED BLOOD CLOTS IN THE LEGS

Popkin, R. J. The Postthrombophlebitic Syndrome, C. C. Thomas, Springfield 1962.

Naide, M. in "Check for Blood Clots," *Science News Letter*, 11 April 1953.

Franz, R. C. "Postoperative Thrombosis and Plasma Fibrinolytic Activity," *The Lancet*, 28 January 1961.

Japanese Thromboembolic Data in: Ueda, H. *American Journal of Cardiology*, September 1960.

Wessler, S. *Transactions of Association of American Physicians*, 74: 111, 1961.

Wessler, S. "Thrombosis in the Presence of Vascular Stasis," *American Journal of Medicine*, November 1962.

*Additional Research Reports:

*McDonald, L. "Dietary Restriction and Coagulability of the Blood in Ischemic Heart Disease," *The Lancet*, 1: 996, 1958.

*Conner, W. E. "The Acceleration of Thrombus Formation by Certain Fatty Acids," *Journal of Clinical Investigation*, 41: 1199, 1962.

*Kudrjashol, B. A. "Experimental Prethrombotic State . . . Induced by an Atherogenic Diet," *Nature*, 7 January 1961.

*Poole, J. F. C. "Effect of Diet and Lipemia on Coagulation and Thrombosis," *Federation Proceedings*, July, Part 2, No. 2, 1962.

*Thomas, W. A. "Incidence of Myocardial Infarction Correlated with Venous and Pulmonary Embolism," *American Journal of Cardiology*, January, 1960.

*Kommerell, B. "The Significance of Blood Coagulation in Atherosclerosis," *Journal of Atherosclerosis Research*, 2: 233, 1962.

*Oshima, K. "Blood Lipids, Blood Coagulation and Anti-coagulants," *Japanese Circulation Journal*, February 1963.

*Ikeda, M. "Incidence of Thromboembolism in Japan," *Japanese Circulation Journal*, February 1963.

Pages 242-249

WHO CAN BENEFIT MOST FROM THE PRUDENT DIET

Dock, W. Editorial: "The Reluctance of Physicians to Admit that Chronic Disease May be Due to Faulty Diet," *The Journal of Clinical Nutrition*, March 1953.

Stamler, J. *American Journal of Cardiology*, September 1962.

Dawber, T. R. *Journal of the American Geriatrics Society*, October 1962.

White, P. D. *Amer. J. Public Health*, April (Part 2) 1957.

Corcoran, A. C. *American Heart Journal*, April 1961.

de Takats, G. in *Health Bulletin*, 22 June 1963.

Kinsell, L. W., Pollack, H. News Item, *New York Post*, 17 April 1962.

Editorial, *American Heart Journal*, July 1962.

National Nutrition Council, *South African Medical Journal*, 17 March 1956.

Gofman, J. W. Coronary Heart Disease, C. C. Thomas, 1959.

Pages 250-279

MYTHS AND MISUNDERSTANDINGS ABOUT HEART ATTACK AND DIET

McFarland, M. D. *J. Germantown Hospital*, February 1962.

Gibson, G. D. in: *Science News Letter*, "African Diet Studied," 7 October 1961.

Dock, W. in Symposium on Arteriosclerosis, B. Schwabe & Co., Basel, 1957.

Bloomberg, B. M. *Circulation*, June 1958.

*Brunner, D. "Alpha Cholesterol Percentages in Coronary Patients with and without Increased Total Serum Cholesterol Levels and in Healthy Controls," *Journal of Atherosclerosis Research*, 2: 424, 1962.

*Schrade, W. "On Hyperlipidaemia and Atherosclerosis," *Journal of Atherosclerosis Research*, 2: 161, 1963.

Labecki, T. D. *American Journal of Clinical Nutrition*, May 1960.

Hirst, A. E. "Editorial," *Medical Arts and Sciences*, Third Quarter 1960.

Shallock, G. *Journal of Atherosclerosis Research*, January 1962.

Watts, H. F. Report at the A. H. A. Conference on the Evolution of the Atherosclerotic Plague, Chicago, March 1963.

Friedman, M. *Progress in Cardiovascular Disease*, March 1962.

Keys, A. "Diet and the Epidemiology of Heart Disease," *Journal of the American Medical Association*, 164: 1912, 1957.

Keys, A. "Lessons From Serum Cholesterol Studies in Japan, Hawaii and Los Angeles," *Annals of Internal Medicine*, January 1958.

Keys, A. "Editorial" "The Risk of Coronary Heart Disease," *Circulation*, June 1961.

Jerushalmy, J. "Fat in the Diet and Mortality from Heart Disease," *New York State Journal of Medicine*, 15 July 1957.

Yudkin, J. "Diet and Coronary Thrombosis: Hypothesis and Fact," *The Lancet*, 2: 155, 1957.

Womack, M. Reported in: *Wall Street Journal*, 18 June 1959.

Portman, O. W. *Archives of Biochemistry*, 59: 224, 1955.

Keys, A. "Cholesterol Depressing Effects of Fruits, Vegetables and Legumes When Substituted for Sucrose and Skim Milk in Human Diets," *Circulation*, November 1959.

Keys, A. *Journal of Nutrition*, 70: 257, 1960.

Uram, J. A. *Amer. J. Physiol.*, March 1958.

Ruffer, M. A. "On Arterial Lesions Found in Egyptian Mummies," *Journal of Pathology and Bacteriology*, 50: 453, 1911.

Ruffer, M. A. Studies in the Paleopathology of Egypt, University of Chicago Press, Chicago 1921.

Shattock, S. G. "A Report on the Pathological Condition of the Aorta of King Meneptah, Pharoah of the Exodus," *Proceedings of the Royal Society of Medicine*, 2: Path. Sect. 122, 1909.

Breasted, J. H. *Science*, 74: 639, 1931.

Terry, L. L. *Heart Newsletter*, June 1963.

Ahrens, E. H., Jr. *"Transactions of the Association of American Physicians,"* December 1961.

Antonis, A. "The Influence of Diet on Serum-Triglycerides in South African White and Bantu Prisoners," *The Lancet*, 7 January 1961.

Antonis, A. Influence of Diet on Serum Triglyceride, Mimeographed Supplement to the above paper, South African Institute for Medical Research, Johannesburg 1961.

Antonis, A. "Serum Triglyceride Levels in South African Europeans and Bantu and in Ischaemic Heart-Disease," *The Lancet*, 7 May 1960.

Ahrens, E. H., Jr. "Dietary Fat and Coronary Heart Disease," *Review of Modern Medicine*, Page 70, 1961.

Bierman, E. L. *Diabetes*, November 1961.

Lee, K. T. *Archives of Environmental Health*, January 1962.

Lee, K. T. *Archives of Internal Medicine*, 422, 1962.

Snapper, I. Editorial "Diet and Atherosclerosis," *American Journal of Cardiology*, March 1963.

*Data on Calcium Requirements:

World Health Organization Chronicle, "Calcium Requirements," July 1962.

*British Medical Journal, "Calcium Requirements," 29 December 1962.

Walker, A. R. P.   Nutrition Reviews, November 1960.

Pages 279-291

BREAKING THROUGH THE CORONARY CURTAIN

Kossmann, C. E.   Heart Newsletter, June 1963.

Gofman Mechanical—Centrifugal Test for Complete Spectrum of All Fatty Globules in Blood. Obtainable from the Institute of Medical Physics, a Non-Profit Scientific Research Laboratory, Belmont, California.

Sherber, D. A.   "Readily Extractible Cholesterol as an Index to Species Susceptibility to Spontaneous Atherosclerosis," Circulation, October 1962.

Horlick, L.   "Serum Lipoprotein Stability in Atherosclerosis," Circulation, July 1954.

Amatuzio, D. S.   Circulation, March 1962.

Michaels, G. D.   American Journal of Clinical Nutrition, January 1960.

*Wilkens, J. A.   "Stabilization of Supersaturated Cholesterol Solutions by Serum Lipid Extracts: A New Serum Parameter Associated With Ischaemic Heart Disease," Journal of Atherosclerosis Research, January 1963.

Berkowitz, D.   "Serum Lipids and Fat Tolerance in Patients Receiving Sippy Ulcer Diets," J.A.M.A., 21 July 1962.

*Additional Reports on the Value of the Fat Tolerance Test in Predicting the Coronary-Prone Person:

*Malamos, B.   "Fat Metabolism in Patients wtih Myocardial Infarction," American Journal of Cardiology, December 1962.

*Tolchowitz, L.   "Cholesterol and Serum Turbidity Measurement in Atherosclerosis," American Heart Journal, June 1962.

*Sklarin, B. S.   "Hyperlipemia," Geriatrics, August 1961.

Klein, E.   Journal of Investigative Dermatology, 33: 91, 1959.

Martarini, I.   Metabolism, November 1962.

Stepanova, M. P.   Federation Proceedings, March (Part 2) 1963.

Eggstein, M.   International Congress Biochemical Problems of Lipids, (III) Oxford, 1958.

Kinsell, L. W. in: Essential Fatty Acids, Page 104, Academic Press, New York, 1958.

Kuo, P. F. *Journal of Clinical Investigation,* August 1959.

Bronte-Stewart, M. B. *The Lancet,* 24 January 1959.

Böhle, E. *Klinische Wochenschrift,* 39: 5, 1961.

Jones, R. J. "Factors Influencing Fat Tolerance Curve," *Circulation,* October 1963.

*Reports Concerning Impairment of Fat Tolerance due to Digestive Enzyme Exhaustion and Atherosclerosis:

*Marks, I. N. "Gastric Secretion and Alimentary Lipaemia in Ischaemic Heart-disease," *The Lancet,* 24 November 1962.

*Tietz, N. W. "Pancreatic Secretion and Fat Tolerance," *Circulation Research,* January 1960.

*Bassett, D. R. "The Fat Tolerance Curves of Patients with Hyperlipidemia and Atherosclerosis," *American Journal of Clinical Nutrition,* March 1963.

*"Electron Microscopy and Biochemical Studies of Chyle, Serum, and Liver after Fatty Meals," *Nutrition Reviews,* July 1963.

*Reports Concerning Laboratory and Instrument Tests:

*Seide, M. J. "Laboratory Control of Coumarin Therapy: The Clinicians Dilemma," *Ann. Int. Med.,* October 1962.

*Starr, I. "Histories of Over 200 Persons, Originally Healthy, Followed until Death or for 20 Years after Their First Ballistocardiograms," *Circulation,* October (Part 2) 1959.

*Rosa, L. M. "The Precordial Accelerogram in Ischemic Heart Disease," *American Journal of Cardiology,* April 1962.

*Agress, C. M. "The Vibrocardiographic Exercise Test for Coronary Insufficiency," *American Journal of Cardiology,* April 1962.

Raab, W. "Prevention of Degenerative Heart Disease by Neurovegetative Reconditioning," *Public Health Reports,* April 1963.

Pages 292-301

ANTICOAGULANTS AND HEPARIN

Griffith, G. C. "Long Term Intermittent Heparin Injection: Preventive Therapy," California Medical Assn. Convention, April 1962.

Griffith, G. C. Address at First International Heparin Conference, October 1963.

Wagner, R. T. in Medical Report: "Heparin Called Therapy of Choice," *Medical World News,* December 21, 1962.

*Hughs, M. L. "Comparison of Continuous Long-term Heparin and Oral Anticoagulant Therapy," *American Heart Journal,* May 1963.

Pages 301-307

HEART ATTACK VULNERABILITY

Burch, G. E. "Hematocrit, blood viscosity and myocardial infarction," *American Journal of Medicine,* February 1962.

Eisen, M.E. "The effect of smoking on packed red cell volume, haemoglobin and platelet counts," *Canadian Medical Assn. Jour.* 75:520, 1956.

Knisely, M. H. in The Etiology of Myocardial Infarction, Little Brown, Boston, 1963.

*Swank, R. L. "Blood viscosity in cerebrovascular disease. Effects of low fat diet and heparin," *Neurology,* August, 1959.

Recommended Reading

DIETARY BOOKS

EAT DRINK AND LOWER YOUR CHOLESTEROL
Dr. F. T. Zugibe   McGraw-Hill, 1963

LOW FAT DIET—REASONS, RULES AND RECIPES
Dr. Roy L. Swank   University of Oregon Press, 1959

LOW-FAT WAY TO HEALTH AND LONGER LIFE
Dr. Lester Morrison   Prentice-Hall, 1958

EAT WELL STAY WELL
Dr. Ancel Keys   Doubleday, 1959

REDUCE AND STAY REDUCED
Dr. Norman Jolliffe   Simon and Schuster, 1957

DIETARY PREVENTION AND TREATMENT OF
  HEART DISEASE
Dr. J. W. Gofman   Putnam, 1958

EAT WELL AND LIVE LONGER
Dr. Emil Conason   Crown, 1958

LIVE HIGH ON LOW FAT
Sylvia Rosenthal   Lippincott, 1962

THE LOW FAT, LOW CHOLESTEROL DIET
Dobbin, Goffman, Jones, Lyon & Young   Doubleday, 1951

SUPPLEMENTARY PAMPHLETS

Planning Fat-Controlled Meals
for Unrestricted Calories
                        1963
Dietary Fat and its Relation   American Heart Association
to Heart Attacks and Strokes   424 East 23 Street
                        1961 New York 10, New York
What We Know About Diet
and Heart Disease

REFERENCE BOOKS

Dr. H. Engelberg *Heparin*
    C. C. Thomas, Springfield, 1963

Dr. C. Moses *Atherosclerosis Mechanism as a Guide to Prevention*
    Lea and Febiger, Philadelphia, 1963

IMP Handbook #1 *Screening Diagnosis Control in Coronary Heart Disease*
    Institute of Medical Physics, Belmont, Calif., 1962

Dr. A. L. Miasnikov *Atherosclerosis*
    National Institute of Health, Bethesda, 1962

Dr. R. L. Searcy, L. M. Bergquist *Lipoprotein Chemistry in Health and Disease*
    C. C. Thomas, Springfield, 1962

Dr. S. Garattini, Dr. R. Paoletti *Drugs Affecting Lipid Metabolism*
    Elsevier, Amsterdam, 1961

Dr. A. N. Brest, Dr. J. H.Moyer *Hypertension, Recent Advances*
    Lea and Febiger, Philadelphia, 1961

Dr. R. L. Swank *A Biochemical Basis of Multiple Sclerosis*
    C. C. Thomas, Springfield, 1961

Henry Ford Hospital, International Symposium, *Blood Platelets*
    Little, Brown, Boston, 1961

Dr. I. Snapper *Bedside Medicine*
    Grune & Stratton, New York, 1960

Dr. J. W. Gofman *Coronary Heart Disease*
    C. C. Thomas, Springfield, 1959

Dr. D. Kritchevsky *Cholesterol*
John Wiley, New York, 1958

Dr. L. N. Katz, Dr. J. Stamler, Dr. R. Pick *Nutrition and Atherosclerosis*
Lea and Febiger, Philadelphia, 1958

Dr. A. D. Morgan *Symposium on Arteriosclerosis*
B. Schwabe, Basel, 1957

Dr. A. D. Morgan *The Pathogenesis of Coronary Occlusion*
C. C. Thomas, Springfield, 1956

National Research Council *Symposium on Atherosclerosis*
National Academy of Sciences, Washington, D.C., 1954

Dr. W. Raab *Hormonal and Neurogenic Cardiovascular Disorders*
Williams & Wilkins, Baltimore, 1953

Dr. E. V. Cowdry *Arteriosclerosis*
Macmillan, New York, 1933

Dietary Aspects of Cardiovascular Diseases SELECTED REFERENCES   1960
U. S. Department of Health, Education, and Welfare
Washington 25, D. C.

The Regulation of Dietary Fat   1962
Council on Foods and Nutrition

Fats in Human Nutrition WITH PARTICULAR ATTENTION TO *Fats Cholesterol and Atherosclerosis*   1957
American Medical Association
Chicago 10, Illinois

Index

If you have enjoyed this book, you will want to read other inexpensive Pyramid best-sellers. You will find them wherever paperbacks are sold or you can order them direct from the publisher. *Yours For The Asking:* a free, illustrated catalogue listing more than 700 books published by Pyramid. Write the publisher: PYRAMID BOOKS, Dept. K-99, 9 Garden Street, Moonachie, N. J. 07074.

LATEST PYRAMID BESTSELLERS

DOSSIER IX, Barry Weil	N-2243/95¢
HOWARD HUGHES, John Keats	V-2220/$1.25
THE DANGEROUS MONTH OF MAY, Edward Henry Russell	N-2221/95¢
THE STRIKER PORTFOLIO, Adam Hall	N-2197/95¢
THE COEDS, Alison Lord	T-2160/75¢
AND TO MY NEPHEW ALBERT, David Forrest	T-2185/75¢
THE CROSS AND THE SWITCHBLADE, David Wilkerson	N-2189/95¢
LOVING, J. M. Ryan	N-2188/95¢
A KISS BEFORE DYING, Ira Levin	T-2158/75¢
SAM'S SONG, Shirley Schoonover	N-2140/95¢
THE PROMISE OF SPACE, Arthur C. Clarke	V-2157/$1.25

NOTE: PYRAMID pays postage on orders for 4 books or more. On orders for less than 4 books, add 10¢ per copy for postage and handling.

— — WHEREVER PAPERBACKS ARE SOLD OR USE THIS COUPON — — —

PYRAMID BOOKS
Dept. K234, 9 Garden Street, Moonachie, New Jersey 07074

Please send me the BESTSELLERS I have circled below. I enclose $_____

N2243	V2220	N2221	N2197	T2160	T2185
N2189	N2188	T2158	N2140	V2157	

NAME_____

ADDRESS_____

CITY_____STATE_____ZIP_____